Are Your Kids Running on Empty?

Better Food Choices Can Make the Winning Difference

Ellen Briggs, Food Consultant
Sally Byrd, N.D.

MHP
Many Hands Publishing

Library of Congress Cataloging-in-Publication

A CIP catalog record for this book can be obtained from the Library of Congress.

Editorial/Production Supervisor: Erica Orloff
Composition/Typesetter: Carol Shields
Proofreader: Maryanne Orloff
Art Director/Cover Design: David Rhodes

Many Hands Publishing
P. O. Box 1221
Deerfield Beach, Florida 33443

Printed in the United States of America
First Paperback Edition

ISBN 0-974-66530-4

The information in this book reflects the authors' experience and is not intended to replace the advice and counsel of your personal pediatrician. Any use of the information in this book is at the reader's discretion. This book is intended to be informational only and by no means should be considered a substitute for advice or instructions from a medical or health professional. Always consult with your physician or other appropriate health professionals in matters relating to individual health and any symptoms requiring medical attention. The authors and publisher expressly disclaim any and all liability and responsibility for any adverse effects arising directly or indirectly from the use or application of the information contained in this book.

It is important to note that amounts quoted throughout this book, whether they represent the number of fat grams in a packaged product or the amount of sodium found in a fast food restaurant's pizza slice, were well researched utilizing product labels, manufacturer and fast food chain websites, and other research sources such as books, newsletters, and articles. Hours were spent to assure the greatest degree of accuracy. There is a small variance from end product to end product due to variables such as different manufacturing procedures and different hands that help create the finished product. Having taken this into account, we are confident that the numbers used in this book offer a well-assessed picture of the product contents mentioned.

Dedication

To our mothers, Mary and Jeanne,
who practiced what they preached:
God-made foods are better foods.

ACKNOWLEDGMENTS

Together we thank so many people, so many hands that have blessed this project.

To all the moms who opened up their kitchens to help us in this endeavor: Kim, Robin, Lesley, Becky, Robin, Linda, Peggy, Virginia, Sharon, Michele, Marian, Teri, Margaret Anne, Ruth Ann, and Judy. To a gifted chef, Michael.

To all the Kid Kritics who taste-tested recipes and food products. Their honesty and candidness has given this project credibility: Will, J.P., Adrian, Justin, Carter, Everett, Ella, Sam, Zachary, Austin, Christina, Katie, Will, Amy, Tessa, Nicole, John, Robert, Caroline, Grace, Alexus, Nicole, Carter, Terry, Tyler, Lauren, Goldie, Matt, Christina, Joseph, Sarah, Marsha, Missy, Wendy, Sebastian, Adam, Susan, Janice, Chelsey, Jessie, Seth, Joey, Michael, Philip, Natalie, Steven, Nick, Blake, Ryan, Shawn, Brittany, Steve, Chris, Lauren, Thomas, Ashley, Alex, Jonathan, Caitlyn, Stephen, J.T., Kriya, Mike, Ian, Matt, Sonali, Chelsea, Nick, Jade, Martin, Enrique, Haley, Marcello, Alex, Jessica, Bret, Brittany, Amanda, Jeffrey, Samantha, Zachary, Briana, Lauren, Allie, Sophie, Iris, Randy, Julia, Brian, Andres, Daniel, Felipe, Jennah, Meredith, Jason, Laura, Lauren, Chad, Zach, Shannon, Emerson, Cal, Colton, Austin, Ethan, James, Morgan, T.J., Al, Juan, Devin, Megan, Max, Sonali, Devin, Kyle, Devin, Anders, Adam, Sarah, Heather, J.T., Jackie, Chad, Danny, Gregory, Elizabeth, John, Patrick, Blair, Brittany, Christopher, Sarah, Michelle, Jessie, Field, Ian, Kaitlyne, Tessa, and Jill and the many more not listed before this printing!

To those who provided their facilities for taste-testings: many helpful families, Chapel of Saint Andrew's (wonderful kitchen and taste-testing venue!), the Saint Andrew's School.

To all the food and drink manufacturers who willingly sent food and drinks to us so they would be evaluated by the Kid Kritics.

To Janet Zand, LAc, OMD for her consistent encouragement and for writing the Foreword. Doctors Hyla Cass, Jesse Lynn Hanley, and Katharine Hession for their enthusiastic professional endorsements.

To David Rhodes, the artist who created the graphics, covers, and so much more.

To Sara Goodman, for her dedication and brilliant legal mind. We feel so blessed by your nurturing commitment.

To Erica Orloff, an incredibly in-tune editor, who patiently mentored us every step of the way. Without her, the book, CD-ROM, grocery list, and poster would not have been birthed.

To Kelvin, who said this book had to be written, believed in our ability, and felt passionate about the health of children.

As one, we thank our Lord and Savior Jesus Christ, for steering us to do God's will, opening doors, and walking us through the challenges of this project. It is our joy to honor you!

While reading *Are Your Kids Running on Empty?*™ you may notice that we were especially impressed with three authors for their works invaluable information concerning children's nutritional health.

Fred Pescatore, M.D., *Feed Your Kids Well*
Joseph C. Piscatella, *Fat-Proof Your Child*
Eric Schlosser, *Fast Food Nation*

Too few books have been written on the food issues of children. Dr. Fred Pescatore and Joseph C. Piscatella have thoroughly addressed this subject in their well-researched books. When we discovered *Feed Your Kids Well* and *Fat-Proof Your Child*, we realized both books offered wells of information pertinent to *Are Your Kids Running On Empty?* Hence we chose to refer to Dr. Pescatore and Joseph Piscatella's works as valuable sources to you, the reader. Their well-written health and diet books may be of interest to you as well. Look for them in bookstores or on the internet.

Eric Schlosser alerted the public to the truths about the fast food industry with his memorable book, *Fast Food Nation.* If you have not read it yet, it is a must-read. We believe he has revealed more information about the practices of the fast food restaurant giants than anyone else. His research is so compelling that we had to share several relevant parts with you. Mr. Schlosser's recent release targets another subject all together. It, too, can be found in bookstores or on the internet.

Both of us extend a sincere thank you to each of these authors. We so appreciate their dedication to the health of children. It is with pleasure that we bring their works to your attention.

Ellen Briggs and Sally Byrd

Credit Notices

FOREWORD

Are Your Kids Running on Empty? is a much needed and timely book. The health of the average child today is often compromised, in large part due to their diet. Health professionals are seeing the consequences of low-nutrient diets in the forms of disease and behavioral problems. The obesity epidemic is at dangerous levels. In my practice, I am seeing more childhood obesity and diabetes than ever before.

This book presents the truth about why kids are running on empty even though they are eating all day long. It clearly spells out which foods are not good for your children and makes identifying healthy foods easy. With every challenge you face, these authors provide you with solutions, ones that your children will like. There is a realistic emphasis on working toward making Better Food Choices.™ You can tell that Ellen and Sally are moms. They know it takes time to change. They know that when you take a favorite food away from your child, you must be able to replace it with something that they want to eat — something good. The Better Choices Grocery List™ serves as a shopping bible. Every product listed has been scrutinized for better choices of ingredients. Many have been taste-tested by Kid Kritics and given their seal of approval.

The recipes found in the CD-ROM, *Mom, I'm Hungry. What's for Dinner?*, are planned for busy moms and dads. No more than ten ingredients (thank you!) with the limit of twenty preparation minutes makes me think I can find time to cook these for my family. I love the fact that I can print out recipes and the Better Choices Grocery List from my office!

Little has been overlooked by these authors. Use this as a reference book. Use their helpful tools. It can make a winning difference.

Janet Zand, LAc, OMD
Author: Smart Medicine for a Healthier Child

INTRODUCTION

MEET ELLEN! From the very beginning my mother was committed to feeding my father, two sisters, and me well. In those days, most foods were freshly prepared; there were no frozen foods. Boxed, jarred, and canned foods filled only a few shelves in local grocer's store. There were no supermarkets. I clearly remember when the Grand Union opened a "big" store in the neighboring village. After frozen foods hit the market, I vividly remember when TV dinners were introduced to the public. WOW! My eyes popped out when I saw one, the only time there was one, in our icebox. Though I often yearned for my mother to run out and buy packaged foods, such as cookies, candy, soda, today, I so appreciate her tenacity and example of good eating habits. They have influenced me always, even during my single days when I could eat whatever I wanted. Yes, I ate whatever I wanted but paid the price. While drinking gallons of Tab as a food replacement, I became overweight. Then one day my throat began closing up so tightly that I couldn't breathe. I was sent to a great doctor who took me off caffeine cold-turkey. For three weeks I had the worst nail splitting headache you can imagine. Ever since, caffeine and sodas have been off my list. If I ever question my mother's wisdom, I have only to reflect on her long healthy life that ended when she was just shy of 91 years. She set the standards for all of us with her diet of fresh fruit, vegetables, whole grains, eggs, fish, poultry, some beef, good dairy (buttermilk!), and occasional treats. I pray my family and I can enjoy such an active and full life.

God began preparing me for this mission by blessing me with the healthy wisdom of my mother and my father's extraordinary example of integrity and commitment. Over time, God moved me along a path that eventually led me to my husband, Robert. His faith in me has been persistent. My two children, Deirdre and Justin, have reinforced the value of well-fueled minds and bodies. Both have challenged and inspired me.

Between the two of them I have spent many hours at studios, pools, tennis courts, and an array of sports fields. Many more hours have been spent listening to music lessons followed by recitals and concerts. For over thirty-three years I have nurtured them through schools with just a couple years left to go. (Justin was born the month Deirdre first attended college!) My understanding of the challenges kids face academically, athletically, and artistically has grown. When Justin was a young competitive athlete it became necessary to provide him better nutrition solutions in order to support his physical and mental needs. I began by researching the food industry. Talking to parents, faculty, and administrators at his school provided additional valuable information. What became evident was that parents expected and relied on the school to orchestrate academic excellence. When it came to athletic excellence they were anxious to know how to fuel their kids to be winners. I took this cue and began further researching this subject. Everywhere I turned, mothers expressed frustration over the challenge of finding winning foods that their kids would eat! It also dawned on me that whenever moms did seek nutritional advice from health professionals, all it took was a walk into an unfamiliar health-food store, and/or one trial of a new food that tasted like cardboard, to end their effort to serve their families healthier foods. This was the dawning of the awakening. The world did not need another nutritionist, it needed a personal food-shopping consultant. Moms began going with me to grocery stores for walkabouts where they were introduced to Better Food Choices. Their positive results inspired more research. It became apparent that there was a crying need to package the information I was gathering. Soon I began the journey of writing a book on how to fuel young athletes. Personal challenges, including the passing of my mother, put a halt to this for a couple of years. Then a friend told her husband, Kelvin, about my passion. He came to me and said, "You must put this together. You must finish this." These were profound words, as I then knew the power of the Lord's will. After reorganizing my thoughts, I called Sally and asked her to partner with me in writing *Are Your Kids Running On Empty?* Thankfully, she said yes. Both of us were motivated by the food misinformation stream and disturbing eating trends, disease statistics, and increasing spread of behavioral disorders among the young. Neither of us knew how to write a book or what we were getting into! By the grace of God, after a national search for an editor, Erica came into our lives, who we later discovered lives just around the corner from me! As Sally and I began writing *Are Your Kids Running on Empty?* we created the *Kid Kritics* taste-tests in order to give credibility to our recommendations. From there the cookbook and grocery list evolved. So did the booklet for a fast read and the *Fuel Your Dreams*™ poster. Together, Sally and I ran with this project!

MEET SALLY! I grew up in Connecticut, the oldest of five girls. My dad was a strict Italian overachiever, and, my mother was a creative and assertive health food advocate. Mediterranean cuisine of fresh God-made foods filled our mouths, daily. Sardines and artichokes, included! That is all I knew and I loved it! Then I went to school. My mother filled my lunch box with sandwiches made of whole grain bread, fresh cut lean meats, fish, veggies, sprouts, and non-hydrogenated nut butters that didn't spread very well. She added yogurt and trail mixes. That's when I learned how different my upbringing was from other kids. As you can imagine, some kids were merciless. I was painfully ridiculed for being a health-food nut.

My mother carried this source of embarrassment into my play-date world. My parents had a large vegetable garden with all sorts of foods — eggplant, broccoli, fennel, berries, asparagus, fruit trees, and herbs. Mom was a beekeeper and provided us with a constant supply of raw honey and bee pollen. I was always afraid to have kids over in case she would be wearing her 'bee outfit' or trying to get us to work in the garden or at the food co-op where we purchased many of our natural foods. In my eyes, this was not a kid-friendly place. No processed foods were found in our house. Coke was only purchased as a household cleaner. None of us ever drank it. It is one of the best rust-removers on the market. We used it to clean our bikes! To this day, I have never sipped a Coke.

When I was a teenager, I rebelled. Whenever I could, I ate at McDonald's and always ordered milkshakes. It wasn't until I went to college that I began to appreciate health foods and looked forward to my mom's care packages of protein powders, nut butters and dried fruit. By then, health foods were beginning to catch on and my friends were curious. When my environmental degree proved useless in the 1980s job market, I found jobs in health-food stores. A new career blossomed. A passion began developing inside of me; I wanted to know more and educated others on the perils and solutions of the world's current food supply. The more I learned, the more I understood the benefits of making Better Food Choices. Eventually I became a board-certified Naturopath and a licensed body worker. Now, I consider myself a Nutritional Missionary for adults and children.

My children, Everett and Carter, are very healthy productive teenagers. Rarely have they been sick. Both were raised with Better Food Choices than most of their friends. Both know the difference. Most kids do not. I know that at times this has not been easy for them. However, they agree that a healthy foundation has been set and it is up to them to continue their own personal health regime. As a child of my parents, I learned the hard way. Through better-balanced choices, you can make it comfortable for your kids to take nutritious, normal looking, and good tasting lunches to school!

Unfortunately, today kids are subjected to landmines of environmental and manufacturing practices that threaten our mental and physical health. Our kids are growing up in suburban sprawls with streets filled with moving cars, superstores filled with processed foods supported by chemically driven and over-farmed farms, houses, and yards cleaned and fertilized with chemicals, air and water that are challenged by chemicals, and rooms electronically loaded with televisions, sound systems, and the internet. They are subject to physical and mental overload. Already, we are seeing the consequences of this.

As parents, we have options to lighten our kids' toxic loads and give them the defenses needed to counter these challenges. During their primary years, we can control and influence what our kids put into their mouths. Your kids can eat yummy foods that will fuel their minds, bodies, and dreams. This is what *Are Your Kids Running on Empty?* and its CD cookbook are all about! Your kids and their dreams. The *Kids Kritics* taste-testers continue to help us find the foods and drinks filled with nutrients that taste good. The natural food and traditional supermarkets stock these foods and drinks, making it easier for every mother to conveniently find them on the shelves. Taste-tested recipes have been written and rewritten to meet the demands of moms, as all moms are working moms with little or no spare time. The *Food Circles* has been designed to replace the Food Pyramid. It is easier to read and makes more sense. It includes our most important fuel, water! *Counting Colors*, another guideline that is simple to follow, is a fun way to entice your kids to eat more fresh fruits and vegetables. *Five days on, two days off*, the suggestion of eating nutrient-filled foods and drinks for five days, from Sunday afternoon to Friday afternoon, and then having treats on the weekend works! This eating pattern helps keep your kids' minds focused during the school week while not feeling deprived of junk foods since they eat them on weekends. The *Better Choices Grocery List* is your shopping list guide. We have scrutinized all the foods listed by category for content. Either through the Kid Kritics taste-testings or common knowledge, we know most kids will eat those listed. Because the list is so long, we have published the *Brands to Trust*™ grocery list that can be carried in your bag. You will find this helpful when choosing which ketchup brand to buy. Better choices it the key phrase when describing this venture. We know it is unrealistic for moms to fuel their kids perfectly. We don't! However, it is true that by making better food and drink choices, you may give your kids better odds in reaching their potential and living healthy happy lives. This is the goal. Better Food Choices.

For those of you who want the information in a chapter but are too busy for a full read, we have positioned *Chapter Quick Facts* at the beginning of each chapter. Their purpose is to serve as your reading barometer for the following chapter. Quickly scan them for some key facts. When time allows, curl up in bed and explore the world of Better Choices.

Table of Contents

1

Are Your Kids Hungry?

Chapter Quick Facts

- ▶ Your kids may be running on empty because most foods they eat are void of nutricnts.
- ▶ By definition, food is a substance consumed by an animal or human to keep it alive and enable it to grow. Many foods you buy at the store are invented and altered in laboratories. Many fail to meet the definition of food.
- ▶ Living food can be defined as food containing its naturally occurring living enzymes. Many processed foods are dead foods that are indigestible and void of nutrients.
- ▶ Meet the Junk Food Generation. Kids mostly eat nutrient-stripped processed foods that contain some appetite stimulating additives. The average child consumes about 275 pounds of nutrient-empty sugar a ycar! At least 36 percent of the caloric content of food in today's kids' diets is fat, usually the bad kind.
- ▶ Four percent or less of kids ages 2 to 12 eat 5 servings of life-giving, fiber-filled fruits and vegetables.
- ▶ Your children's bodies can be full of "food" and still be empty of the nutrients they need to run efficiently. Chances are your kids are truly hungry.

Are Your Kids Hungry?

"Mom, I'm hungry!"

"Can I have a snack? What's for dinner? Can we stop at McDonalds?"

Sound familiar? Does it seem like your kids eat all day long? If your kids are like most, on a typical day they have devoured toaster pastries, bagels, cheese, cereal, bread, pasta, fries, chips, cookies, ice cream, pizza, salad, chicken, hamburgers, candy, juice, sodas, and more. How could they possibly be hungry?

Kids Eat Empty Food

"Empty foods" are foods that are missing naturally occurring nutrients originally found in whole, God-made, foods. Though the origin of some processed foods are whole foods, they often end up being "empty" because the original nutrients are either compromised or removed during processing. The birthplace of many processed foods is a food science laboratory. The creators are food engineers who invent ingredient variations. Take a minute to read a cereal box label, especially one targeted for kids, to see if you can identify any whole grain foods on the ingredients list. It is fair to question whether some processed foods even meet the definition of food. *Webster's New World Dictionary* defines food as:

- Any substance taken into and assimilated by a plant or animal to keep it alive and enable it to grow; nourishment, nutriment.[1]

The key words here are *keep it alive and enable it to grow.* Many foods your kids eat fail to fit this definition of food. Margarine is a good example. It was originally created as an inexpensive source of "nutritional" fat to feed the poor classes of people during the time of Napoleon III (1867). Even then, many viewed margarine as being hazardous to your health. This form of fat has been formulated and reformulated in food science laboratories. Unlike butter, margarine is not made from cow's milk. Thus, it does not have a foundation of milk's original natural ingredients. Instead, margarine is often composed of many multisyllable, hard-to-pronounce chemicals. Plus, through the magic of food engineering, disease causing trans fatty acids have been added.

Look at what happens when we apply the definition of food and nutrition to margarine. Does margarine keep you alive? In fact, scientists have proven it contributes to serious heart disease. Does margarine replace worn or injured tissues? Again, it is known to be detrimental to the cardiovascular system. Does margarine promote growth? If you consider growth as adding saturated fat cells to your body that increase your girth, the answer is yes. If you believe that the use of growth in this definition means the addition of healthy cells for your blood, muscles, brain, bone, and organ tissues, the answer is no.

Not only does margarine seem to be an empty food, we can question whether it is a food at all.

Processed Foods: A Double-Edged Sword

The good news is that processed foods have become quick and easy answers to meal preparation for our families. The bad news is that, "About 90 percent of the money that Americans spend on food is used to buy processed food."[2] Most of the remaining 10 percent of this money is spent on beef and poultry. That does not leave much left to buy fruits and vegetables. Take a look at the items in your grocery cart and those of others next time you shop at your local supermarket. Most are filled with bags, boxes, and cans, not produce.

Paul Stitt, food biochemist, owner of Natural Ovens (a baking company) and author, has witnessed food-manufacturing processes of what he calls the food giants. He saw it from the inside when he worked for a major food corporation. His quote tells us like it is: "Processed foods are foods that have been changed — foods no longer in the form in which they are found in nature ... they are stripped of their nutrient value in the refining process."[3]

Doctor Fred Pescatore reveals: "During processing, natural vitamins and minerals are taken out of the food. At best, they are replaced with chemical versions that the body cannot readily or completely absorb and thus are nutritionally useless. At worst, these natural nutrients are not replaced at all."[4] Frequently, your kids are eating the results of expensive chemistry lab tests, nutrient-depleted non-foods.

So while processed foods are providing you and your family quick and easy meals that stir up few complaints, these foods are coming up empty of the very nutrients your kids need to grow, be healthy, and productive. Now are you beginning to see why your kids are hungry? About 90 percent of your food budget is spent on foods void of nutrients needed to fuel their engines, engines that are designed to run in high gear.

White Flour Versus Wheat Flour

Food biochemist, Paul Stitt, explains the difference.

> Wheat flour is one food that is especially ravaged by processing. In the refining process, more than half of each of the most essential nutrients is sold for making pet food. The milling process destroys 40 percent of the chromium present in the whole grain, as well as 86 percent of the manganese, 89 percent of the cobalt, 68 percent of the copper, 78 percent of the zinc, and 48 percent of the molybdenum. By the time it is completely refined, it has lost most of its phosphorus, iron, and thiamin, and a good deal of its niacin and riboflavin. Its crude fiber content has been cut down considerably as well. White flour is wheat flour that has been plundered of most of its vitamin E, important oils and amino acids. Yet, all of these nutrients are needed for a satisfied, healthy body. While whole-wheat flour is one of the most nutritious foods, processing sees to it that the white flour found in most products is nutritionally worthless.[5]

Refined soft white bread first started being marketed to the consumer after World War II. The message was white bread is the best choice. The bad news is that over years of costly marketing and advertising campaigns, the consumer has been duped into believing this untruth. In addition to commonly consumed white flour products such as bread loaves, hamburger and hot dog buns, and rolls, white flour is also used as cheap filler in hundreds of other foods. Doughnuts, crackers, cookies, cakes, refined pastas, pizza crust, and a myriad of other baked goods are made from whole-wheat flour that has been stripped of its nutrients. What percentage of your son or daughter's diet consists of white flour products? But you thought white breads were enriched and vitamin-fortified. You thought right. The downside is, the synthetic nutrients used to enrich adulterated foods are generally more difficult for the body to absorb. Furthermore, nutrient enriched products contain significantly fewer vitamins, minerals, and fiber than originally found in whole grain wheat flour. How can a food that was stripped of about thirty naturally occurring nutrients and then sprayed or injected with lesser amounts of about five man-made nutrients be better for your kids? Even many wheat flours have been pillaged of its nutrients, any color left is bleached out with harsh chemicals. This is done to please the buyer's eye.

Now you are beginning to see why your kids can eat some foods and still be hungry? And there's more.

Dead or Alive?

Living food can be defined as food containing its naturally occurring living enzymes. Enzymes are specialized protein molecules that are necessary for the existence of life and food digestion. Scientists have confirmed that enzymes stimulate and monitor nearly all of the biochemical reactions that occur in the body. Your child's body makes some but not all of these 2,700 enzymes. Saliva is the front line and most immediate source of digesting enzymes. As your son or daughter chews food, enzymes are mixed into this food where it begins the first step of breaking down into digestible nutrients. In the stomach, more enzymes are available to further the digestive progression. The process of transforming foods chewed and swallowed into digestible nutrients is precise, job specific, and complicated. It requires the involvement of enzymes naturally contained in the body plus those found in the foods being eaten by your son or daughter.

Raw foods are living foods. They are naturally designed for active human digestion and absorption. Fresh vegetables and fruits are filled with living enzymes. So are raw nuts, seeds, and grains. Even when lightly cooked, at no more than 118 degrees Fahrenheit, whole foods retain their living enzymes, and are easily digested and efficiently absorbed high-octane fuel for your growing active kids.

Unfortunately, not all foods you buy at the grocery store can be digested efficiently, as they are not living foods. They are often void of the digestive enzymes needed to act in concert with the enzymes your child's body produces. Some food manufacturers have gone further and designed foods that by-pass the digestive process to avoid the absorption of fat. WOW potato chips, made with the synthetic ingredient Olestra, are a good example. Olestra is an artificial fat tasting additive invented and designed to make the chewed chips slide right on through the stomach and colon, exiting out of the elimination tract without being digested. It has been linked to diarrhea and other uncomfortable digestive conditions. Prior to August 2003, the FDA required products containing Olestra to have warning labels stating that the synthetic chemical might cause cramps and diarrhea. It is important to note that when your kids have diarrhea, they also lose other stomach contents such as nutrients, friendly bacteria, and water. In August 2003, after reviewing a six-week study of 3000 participants, the FDA lifted this warning label requirement. It concluded that if Olestra caused digestive problems, the effects were mild and rare. Our question to you is whether risking diarrhea and possible stomach cramps for the temporary pleasure of consuming these chips worth it? There are other chips on the market that use more digestible ingredients with a limited fat content. (Please see the Better Choices Grocery List™) We recommend that you be on the lookout for Olestra on ingredient lists and pay close attention to whether or not your kids have any digestive discomforts.

Most processed foods are exposed to high degrees of heat when manufactured. Consequently, any living enzymes and nutrients that originally existed are usually lost in the process. Toaster pastries and cheese that squirt out of tubes are two products that come to mind. Hundreds and hundreds of lab-made, enzyme-scarce foods fill the grocery stores. Because they are enzyme-empty, undigested particles may be left to collect in your son or daughter's colon. Researcher, Sam Graci, says they sit there and build up like layers of snow, eventually inviting disease. When kids eat too much "dead" food, their bodies resort to pooling enzyme resources from other organs and tissues in order to help break down what has been consumed. This practice of robbing enzymes from other parts of the body may stir up systemic imbalances that may result in weakened immune systems.

Many well-intended moms who do buy fresh living foods for their kids often overcook them by using high temperatures. As previously noted, when naturally rich enzymatically-alive foods are exposed to excessive heat (over 118 degrees Fahrenheit), they are killed. Excessive heat can also destroy other important nutrients such as vitamins and minerals. Vegetables cooked until they are soggy and flame-grilled hamburgers have probably had their respective living enzymes and nutrients annihilated. They then become dead foods.

By serving kids more living foods than "dead foods," you are taking a big step in gradually improving the selections of food you feed them. The nutrients found in these foods they eat will be digested, transported into the blood, and distributed throughout the body. For example, replace a sugar-laden grape-flavored drink with 100 percent real grape juice or best yet, fresh (frozen) grapes. Fresh grapes are filled with living nutrients. To quench any additional thirst, give your kids some ice-cold water. Quick and easy to prepare processed foods may ease your life in the short term but many of them may pave the way to medical chaos for your children in the long run. Clearly, kids eating "dead foods" are running on empty. Fill yours up with enzyme-filled alive foods!

Smells, Looks, Tastes

In this order, your kid's mind decides whether to take a bite. If food does not pass the smell test, forget it. If it smells good but looks bad, you are in trouble. Both positive smell and look appeal triggers the production of enzyme-filled saliva that is required for the first stage of digestion. To entice kids to eat food, it is necessary to make it smell, look, and then taste good. Fresh out of the oven chocolate cake made from a boxed product smells, looks, and tastes delicious. If your kids had the chance, they might eat the whole cake before it cooled. Warm doughnuts make kids' mouths water. These food manufacturers are experts at stimulating kids with smells, tastes, and looks. The end result is that kids love to eat lab-invented synthetic processed foods and drinks. Today's statistics say kids are eating endless amounts of these foods. Manufacturers, distributors, and retailers take this fact all the way to the bank!

Are Kids Addicted to Certain Foods?

Addiction is defined as a compulsive need to use a habit-forming substance that results in physiological withdrawal symptoms. Tobacco and drug addiction withdrawal symptoms are scientifically documented and well understood. The tobacco industry has been called on the carpet for its participation in setting up consumers to become addicted to their products.

Many believe that repeated consumption of a particular food in the quest of satisfying an ever-present drive for it raises questions about food addiction. The behavior is compulsive. The withdrawal symptoms are real. Have you ever noticed the behavior of people when they can't get their hands on something they are craving? Don't they become irritable, and short-tempered? Complaints of headaches add to the craving distress. These are just a few of the typical withdrawal symptoms experienced by kids who feel a driving need to eat certain foods.

Food engineers are brilliant inventors of foods that your kids find difficult to stop eating, foods that directly appeal to kids' sense of smell, sight and taste. It has been reported that food manufacturers spend megabucks creating food formulas that incite the "eat the whole bag" syndrome. Most kids have no problem finishing off a bag of chips, popcorn, or candy. Boxes of cookies disappear with only remnants of crumbs as evidence of their existence. Frequently, twelve-ounce and larger sized bottles of soda are emptied in record time. Often, one is not enough. Keeping your cupboards and refrigerator stocked with appetite stimulating foods and drinks can be a challenge. "Mom, we're out of soda." "Mom, where did all the cookies go?"

Artificial ingredients may be a source of appetite stimulants. They are found in mountains of cereals, cookies, and other treats. Ask most anyone who regularly eats packaged artificially-flavored chocolate and vanilla cookies if they find themselves eating the whole bag at one or two sittings. We know that addictive caffeine is found in cocoa beans, the source of chocolate. However, the amount of cocoa found in one of these packaged cookies is minimal next to the amount of simple carbohydrates (sugar) and artificial ingredients. It is hard to know exactly what drives kids to eat so many at one sitting. It is fair to assume that answers lie in the manufacturer's secret recipe.

Take a minute to stop and think of foods your kids eat and drink that make them want more. Does soda come to mind first? Soda manufacturers are skillful at driving soda drinkers to drink more soda. Contrary to popular belief, sodas are not thirst-quenchers. Most sodas are formulated to make your kids thirsty! An 8-ounce serving of most sodas contains at least 20 grams of sodium (five teaspoons), and several popular brands contain as much as 35 to 50 grams which may add up to about 12 or more teaspoons! It is known that sodium stimulates the desire for liquids! Sodium sends the message that you want more. Check for sodium chemicals in the ingredients lists and nutrition facts of the sodas and foods your kids are drinking and eating to see how much your kids are consuming.

Thanks to today's food science, repetitive food and drink cravings is a common phenomenon. "Instead of (food) being eaten when we are physically hungry, food is now consumed to satisfy artificial cravings generated by a brain that isn't working right and whose receptor sites beg for synthetic stimulation from chemicals. We eat, but are never satisfied. We're full, but we aren't contented."[6]

The science of adding unhealthful chemicals into processed foods is not uncommon among food manufacturers. We, the consumers, parents and our children, are vulnerable and many are, or will be, suffering the consequences. Yes, our kids are eating a lot, but they are still hungry and thirsty.

Processed Foods Fatten Profits

As in all businesses, manufacturers of "foods" are focused on profits. Their primary interest is to produce a product for the lowest cost, that the public will buy repeatedly, for the highest price. In the food industry, health concerns may get lost in this business formula.

Surprisingly, the cost of manufacturing, distributing and stocking processed foods is frequently more cost efficient than providing the real thing. Let's use whole-grain wheat flour versus bleached white flour as an example. As previously mentioned, when the whole-wheat grain is stripped of its nutrients, the germ and other "waste" products are either used to make other products or are sold to other companies for their use. (Dogs often end up with the best part of the whole grain in their food!) What is left is used to manufacture a variety of flour–based products such as bread. By dissecting whole grain into multiple ingredients, more products and more money can be made.

Enzyme-depleted flour becomes less perishable making it a manufacturer's welcomed penny-saver. When flavors, colors, preservatives, and other additives are added, white flour becomes a product with a longer shelf life. They become well-preserved foods that do not have to be thrown away or replaced for a very long time. Making long shelf-life foods is a high priority for food manufacturers, distributors, and retailers. The longer a food can be stored without deteriorating, the cheaper the cost of doing business. With the handling requirements simplified, transportation, storage, and retail facilities become easier and less expensive to run and maintain.

This practice of manufacturing enzymatically-dead foods that have been doctored with preservatives is also prevalent in the fast-food industry. Try taking a fast-food hamburger and leaving it on your kitchen counter. Tuck it away in a corner. How long do you think you can leave it there without finding a bug eating it or a fungus growing on it? Experimenters will attest it can maintain its "just off the grill condition" for many, many moons. Some products are designed to last for a year or longer. Try to imagine what happens when such foods enter your kids stomach and colon. Will they sit there, undigested, for a long time? Some scientists say yes.

In summary, most preserved food is processed, indigestible dead food. Undigested food cannot be absorbed into the blood. The nutrients you thought were fueling growth and energy may not be filling your child's nutritional needs. The result is that your kids feel hungry and eat more food, probably more processed food. The more processed foods they eat, the more you spend. Convenience comes with a price. Processed foods with additives are not only fattening manufacturers' profits, it is likely that they are fattening your kids, too. What's good for business is not necessarily good for your son or daughter's health.

The Junk Generation

Advertising, especially on television, sells junk foods all day long. Approximately 90 percent of the food commercials kids watch promote junk food. Some of these are viewed at school on Channel One, thanks to lucrative deals cut by the school administration with food and drink corporations such as soda companies. As a result, most children and young adults eat junk food from morning to night. Sodas, candy, chips, candy cereals, plus fast foods that are also labeled by food experts as junk food, are created and repeatedly marketed as irresistible to kids. In fact, both the advertising and the products may be addictive.

Junk Food

Are you sitting down? This is not a pretty picture.

A common fast food restaurant's large order of French fries contains 25 fat grams. Adding a cheeseburger throws in another 46 grams of fat, totaling of 71 grams of fat.[7] At 9 calories per fat gram, this combination produces 631 calories from the fat alone. Kids love the mouth-feel and taste of fat. Fast-food chains give them plenty of it. But there is more. Sugar calories found in the fries, plus the spoonfuls of sugar usually found in the ketchup and buns most kids eat with their burgers and fries, have not been added to the above total of calories. With them, calorie counts skyrocket. We are placing fat and sugar in the same fat category because unused sugar calories are stored as fat in the body. (This is a major reason why so many kids in America are woefully overweight.) Add to this ugly picture the fact that the contents of fast food burgers and French fries include a measurable amount of processed ingredients. Plus they are cooked on and in extremely hot, trans fatty acid producing oils. Since these burgers and fries have been depleted of many whole nutrients, we classify them as "empty foods." Without a doubt, this fast food order qualifies as a major junk meal.

Junk Facts

- "A traditional McDonald's burger with a 16 ounce Coke and a small order of fries carries 627 calories and 19 grams of fat. Upgrade to a Big Xtra! with cheese, and 'super size' the drink and fries. Now your lunch packs 1,805 calories and 84 grams of fat."[8]

- Soda has been rightly coined as "liquid candy" by the Center for Science in the Public Interest. Coca Cola (12 ounces) has around 10 teaspoons of sugar. Mountain Dew (12 ounces) has about 11 teaspoons of sugar. Hi-C Grape Juice (8 ounces) has around 8 teaspoons of sugar. That's a lot per serving.

- Most cereals should be called candy cereal. The amount of sugar in ½ cup, an average serving size, is about 3 or 4 teaspoons.

- Candy is made of processed sugar and dyes. A 1.5-ounce bag of plain M&Ms contains around 7½ teaspoons of sugar. Eighteen pieces of Gummi Bears also has about 7½ teaspoons of sugar! Artificial dyes are used to color these and most other candies.

- Candy, desserts, sodas, doughnuts, fruit drinks, and refined flour products such as white pasta, white bread, and pizza crusts are primary sources of sugar consumption by kids. As you know, they eat plenty of it.

According to studies conducted at Washington State University, the average child consumes more than 12 ounces of sugar a day – or about 275 pounds a year![9]

That's over 20 pounds of sugar a month! Does this seem impossible? Start adding up the amount of sugar your kids are eating and drinking for breakfast, lunch, snacks, dinner, and after dinner snack. Include the artificial sugars, too. You will be amazed. Even if your kids ate half this amount, one 10-pound bag a month, they are still stimulating their bodies and minds with way too much sugar. Also recall, that unused sugar is stored as fat. The consequences are now visible.

- Since 1990, Type 2 Diabetes (Adult Onset) has jumped by 33 percent nationwide.[10]
- One in three children is overweight, if not actually obese, and the numbers continue to grow.[11]

Diabetes is closely linked to obesity. The incidence among children and young adults of Adult Onset Diabetes (Type 2), obesity, ADD, ADHD, and auto-immune diseases is on a worrisome rise. Obesity among children is on the epidemic scale. Hopefully these facts have caught your attention. The health consequences facing junk generations of kids are monumental. Junk foods, for the most part, are toxic-filled and provide lots of nutrient-empty calories. No wonder kids are hungry.

Food Pyramids: The Myth and Reality

The current Food Pyramid, designed by the USDA (United States Department of Agriculture), recommends the following for a daily diet.

6-11 servings from the bread, cereal, rice, and pasta group
3-5 servings of vegetables
2-4 servings of fruit
2-3 servings from the milk, yogurt, and cheese group
2-3 servings from the meat, poultry, fish, dry beans, eggs, and nuts group
Fats, oils, and sweets are to be eaten sparingly.

If you believe that most of us are following this food consumption guideline, you believe a myth. If you believe that kids come close to eating according to this guideline, you are dreaming. The reality is that kid's daily diets do not even come close to meeting the recommended number of servings of this pyramid's food groups.

> Research has revealed that "96% of kids ages 2-12 do not eat 5 servings (fruits and vegetables) per day."[12]

The number-one-vegetable eaten by kids today is French fries followed by ketchup and iceberg lettuce. Since tomatoes are really fruit, iceberg lettuce moves up a notch. Some want to count fruit juice as a fruit. However, is it sugar-filled and is missing important fiber content, which slows down the rate of sugar absorption within your kid's blood stream. One hundred percent fruit juice at best provides a fiberless fruit source. But at least it is better than the sugar-laden fruit drinks that fill the grocery store shelves.

Kids are eating according to their own food pyramid. Studies show that fat, oils and sweets, and the bread, cereal, rice and pasta groups make up the lion's share of this pyramid. Meat, poultry, fish, dry beans, eggs, and nuts are on par with milk, and cheese. Located at the top of the Junk Generation Food Pyramid are the fruits and vegetables groups. It is a lucky day when kids eat more than one serving of a fruit and vegetable.

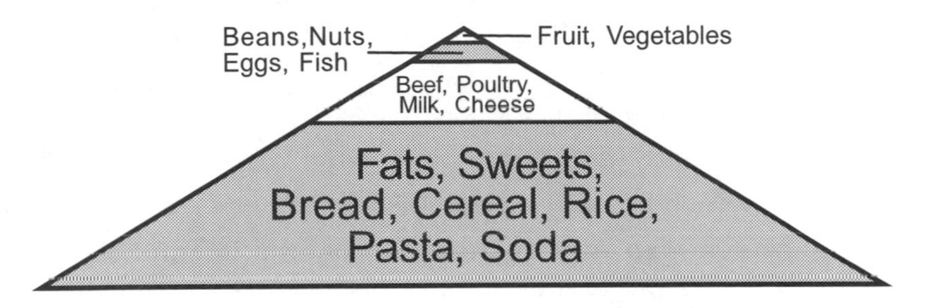

This mix of nutritionally deficient foods supplies an excessive amount of empty fuel for kids. A car requires proper fueling in order to run well. If you put a low-grade fuel into your new high-tech Porsche, your car's performance would be reduced proportionately. If you poured a mixture of middle-octane gasoline and soda into your SUV, your car's engine may not run at all, even though its tank gauge would register full. If you filled your car's gasoline tank with just soda, again, your car would be full of liquid, but it will be empty of the fuel ingredients needed to run.

The high-tech bodies of your kids also need proper fueling in order to run efficiently. We are what we eat. Actually, we are what we digest (enzymes!). Junk in, junk out. Better said, put junk in, get junk results.

Food Circles: A Better Food Guideline

The concept of a circle within a circle illustrates the relationship among all the food groups that fuel your kids. The Food Circles™ are meant to replace the USDA Food Pyramid. A simpler and more meaningful food guideline graphic was needed.

Food Circles are designed to simplify the complex question of how much of each food group should be served to kids. The recommendations made will fill them up with high-octane fuel that may steer kids away from some of the anti-fuels. The reality is that kids won't change their eating habits over night. But, step-by-step, they will feel more comfortable with moving in the right direction. Start with water! These Food Circles are for kids. (See Food Circles below.)

What Is a Serving Size?

Most moms do not know what size a serving is for an adult or a child. Knowing sure makes a difference. It is key to preventing over- or under-feeding of a food. Here are two ways to describe a serving size:

- 1 serving equals ½ cup on average
- 1 serving size equals about a medium handful of the child eating it. (Mom or dad's hand would be too big.)

The benefit of using a customized medium handful serving is that it allows for the difference of size of each kid. A medium handful for a seven-year-old girl is rightfully smaller than one for a twelve-year-old boy. A seven-year-old girl does not need to eat the same amount of chicken as a boy who is on the precipice of being a teenager. The medium handful size is our preferred serving measuring tool.

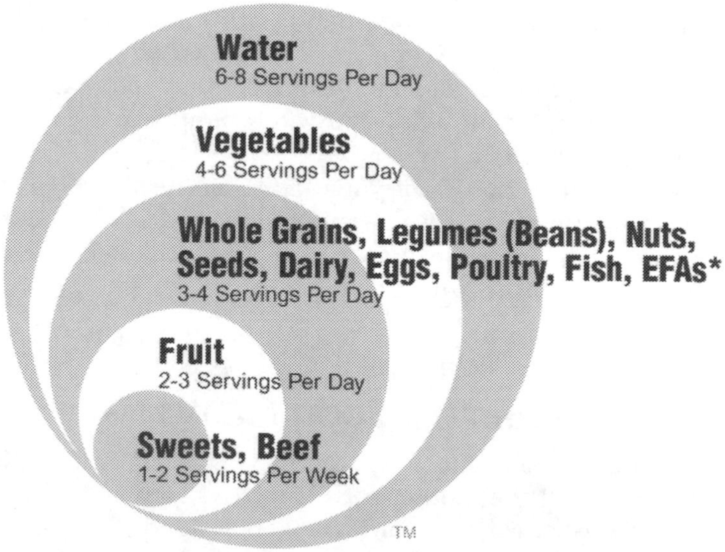

Water
6-8 Servings Per Day

Vegetables
4-6 Servings Per Day

Whole Grains, Legumes (Beans), Nuts, Seeds, Dairy, Eggs, Poultry, Fish, EFAs*
3-4 Servings Per Day

Fruit
2-3 Servings Per Day

Sweets, Beef
1-2 Servings Per Week

TM

ONE SERVING equals each child's own handful.
SERVING SIZE EXCEPTIONS: Water – 6-8 ounces, EFAs/Seeds – 1 teaspoon, Eggs – 1, any size
*EFAs - Essential Fatty Acids (refers to oils only)

Food Circles Explanation

Every food category in a circle is assigned a specified number of daily servings recommended for that circle. For instance, it is recommended that your son or daughter should eat three to four servings of legumes (beans), whole grains, nuts, seeds, essential fatty acids (plant oils), fish, poultry, and eggs per day. People ask if this means their son or daughter must eat three to four of each kind of food listed in the circle. The answer is no. However, three to four servings of just eggs or chicken a day is also not sufficient. Eggs for breakfast, fish for lunch (tuna sandwich), and chicken and salad (olive oil) for dinner, all in one day makes sense and is possible, especially for an active boy or girl. Use your common sense. Ideally, it is best for your kids to eat servings from most of the food categories listed for each day. Simply work toward this goal.

Water has been added and occupies the largest circle, positioning it as the most important food group. It is. Water is fuel.

BASIC WATER FORMULA

Drink ½ body weight in ounces, per day

Example: 64-pound girl's weight divided by 2 = 32 ounces per day. 32 ounces = 4 cups of water

This easy formula accounts for the size of each boy and girl. Active kids, especially those located in warm climates, need more water. Kids love to drink out of water bottles. Keep them handy and they will probably drink more water!

Vegetables provide very important nutrients needed for optimum health and fitness. Four to six servings per day would cover basic nutritional needs while more may be required for an active child. (Yikes! you say.) A child size medium handful of lettuce on a sandwich at lunch, baby carrots for a snack, salad and peas at dinner adds up to four servings. Using the child-customized handful serving measurement make this more plausible.

Essential Fatty Acids are critical for a well fueled body and mind performance. Three to four servings per day of EFA oils such as olive, fish, flaxseed, sesame, and canola, are essential for your growing kids. One serving size equals one teaspoon. Raw nuts and seeds, egg yolks, cold-water fish, and legumes (soybeans) also supply EFAs. However, in the Food Circles EFAs refers to only the oils.

Whole Grains, Legumes (beans), Nuts, Seeds, Dairy, Eggs, Poultry, and Fish provide a balance of important nutrients and good fats when on a three to four servings a day program. An egg with whole grain toast for breakfast, tuna sandwich on whole grain bread for lunch, ice cold crunchy nuts and seeds sprinkled on yogurt for a snack, chicken served with a black bean and rice recipe for dinner, easily fills this serving recommendation.

Fruit servings should equal two to three per day. Fruit juice without pulp does not really count. It contains a lot of sugar without the benefit of fiber. Better choices are low-sugar and high-fiber fruits like berries and kiwis. A handful of berries on cereal or waffles at breakfast, tangerine sections at lunch, and slices of apple for a snack will do it. That's three servings!

Sweets and Red Meat fall into in the smallest circle, as they are the least frequently needed food group. Both are sources for sugar, animal fats, and trans fatty acids. One to two servings a week are enough. Your challenge will be to limit the servings of sweets and burgers!

These Food Circles are a guide for you to follow. It takes time to change the eating habits of anyone. Kids will be receptive to good-tasting replacements for the low-nutrient and high-fat sugar foods they are eating. This book offers a Better Choices Grocery List, recipes, and tips to help you move in that direction.

In 2001, *USA Today* learned that among the parents interviewed, a resounding 96 percent were "very concerned" about their child's health. It was their number-one concern. Education was second by a squeaker, 95 percent. The odds are that you are one of these caring and concerned parents. Health, academic grades, athletic achievements, creative performances, and social behavior are all jeopardized for kids whose bodies are running on empty.

Follow the Food Circles and lead your kids into a healthier and more productive lifestyle. Use the Better Choices Grocery List for better results.

2

Label Roulette

Chapter Quick Facts

- Do you feel like you are gambling when grocery shopping for your kids because you don't always know what you are buying? Aren't the labels confusing?
- The Food and Drug Administration (FDA) requires food labeling for most prepared foods. Nutrition labeling for raw produce and fish is voluntary.[1] The words *most* and *voluntary* leave the door open for confusion.
- Boxed, bagged, and canned food products are decorated with brand names, marketing messages, and information printed to seduce you. New, Improved, Lite, Fat-Free, Low Sugar, All Natural are just some of the sell words.
- Some phrases are misleading: "95% Fat-Free." The percentage represents the weight of a product. Most or all of this product's weight is from fat-free water. The other 5 percent may be filled with fat adding up to a lot of calories.
- The numbers don't add up on the Nutrition Facts.
- The Ingredient Lists, your best source of food content facts, are usually so small that you can't read them.
- For the health of your children, read this chapter's guide to reading labels. Or, use the short cut, the Better Choices Grocery List™.

LABEL ROULETTE

Have you ever played roulette? The wheel spins and you haven't a clue where it is going to stop. The unknown result makes it a gamble, a risky undertaking.

Do you feel like you are gambling when grocery shopping for your kids because you don't always know what you are buying? Is it real? Is it fattening? Is saturated fat the good or bad kind? Is it filled with sugar? Is it the good kind of sugar or bad? Is the sodium count too high? How much protein is too much? Should I be counting the calories? Natural, is that good? Does new and improved mean the other wasn't so good? What is the truth and what is not? How the heck are you suppose to know? When you buy food for your kids, do you sometimes not have a clue what all the words on the package really mean, or, do you know for sure what exactly is in the package? Do you sometimes buy one brand of margarine one week and switch to another brand the following week hoping it is a better butter alternative. How many times have you tried different brands of bread because you are not really sure how healthy each one is? How many times have you tried different cereals, become frustrated, and gone back to feeding your kids what they like, knowing it is probably not very good for them?

Welcome to the Label Roulette Anonymous Club with a membership of millions! There are no initiation fees or monthly dues, and the benefits include, a quick and easy guide to label reading, and the Better Choices Grocery List! No longer do you have to be at the mercy of the manufacturers' game of Label Roulette! Kick the gambling habit with knowledge. Educating yourself is key to making good decisions. If you want to understand more, read on. If not, go to the supermarket with the Better Choices Grocery List. We have already scrutinized the labels for these products. However, if your kids do have food sensitivities (allergies) we advise you to finish reading this chapter.

Label Truths and Pitfalls

Who wrote the label laws? Who designed the Nutrition Facts? Who allows the ingredients list requirements to be filled with loopholes? You can look at the Food and Drug Administration (FDA), United States Department of Agriculture (USDA), and Congress for the answers. What makes it confusing is that the USDA is responsible for the regulation of meat, poultry, liquids, and eggs that are frozen. The FDA is responsible for fish, dairy, and all other foods, including fresh eggs. No doubt, conscientious government employees worked hard alongside experts to determine how to best reveal and regulate the contents of food and drink products we buy. However, we have arrived at the conclusion that the food labeling laws and regulations are the victims of the decisions-made-by-committee syndrome. It appears that too many interested parties (lobbyists, lawyers, and politicians!) stood their ground to favorably position their clients' and constituents' financial interests. This situation seems to have opened the door to omit or camouflage some facts. Sometimes, the health of the consumer appears to have been pushed aside in order to placate some big businesses. Not surprising.

The FDA (Food and Drug Administration) who is responsible for label contents including the Nutrition Facts won't agree with our commentary. They describe food labeling as follows:

> Food labeling is required for *most* prepared foods, such as breads, cereals, canned or frozen foods, snacks, desserts, drinks, etc. Nutritional labeling for raw produce (fruit and vegetables) and fish is *voluntary*.[2]

So there you have it. The words most and voluntary already leave the door open.

If you read the Food Labeling Guide document, you find yourself impressed with the detailed verbiage. Problem is, some meanings are connected to others, several layers deep, and before you know it, you become confused by the double-negative, double-talk disorder. We will tell you that even with our amount of research and experience, it is still difficult for us to decipher the truth about the foods we are buying for our kids. In this chapter, we try to simply explain the facts so you can make better decisions when selecting foods. The best defense in this situation is to be well versed on how to read each line, and, read in-between the lines of the information placed on packaging. If this seems too cumbersome, brain taxing, and time consuming, retreat to using the Better Choices Grocery List and shop with confidence.

Food Watch: Read the Label!

Boxed, bagged, and canned food products are decorated with brand names, marketing messages, and facts. In a very small space, a lot is written with the purpose of making you a loyal consumer.

When scanning a label, consumers first eye the brand names, which identify the product. As we write a grocery list, most of us list the brand names. Next, we eye the marketing messages; phrases that are strategically positioned on the box, bag, or can to lure us into buying the product. NEW, New & Improved, Lite, Fat Free, Low Sugar, All Natural are just a few of the long list of sell words. Manufacturers spend a lot of time and money zeroing in on the banner phrase that will catch your eye. Sub messages such as original, enriched, America's favorite (French's mustard), Generous Cuts (Pepperidge Farm croutons), and Win $1000 (El Paso Taco Shells) are there to grab your attention and your dollars. With the phrase, America's favorite mustard, they want you to believe that most everyone loves it and so should you. Generous cuts implies that the enclosed crouton squares are larger than most suggesting that bigger is better, another psychological sell message. And then there is the often-used win-a-prize appeal. Win $1000? You bet! I'll buy your taco shells rather than the other brands sitting on the same shelf. None of these phrases give you clues to the nutritional value of these foods.

All marketing phrases must meet the guidelines set by the FDA. You expect them to be accurate. Yet, how can a product such as some popular fruit yogurts be labeled sugar-free when they contain fruit and even some artificial sugars. Many products fall into this category. This same problem applies to fat and sodium labeling. Natural can mean most anything in today's market. Your definition may be very different from the food manufacturers. It is not uncommon to find synthetic ingredients such as lab-made dyes, in a product that feature "Natural" on the label. This is not prohibited. Food manufacturers know how to play the game. However, you can outwit them by knowing the facts.

Ingredients: Your Window to the Truth

When you can identify all of the ingredients used to make a packaged food, you can be assured of what you are serving your family. However, what you cannot see may be what you get. How many times have you tried to read ingredient lists and find it is almost impossible? Often they are printed in color combinations that make reading it next to impossible: blue letters on red, black on brown, white on yellow. Who can read those? How about the lists printed with laser-thin miniature letters squeezed together so closely that even magnifying glasses can't help you decipher the letters much less the words? Food packaging designers are becoming very clever at camouflaging the ingredients. Often, they are buried in a foldover which you usually tear up when you open the package. Hmmmm. Ingredients are listed in descending order, by weight, not volume. Thus the ingredient weighing the most is listed first, the lightest is listed last. Of course, what is listed last probably has the least amount volume contained in the product. This is why you hear people saying what is listed first has the most and what is listed last has the least amount in the bag, box, or can. More often than not, this applies. It is a safe rule of thumb.

There are several popular brands of dehydrated chicken noodle soups with claims of real chicken broth filled with real chicken chunks and extra noodles. As a teaching tool, let's examine a typical list of ingredients found in these soups. Though reading this may seem a bit laborious, you may find it enlightening as it demonstrates how to determine the value of a food product. Here are typical ingredients found in a dried packaged chicken noodle soup in larger letters for easy reading.

INGREDIENTS: Enriched Egg Noodles, Corn Syrup, Salt, Yeast Extract, Chicken Fat, Chicken, Monosodium Glutamate (MSG), Maltodextrin, Natural Flavors, Cornstarch, Parsley, Chicken Broth, Onion Powder, Color Agents.

Now let's examine the contents of this soup.

1. ENRICHED EGG NOODLES. Note they are enriched which sometimes may indicate the use of bleached white flour. The bleaching process can deplete the flour of its original nutrients. In cases where it has been bleached these noodles are less nutritious. Some synthetic nutrient replacements are usually not as easily absorbed in the body.
2. CORN SYRUP. This is a highly processed form of sugar. It is the second ingredient listed which means there is more corn syrup than chicken in this soup.
3. SALT. In fact, the sodium content is noted as a whopping 680 milligrams per one-cup serving. This exceeds the entire daily recommended amount of sodium for children aged between five and fourteen.
4. YEAST EXTRACT. Yeast extract may have been added as a fermenting agent. Yeast is derived from microscopic fungi. It is a possible MSG source. Some people have allergies to this ingredient.
5. CHICKEN FAT. Out of 14 ingredients, chicken fat is number 5. There is more chicken fat than chicken in this soup. The taste of fat sells.

6. DRIED CHICKEN. The small amount of chicken found in this soup is dehydrated which can reduce its nutrient value.
7. MONOSODIUM GLUTAMATE (MSG). A lab-manufactured form of salt, MSG was formulated as a flavor enhancer as well as an appetite stimulant. Consequently, it is hard to eat just one bite of anything containing MSG.
8. MALTODEXTRINE. This is a lab-made form of sugar used to add flavor and texture. There is no known toxicity. Because it is found in many processed foods, it adds to the over consumption of sugar.
9. NATURAL FLAVORS. Invented as a catchall term, natural flavors leads consumers to believe that the use of the word *natural* makes it acceptable. In fact, we, the consumer, do not know what those natural flavorings are because they are not identified anywhere on this package. This is permitted and is not contrary to any FDA regulations. "Natural flavorings may contain anywhere from 20 to 60 percent MSG."[3]
10. CORNSTARCH. Cornstarch is simply another concentrated form of corn sugar, derived from chemically processed corn. Note: another sweet corn by-product, the sweetener corn syrup, is already listed as ingredient number two.
11. PARSLEY. Fresh parsley is filled with potent nutrients in its natural, unprocessed state. This dried parsley will also contain some beneficial nutrients.
12. CHICKEN BROTH. Because it is not listed among the top five ingredients, there is not very much chicken broth in this product.
13. ONION POWDER. Another processed, dried and finely powdered seasoning. Onions, in the raw state, are filled with healthy nutrients. Dried and powdered versions have fewer.
14. COLOR AGENTS. When there is "real chicken broth" in a product, dyes are not needed to make it look real. Can you see your mother or grandmother adding any colors to her homemade soup?

Now, let's compare this packaged dehydrated chicken noodle soup to a typical homemade chicken noodle soup recipe. Please read the following ingredient list.

> Chicken broth (made from chicken parts simmered in water), Noodles (made from real chicken eggs and seminola wheat flour), Chicken (not dehydrated), Onions (not dehydrated), Salt (sea salt), Pepper, Parsley (not dried).

This soup is going to best fill your kids with nutrients. Most of us have little time to prepare chicken noodle soup from scratch. There are good alternative canned soups made with real whole food ingredients. These can be found on your grocery store shelves. (Please see Better Choices Grocery List)

Try and take time to read ingredient lists. It is your best guideline to the nutrient value of food products. Here are a few easy to read tips.

Ingredient Quick Tips. When deciding whether to buy a product, go right to the ingredient list. If the list is long, forget it. It is a signal that there are probably several synthetic, non-whole food ingredients. Many breads and cereals found on grocery store shelves fall into this category.

If you cannot pronounce some of the ingredients listed on a product, you can suspect that it was created in a lab, not by nature. Most sodas and cookies are good examples of laboratory made foods.

Watch for what is listed in the first few ingredients. In real homemade chicken noodle soup recipes chicken broth, water, and noodles were listed as the first of three ingredients. In the dehydrated chicken soup ingredient list, chicken broth is the eleventh out of fourteen ingredients!

There are questions raised by some ingredient listings. The use of the term "natural flavors" is one example, as no more information is given about them. This can be of special concern to those with food sensitivities, allergies, and restrictions because of medications. Some children have conditions that can make them vulnerable to reactions. It is better to stay away from foods with unidentifiable ingredients.

The above overview of one product demonstrates the purpose of reading the ingredient list from the beginning to end. You probably believe you are feeding your kids foods filled with nutrients which will help them grow, plus repair and replace damaged tissues. It is disconcerting for all of us to learn that the contents of the package may be void of nutrients and contain synthetic ingredients. Now you can see why your kids may be running on empty even after you have just fed them!

If you want to learn more about packaging and food products, read on. If not, be satisfied with just reading the ingredient list.

"Nutrition Facts" Are Confusing

Does the chart of nutrition facts, found on food labels, make you wonder what they were thinking when they created it? Was it designed to please the food industry more than consumers? Many of us feel inadequate and uneducated when reading "Nutrition Facts". They are not clear.

If you stop to add up the numbers of different kinds of fats or sugars and carbohydrates, you often see that your total does not add up to what is printed on the box. For example Reduced Fat Wheat Thins has 1 gram of saturated fat and 1.5 grams of monounsaturated fat, which only accounts for 2.5 grams of the total reported 4 grams of fat. What is the identity or source of the other 1.5 grams of fat? This discrepancy is commonly found in the "Nutrition Facts" of many other food manufacturer's products. The Food Labeling Law allows manufacturers to round up or round down the number of grams of fat, carbohydrates (sugar), protein, cholesterol, and sodium. The amount varies significantly in some categories. This can lead you to believe the contents are better for your kids than they are, especially for those who eat more than one serving at a sitting. The practice of rounding up and down does not help you, the consumer. You are left with unknowns. The differences can add up to measurable quantities.

The following breakdown of "Nutrition Facts" is for those of you who want a detailed explanation, using Wheat Thins as an example. For those who do not, skip over this section.

The Anatomy of "Nutrition Facts"

Serving Size: First and foremost, read the top line, serving size. Everything written below is based on this fact. (Note: "g" stands for grams, a weight measurement.) *One serving of Reduced Fat Wheat Thins is 16 crackers (29 grams).*

Servings Per Container: This tells you how many servings are in the box. *In Reduced Fat Wheat Thins there are "about" 9 servings.* (If your child ate the whole box, the approximate total would be 16 x 9 = 144 crackers.)

Amount Per Serving refers to all the categories below. Again, remember what one serving equals.

Calories: Calories are the result of what you eat. Here is an explanation. Technically a kilocalorie, or calorie, is a unit of heat energy produced when a nutrient is burned. When 1 gram of carbohydrate is metabolized, 4 calories of energy are produced. Proteins also produce 4 calories of energy per gram. Fats, the great hoarder of energy, produce 9 calories when 1 gram is metabolized. "Contrary to what the food and diet industry would like you to believe, we do not actually 'eat' calories. When we ingest nutrients we do not ingest energy, we ingest 'potential' energy, which becomes energy once it is metabolized."[4] In other words, if you eat 1 gram of fat, you produce 9 calories of heat energy units which must be used or it is stored as fat. In fact, all energy units must be used or they are stored in your body, usually as fat. *One serving of Reduced Fat Wheat Thins lists calories: 130*

Calories from Fat: This number tells you the number of calories, or potential energy units, drawn from a fat source in the ingredients, in one serving. *Calories from Fat in Reduced Fat Wheat Thins is listed as 35.*

% Daily Value*: This fact is listed under calories on the right side of the boxed in area. The asterisk refers to the fine print below that defines daily value. The FDA has based the Percent Daily Values on a 2,000 or a 2,500 caloric daily diet. In fine print, below, you will find a table of recommended number of grams of fat, saturated fat, cholesterol, sodium, total carbohydrates, and dietary fiber for a 2,000 and a 2,500 caloric daily diet. Protein is not included. Too bad, protein recommendations would have been a helpful added fact. IMPORTANT: These daily values are designed for an average adult's weight, not a child's. "An adult diet is no more suitable for a child than is a television program or movie that has been designed specifically for mature audiences."[5] Pediatric physicians, dietitians and nutritionists can be very helpful in adjusting nutritional requirements for children. *One serving of Reduced Fat Wheat Thins (16 crackers) fills 6 percent of the recommended daily value for fat of an adult.* Since recommended servings for a child are not noted, you must calculate this adjustment yourself.

Total Fat: This is a report of the total fat grams in one serving of the product. Following is a summary of the different kinds of fats found in the product. *In Reduced Fat Wheat Thins there are 4 fat grams.*

Saturated Fat is just as it sounds, fat filled to capacity. This ladder-like chain of fat has all of its carbon atoms occupied with hydrogen atoms. It is literally saturated with hydrogen. The source is almost always meat and dairy products.

Polyunsaturated Fat is a ladder-like chain of carbons that are missing hydrogen atoms. Some are harmful. Some are not.

Monounsaturated Fat "... fall halfway between saturated and polyunsaturated fatty acids and have one (mono-) empty space (in the chain) where a carbon atom is missing a hydrogen atom."[6] This is considered to be the good fat. *In Reduced Fat Wheat Thins there is 1 gram of Saturated Fat, 0 grams of Polyunsaturated Fat, and 1.5 grams of Monounsaturated Fat.* You are right, the amount of fat totals 2.5, not 4. You can attribute this discrepancy to the practice of rounding up and down.

Cholesterol: Cholesterol is a waxy substance that research concludes contributes to the hardening of the arteries by accumulating in the walls of the blood vessels including those housed in the heart. There are two categories of cholesterol:

HDL (high density lipoprotein) cholesterol is the good kind that can sweep the bad kind out of the arteries.
LDL (low density lipoprotein) cholesterol has the bad reputation, as it is known to clog arteries.

Whether the cholesterol is the good or bad stuff (HDL or LDL) is not noted on "Nutrition Facts." This information would be very helpful for all consumers. *Reduced Fat Wheat Thins lists 0 grams of cholesterol in 1 serving.*

Sodium: One is left to assume that this sodium is NaCl, sodium chloride, better known as table salt. Not necessarily. There are many kinds of sodium. Each one is different. The distinctions of each should be made clear to you just, as is done for fats. Some sodium sources are health giving, some are the opposite. *One serving (sixteen crackers) of Reduced Fat Wheat Thins has 260 milligrams of sodium.*

Total Carbohydrates: All sugars are carbohydrates. All carbohydrates are sugars! There are three types of carbohydrates:

Monosaccharide (fructose, glucose, high fructose corn syrup, honey)
Di and oligosaccharide (sucrose, lactose, galactose, dextrose, maltose)
Polysaccharide (starches and fibers)

Dietary Fiber, a sub list of carbohydrates, is the indigestible residue of a plant carbohydrate. Fiber is critical for the health of the digestive tract. *1 gram comes from fiber in Reduced Fat Wheat Thins.*

Sugars: It is not possible for you to know how many simple or complex carbohydrate are found in a product according to the Nutrition Facts. Although both are units of sugar, the distinction can be significant. Some sources are better for your kids than others. There are over 75 names for sugar. You will find the complete list in Chapter Four, The Anti-Fuels. *Reduced Fat Wheat Thins lists 21 grams as sugar. Reduced Fat Wheat Thins Total Carbohydrates: 21 grams.*

FYI: On this Wheat Thins ingredient list, there are five names for what is considered simple carbohydrates: sugar, cornstarch, high fructose corn syrup, corn syrup, and malt syrup. Malted barley flour may be another source.

Protein: Protein, composed of amino acids, is responsible for the healthy functions of making and repairing, red blood cells, muscles, hair, skin, nails, and hormones. Proteins are in all living things as they provide the building blocks of life. Hence, proteins are found in plant foods, not just meat. Your children are eating more protein than you probably realize. *Reduced Fat Wheat Thins has 2 grams of proteins per servings.*

Vitamins and Minerals: The daily goal for your kids is to ingest 100 percent of the recommended daily value for kids, not adults. Remember, the facts listed on the box are geared for adults. *Reduced Fat Wheat Thins, in one serving, provide 0 percent daily value of Vitamins A and C, 2 percent daily value of calcium, and 6 percent of iron.*

"Nutrition Facts" can be a source of some good information. Once you understand it, it becomes less difficult and more meaningful to read. Unfortunately, the information is not complete. Still, it can be informative when you take the time to read it.

Food Label Laws: Get Real

The Nutritional Label and Education Act, passed by Congress in 1990, is the result of a combined effort of the United States Department of Agriculture (USDA), the Food and Drug Administration (FDA), and Congress. The Food, Drug and Cosmetic Act was revised and is called the FDA Modernization Act of 1997. Many people, some with their own political agendas, had a hand in formulating both Acts. The end result is confusing and too complex to digest. Apparently, the nutrition educators, comprised of scientists from government agencies such as the NIH (National Institutes of Health) disagree. They think their convoluted definitions and guidelines are helpful.

Food manufacturers like to put words on labels to seduce you into buying their product. There was a time when there were few restrictions on which words were permissible, allowing manufacturers to imply a truth that was not true. Eventually, Congress decided it wanted marketing words used on labels to be defined to protect the consumer from fraud. The idea and intent was good. The result leaps over common sense and lands in a muck of nonsense. Here is an example. Healthy is a popular word for food labels. The official descriptive claim for the word "healthy" is broken down into eight different words: healthy, health, healthful, healthily, healthiness, healthfulness, healthfully, and healthier. Each has its own definition as it relates to fat, cholesterol, sodium, protein, fiber, vitamin and mineral content. Plus it is assigned its own commentary for additional requirements. And there's more! Each has its own application for individual foods, meals and main dishes, seafood and game meat. Of course, there are at least two asterisks, one that says that some requirements do not apply to raw fruits and vegetables. Really. For those who are curious, read the Nutrition Label and Education Act, contact the FDA or visit their Website, www.fda.gov.

It is clear that any use of the word health, or any derivatives thereof, on a food label must comply with minimum and maximum nutrient specifications, regardless of how contrived they may seem to consumers. It is also clear that fat, cholesterol, and sodium quantities are monitored. Vitamins A and C, calcium, iron, protein and fiber are considered to be valued nutrients. What is not clear is why the specified fat and cholesterol contents for individual foods and seafood or game meats should be different. In fact, what is the difference between individual foods and game meats? Why is seafood in the same category as game meat? Seafood contains unsaturated fat and game meats contain saturated fat, an important difference. It seems logical that for each, the per-labeled servings should be the same minimum of unsaturated fat and maximum of saturated fat. Also, why is a per-labeled serving of a meal or a minimum dish different than an individual serving? Aren't we looking at a minimum and maximum per serving of any food? Wouldn't it be easier if every labeled serving of a food was equal in amount thereby allowing for the same content requirements? How in the health are you supposed to remember the content requirements of three different healthful, healthy and healthier food categories that will healthily and healthfully provide your kids with healthiness and healthfulness?

Are you ready to scream? If you are not entertained by the absurd complexity of word games of left-brained lawyers, your alternative is the Better Choices Grocery List. If you are, this crazy maze of word definitions goes on. Take a look at "Fresh."

The Descriptive Claim "Fresh" (21 C.F.R. _ 101.95)

Current Status	*Definition*	*Additional Requirements*
'Fresh' (when used to imply a food is unprocessed.)	Raw Not frozen Not thermally processed Not preserved	Use of approved wax/coatings, post-harvest pesticides, certain washes and radiation, or refrigeration does not preclude 'fresh' claims. Pasteurized milk may be labeled as 'fresh.'
'Fresh frozen' 'frozen fresh'	Quickly frozen while fresh. Food may be blanched.	
Quickly frozen	Frozen to center quickly and with almost no deterioration (e.g. blast frozen)	

The dictionary's definitions of fresh are much simpler: Not altered by processing (as freezing or canning). Free from taint: pure. Not stale, sour, or decayed.

The facts are that the additional requirements of waxing and coating of fruits and vegetables are processes. The tainting of foods with post-harvest pesticides involves a process. Radiation is definitely a specialized process. Fresh? Who do they think they are kidding? Blanching is a process dependent upon heat. A method used to "quickly" freeze foods is referred to as a blasting process. Webster's definition clearly points out that the process of freezing disqualifies foods from being labeled as fresh!

See how the food industry has taken the liberty to adjust definitions to suit their needs. They twist and turn the meaning of words. At the same time, you, the consumer, are making decisions based on the common understanding of the meaning of fresh, or light, reduced or free. Light (lite), light from fat calories (lite), light meal and main dishes, light from physical or original product attributes i.e. color or texture, light from sodium, light (lite) in sodium, light in sodium (meals, main dishes, lite), and lightly salted each have their own official definition. Does this not seem a bit ridiculous? Why couldn't the definition of light be food simplified? Because, the food manufacturers want customized ways to positively distinguish one product from another. Unfortunately, the benefits to the consumer get lost in this word warfare. Yes, lawyers and scientists had a hand in legally and scientifically clarifying label word definitions. It appears that they did this to satisfy their powerful food industry clients. However, it is you, the consumer, who ultimately needs to be comfortable with the meaning of these words.

Label Phrases Can Be Deceptive

Read them carefully. Below, we have tried to simplify definitions of some commonly used words found on food labels. Again, please note the "per serving" reference.

FAT FREE: Less than 0.5 grams of fat per serving (not free of all fat).

CHOLESTEROL FREE: Less than 2 milligrams of cholesterol per serving (not free of all cholesterol).

LIGHT or LITE: a food contains at least one-third fewer calories, or no more than half the fat as the original product.

LOW FAT: 3 grams or less of fat per serving.

LOW SATURATED FAT: 1 gram or less of saturated fat per serving.

LOW CHOLESTEROL: 20 milligrams or less and 2 grams of less of saturated fat per serving.

LEAN: Less than 10 grams of fat, 4.5 grams of saturated fat, and 95 milligrams of cholesterol per serving and per 3.5 ounces (100 grams).

EXTRA LEAN: Less than 5 grams of fat, 2 grams of saturated fat and 95 milligrams of cholesterol per serving and per 3.5 ounces (100 grams).

REDUCED, LESS, OR FEWER: The food contains 25 percent less fat than the standard product.

REDUCED FAT, SUGAR, CALORIES: All product labels using the word reduced must be carefully scrutinized. The question to ask yourself is, reduced from what to what? The FDA says reduced is synonymous with less, lower, and at least 25 percent fewer of a list of conditions. On and on and on go the exceptions.

SUGAR FREE and NO SUGAR ADDED: More misleading phrases. As previously mentioned, sugar has more than seventy-five names. However,"... high fructose corn syrup

(HFCS) and other additives of its kind are not classified as sugar by the Food and Drug Administration (FDA) or the U. S. Department of Agriculture (USDA), and products containing them may, therefore, be sold as a 'no sugar added' product."[7] Can you believe it? Believe it.

UNSWEETENED: Watch out. Search the ingredient list for one or more of the thirty-six names for carbohydrates that the FDA does not identify as sugar.

Food Manufacturers Are Clever

How can anyone remember the finite distinctions of label terms when shopping? The phraseology and picky definitions often used skillfully entice you to buy foods that appear not to be too high in fat, sugar, sodium, and cholesterol.

Light Ice Cream! If your kids, like most kids, are fans of ice cream and choose a Light ice cream such as Light Mint Chocolate Chip or Light Vanilla, in one serving (½ cup) they will be eating about 5 grams of fat, 3 of which are saturated fats. Do you know many kids who limit themselves to a fi cup of ice cream? Most kids will eat a cup-sized portion or more. Then the fat gram count increases significantly. Light is a relative term. Be careful about being led to believing that light has a lot less. Remember, there are 9 units of heat energy calories, per gram of fat. Thus, ½ cup of "light" ice cream has 45 fat calories. One cup has 90 fat calories! Though it is less than what is found in regular ice cream, these numbers do add up more quickly than most of us realize.

Note, when food manufacturers reduce a product's fat content, they often increase the sugar content. This is often done to replace the loss of fat taste and texture with the sweet taste of sugar. Most low-fat products are loaded with sugar, some of which is sickly artificial. Reminder: when sugar calories are not used by the body as energy, they are stored as fat inside the body. Increased sugar usually means increased weight.

Fat-Free Meat. How can a ham sandwich be 95 percent fat-free? We all know ham is not lean meat. The truth is that the 5 percent fat refers to the weight of the fat, not the number of fat grams or calories from fat. The other 95 percent of the weight is water! Actually, about 40 to 65 percent of the ham's calories are from fat. This is not even close to being a fat-free food.

Milk. Whole milk has 8 fat grams per cup. 2% milk has 5 fat grams in 1 cup. 1% milk has 3 fat grams in one cup. How does the 2% and 1% milk relate to the 100% whole milk with 8 fat grams? The math does not make sense to most consumers. Yet, we find ourselves trusting the milk producers. Why don't they say it like it is?

Most food product categories are victims of word play. See how food manufacturers can work the numbers to sell you products that are not always what they appear to be? One could look to them for contributing to the recent obesity epidemic among children. They do need to take responsibility for their part. As parents, so do we.

Mislabeling: A Growing Problem

Sorry to report that investigations have revealed product content misrepresentation on labels by food manufacturers. "The Florida Department of Agriculture and Consumer Services food laboratory (since 1999) has found almost 1,000 misbranded products — those with labels misstating the contents."[8] This article goes on to reveal that the USDA and FDA say their foremost concern is food safety, not labeling accuracy. Furthermore, those caught are seldom penalized; there is poor follow up for any adjusted compliance. Most importantly, consumers are not well informed and therefore do not know of such violations. In this report, many products sighted as mislabeled contained many more carbohydrates (sugar) than claimed. Unsuspectingly, some of you may have innocently fed your kids products containing more sugar than you knew. It has been reported, "in a study of 85 ice cream, candy, and bakery companies, The Food and Drug Administration's Minneapolis district office found that a quarter of products that tested positive for peanut allergens did not list peanuts among their ingredients. Peanuts can cause severe, life-threatening reactions in susceptible people."[9] Mislabeling is a national problem.

Government's Loose Reins

Legally, the government allows some variances in label reporting. However, they seem to be a bit extreme. Most products are given a plus or minus 20 percent variance when notating content amount. A 20 percent increase of sugar or fat in a product can be significant, especially on a per serving basis. How about the product that lists a serving as having 0 grams of carbohydrates when it actually contains .099 grams? This is allowed. A few servings of this product can affect a boy or girl who is carbohydrate addicted or has diabetes. All these variations do add up, and may become meaningful over time.

Food manufacturers are not always required to test their foods. Some do. Others simply calculate their estimates. "The average consumer really has no concept that a particular food doesn't have to undergo any testing," says University of Florida food science professor Elaine Turner. "You, as a food manufacturer, don't have to tell the FDA that you're going to create a new food. You just do it."[10] Furthermore, when food manufacturers make a chemical alteration to an existing food product, they are not required to inform you, the consumer. Often they simply splash the words, New and Improved, over the new packaging. Only when the food manufacturer decides to adjust the package design may you discover any unannounced ingredient changes. What happened to FDA approved?

Some ingredients never show up on the list. They are not required to be there. Glucose is one. Glucose is a "cheap" sugar made from processed corn syrup that has been stripped of any existing nutrients. It is almost tasteless and is commonly used as an easy filler for processed foods such as canned fruit and fruit juices, syrups, jams, sodas, candy, ice cream, ketchup, baked products — you name it. The list is long. Without your awareness, odds are that your kids are eating a lot of it. Glucose is the fast sugar, taking only about fifteen minutes to enter the bloodstream. Without notating glucose as an ingredient on a label, you will never know it is in a product. Roulette can be a dangerous game.

Label Spins

What you may see may not be what you get. Pictures and words can give you the wrong impression. Beautiful, colorful photographs of foods filling the front label of a boxed or canned product can make you a believer. The Center for Science in the Public Interest explains why buyers should beware. They point out that a Nissin Cup of Noodles with Shrimp label shows a bowl of soup filled with shrimp, nice plump shrimp. Wrong! Researchers counted anywhere from zero to four teeny shrimp which when cooked, added up to no more than a twentieth of an ounce. They also discovered that Pasta-A-Roni's White Cheddar and Broccoli Rigatoni contained only specks of broccoli. Furthermore, they found NO strawberries or even cream in the box of Quaker Oats Instant Oatmeal Strawberries and Cream. Instead, bits of dehydrated apples had been dyed red. The cream is actually a recipe of maltodextrin (sugar), partially hydrogenated oil, and whey. Fruit Works, a Pepsi product, is really 95 percent sugar and water. Its juice content of only 5 percent pear juice is spiked with vitamins, Red 40 and Blue 1 food dyes, and preservatives. The only strawberries or melon you see are in the lovely colored picture on the label.[11] You've got the picture. Many labels spin a fuzzy picture.

Organic Labeling, Well Done

USDA and Organic Production experts put their minds together and wrote the clear-cut definitions for organic labeling. The Organic Food Products Act, effective in 2002, along with the National Organic Program provide easily understood distinctions for organic foods. There are four categories of organic foods:

- *100% Organic* contains only organically produced ingredients (water and salt excepted).
- *Organic* must consist of at least 95 percent organically produced ingredients (water and salt excepted). The USDA Organic seal confirms this category.
- *Made with Organic Ingredients* contain at least 70 percent organic ingredients.
- Products containing less than 70 percent organic ingredients cannot use the term organic anywhere on the display panel, but may print the organically produced ingredients on the ingredient list.

In addition, the government has agreed on what qualifies food as organic. These are easily understood and are described in Chapter Eleven, "Always Consider the Source."

There are people who are committed to resolving the food labeling issues. Hats off to them. We believe that the FDA and the USDA could write better versions of many of their guidelines. The food manufacturers also need to show a commitment to straight-shooting production, marketing, and labeling practices.

According to *USA Today*, food is the most trusted industry.[12] Unfortunately, there is a great disparity between the consumer's trust and the truth. The good news is that there are food manufacturers who work diligently to provide you with good food with credible labeling practices. Please see the Better Choices Grocery List for food companies and brands you can trust.

For the health of our children, we must read between the lines to make Better Choices.

3

There Are No Calories IN Food

Chapter Quick Facts

- Kids do not eat calories. Their bodies produce them from the food they eat.
- One gram of carbohydrates produces 4 grams of energy. One protein gram produces 4 grams of energy. One fat gram produces 9 grams of energy.
- The number of calories listed on a food label is not necessarily an indicator of a food's value. The food's source of caloric energy is the best measure.
- The continuous consumption of high-caloric food, especially sugar foods, can lead to obesity, diabetes, and other diseases.
- Junk in, junk out. Low-nutrient calories are junk calories. Junk calories can create inefficient, unproductive bodies.
- Nutrient-filled foods produce high-octane calories, resulting in healthy growth and productive performance.
- To more specifically determine the number of calories your kids need to burn daily, use the BMI and RMI formulas. Both are easily explained in this chapter.
- Quality foods beat quantity when choosing energy producing food for your kids.

THERE ARE NO CALORIES IN FOOD

Keep this in mind when filling up your kids!

None, Zero, Zip! The way everyone talks about calories, you would think that we eat them. We don't. Calories are not substances that are eaten. Calories are not particles or molecules found in any food. There are no calories IN foods. When you buy food at the store, you are not buying calories. You are buying the ability to produce calories, a measure of energy. Daniel Webster's definition of a calorie is "the unit of measuring the energy produced by food when oxidized in the body."

CALORIES ARE ENERGY FUELS

During the digestive process, foods filled with carbohydrates, proteins, and fats are metabolized. As they are broken down for absorption, heat is released, and energy is produced. Either this energy is used up through physical activity or it is stored as fat for future use. Different food groups produce different amounts of energy.

One carbohydrate gram - 4 grams of energy.
One protein gram - 4 grams of energy.
One fat gram - 9 grams of energy.

Fat produces twice as many energy units as carbohydrates and proteins; thus it takes twice as much activity to use up fat energy or calories.

Look at the following to see how grams and calories are related in food products. 1% milk "Nutrition Facts": one serving of eight fluid ounces offers 102 calories. When eight ounces of this 1% milk is swallowed and digested, the contents are broken down as follows:

Content	# Calories per Gram	# Grams in 8 oz.	Total # of Calories
Fat	9	2.5	22.5
Carbohydrates	4	12.0	48.0
Protein	4	8.0	32.0
		Total Calories	102.5

In this milk 102.5 units of caloric energy are available for the body to use as needed. What is not used is then stored in the muscles and as fat cells, and a little is put to use in the liver and brain.

Consider the Calorie Source

The number of calories listed on a food label does not necessarily indicate a food's value. The actual source of the calories is really the best nutrient value indicator. Here is an example of how a food with more calories can be a Better Choice. (The following numbers vary slightly from product to product.)

Famous Amos Chocolate Chip Cookies, 1 ounce (4 cookies), produces 151 calories.

7 fat grams = 63 calories from fat
2 protein grams = 8 calories from protein
20 carbohydrate grams = 80 calories from carbohydrates

Natural by Nature Chocolate Pudding, 4.5 ounces, produces 140 calories.

3 fat grams = 27 calories from fat
4 protein grams = 16 calories from protein
25 carbohydrate grams = 100 calories from carbohydrates

Comparison @ 4.5 ounces:

Amount	Product	# fat grams	# protein grams	# carbohydrate grams	# calories
4.5 oz.	Cookies	32	9	90	684
4.5 oz.	Pudding	3	4	25	143

When eating 4.5 ounces of this pudding, your kids would eat 29 less grams of fat, 65 fewer grams of carbohydrates, with a total of 541 less calories to burn than they would eat if they gobbled down 4.5 ounces of these cookies. The Natural by Nature Chocolate Pudding is a Better Choice for a treat! In addition, Naturally By Nature Chocolate Pudding is made from organic whole milk, sugar, skim milk, and cocoa. Plus, tapioca starch, natural vanilla, carrageenan, and sea salt are added for taste and texture. These ingredients contain their original nutrients. Choose your kid's source of caloric energy wisely.

Unused Calories "Turn into Fat"

Young bodies use caloric energy for three purposes: To maintain basal metabolic rate or BMR; that is to operate vital services such as running the brain and keeping the heart beating. To carry out cell activity involved in growth. For daily activities such as walking, working, and playing.[1] The food your kids eat supply energy units that are to fulfill the three purposes. When energy units, better known as calories, are inactive, they are stored, with the intent of being used later. If your children are eating foods that produce more caloric energy than they can use or store in the liver, brain, or muscles, the body will then store this energy as fat. Today, kids are eating more high caloric foods and are moving around less. Their storage of fat is on the rise. This leads to obesity.

The commonly used guideline to identify obesity is a measurement of 30 percent more than his or her ideal weight. Susan T. Borra, President of the American Dietetic Association, said, "Data from the National Center for Health Statistics suggest nearly 25 percent of children and adolescents are overweight or obese, or at risk of obesity."[2] Several sources, including the National Center For Health Statistics report that around 15 percent of children to adolescents are obese. This is about twice as many as in the 1960s. Today's kids are bigger than their parents and grandparents were as children. Fact: the desks designed for kids during the 1940s cannot be used by most of today's kids. Their bottoms won't fit! Also, sorry to say, the clothing manufacturers have adjusted sizing to meet the body changes of today. Jeans made for a kid's size 12 today are made from a larger pattern than 10 to 20 years ago. That means a child wearing a size 10 now, would have worn a larger size, maybe size 12 in the late twentieth century. (Sorry mom and dad, this applies to you, too.) A root cause for this increase in weight and size of kids aged 6 to 17 is the kind of food they are eating, the portions of serving sizes, and increasing inactivity. This behavioral formula expedites overweight malnourished conditions.

Malnourished Kids Have Inefficient Metabolisms

The reality is that the metabolism of a poorly nourished child runs inefficiently. In addition, the brain may send a message, "Not enough nutrients, hold onto the caloric energy, store it as fat." The sad truth is that children with low-nutrient, high-fat, high-sugar diets are more likely to store more fat for longer periods of time. Conversely, well-nourished kids have smoother running metabolisms. The more active they are, the more fine-tuned their engines may be. Their organs, muscles, and bones are better fueled to grow and develop.

Fat Cells Expand and Are Eternal

Fat cells not only grow in numbers, they also expand in size. Once fat cells exist, they will not go away. They can only be reduced in size. The use of caloric energy through the careful choice of nutritional foods and physical activity can help this. However, liposuction is the only way these cells can totally disappear from the body. This procedure can be a dangerous and is not recommended by these authors. Overweight and obese children should be seen by a health professional for weight-control programs.

Junk In, Junk Fat!

There is only so much an engine can do to process and use high-caloric junk fuel. Junk food equals junk fuel. It produces inefficient caloric energy; kids hit highs and lows, and then turn lethargic. Lethargy usually leads to a sedentary lifestyle of watching TV for hours and being brainwashed by an array of over 10,000 junk food commercials. Junk food commercials entice these kids to eat more junk foods. The young actors and actresses used in these commercials look like they are having a great life because they are eating advertised products. Ask your kids this: "How many junk food commercial models do they think eat a steady diet of the junk foods they advertise?" The truth is that a diet of junk food will interfere with the growth of beautiful silky hair, ivory smooth skin, clear bright eyes, and contoured bodies, the beautiful look. (Unfortunately, many of these preteen and teen models aren't eating much of anything, but that is another subject altogether.)

A day of Cocoa Puffs, Pop-Tarts, Lunchables, Skittles, Sprite, Pringles, extra cheese and pepperoni pizza, fries, fast food burgers and Coke is a day filled with unproductive and excessive caloric energy consumption. To use it you have to move it. Even the most active young kids have difficulty burning the almost 2000 calories found in this common daily diet. Now that you know that unused caloric energy is stored as fat you can understand why kids are growing rounder.

Junk Food Is Sludge

Sources of caloric energy from artificial ingredients, refined sugars, and animal fat contribute to an overtaxed digestive system. Many artificial ingredients, which are not naturally designed for human digestion, may create havoc within the human body. Refined sugars are known to over-stimulate organs such as the pancreas, causing it to break down. Over time, unused digested animal fat is known to clog up the circulatory system. Streaks of cholesterol have been sighted in the arteries of children under the age of one. Collectively, junk food is to the human body as sludge is to a drain. The good stuff, water and nutrients, cannot get through the system. Useless calories are creating useless junk fat-filled bodies.

Nutrient-Filled Foods Produce High-Octane Caloric Energy

The metabolism of well-nourished active children is efficient. Their bodies burn clean fuel. Efficiently used calories create useful bodies. Growing bodies require nutrients to build bones and develop muscles, organs, brains, all connecting tissues, and blood.

The motors of well-nourished active kids just keep on humming with productive results. Foods, such as black beans, broccoli, and Brazil nuts, are filled with protein, complex carbohydrates, essential fatty acids, vitamins, minerals, enzymes, and phytonutrients, all of which are high-octane calorie energy sources.

Caloric Energy and Your Kid

Not all kids need the same amount of caloric energy in a given day. Each one is one of a kind God-made miracle. Because of the number of variables (body type, blood type, age, gender, activity level) it is difficult to make a one-size fits all chart.

Find the Desireable Weight for Your Kids

The Body Mass Index (BMI) is a way to measure ideal weight relative to height.

Formula	Example (thirteen year old)
Multiply current weight in pounds by 703	120 lb. x 703 = 84,360 pounds
Multiply current height in inches by itself	66 in. x 66 in. = 4,356 inches
Divide pounds by inches	84,360 lb. by 4,356 in. = 19.4 BMI

Dr. Fred Pescatore, author of *Feed Your Kids Well*, says ideal BMI for kids are:

Ages	BMI
6-8	13-15
9-12	15-17
teenager	19-21

His or Her Caloric Energy Needs

Susan Kalish, author of *Your Child's Fitness*, offers this customized formula to determine how many calories your kids need to produce in order function well.

Resting Metabolic Rate (RMI) (number of calories needed to *maintain* bodily functions).
Multiply your child's desired body weight by 10.
Example: 120 pounds x 10 = 1,200.

To find out what calories are needed per activity level, select the appropriate category and ADD these calories to your child's Resting Metabolic Rate.

Sedentary child
Multiply desired weight by 3.
Example: 120 pounds x 3 = 360 more calories
Add the RMI 1,200 calories for a total of 1,560 calories needed to sit around after school.

Moderately Active child
Multiply desired weight by 5.
Example: 120 pounds x 5 = 600 more calories
Add the RMI 1,200 calories for total of 1,800 calories needed to ride a bike around the neighborhood a few days a week, after school.

Very Active child
Multiply desired weight by 10.
Example: 120 pounds x 10 = 1200 more calories
Add the RMI 1,200 calories for a total of 2,400 calories needed to play team soccer four or more days a week, after school.[3]

All factors are important when looking for the best guide for your child. Do remember that though reliable, this guideline is not perfect. Children do have different-sized bone structures and other genetic variables. For a more exact calculation of the best caloric formula for your kids, consult a health professional.

Quality Beats Quantity

As has been repeated, repeatedly — on purpose — quality beats quantity when choosing foods for your kids. Here is an example.

Foods low on nutrients, high in calories.
One Big Mac ....590 calories
One French fries (sm.)... 210 calories
One Coke, 8 ounce..........97 calories
897 calories

This meal adds up to 897 calories, of which approximately 400 calories (about 45 percent) are from trans and saturated fats. Unfortunately, most of these calories come from processed, denatured foods.

Quality replacement meal
Salmon, 3 oz..................157 calories
Potato, baked.................220 calories
Butter, 1 pat.....................36 calories
Peas, 4 oz.........................63 calories
Milk, 1%, 8 oz................110 calories
586 calories

This meal is loaded with nutrients and adds up to 586 calories, of which about 117 calories (20 percent) are from fat. Your kids will thrive on these whole foods. And, they won't feel hungry as fast as they would be if they had eaten a Big Mac, fries, and Coke.

The salmon meal is easy to cook! Pour Italian dressing over the salmon and grill it for 10 to 12 minutes. Bake the potato in a microwave (15 minutes) if you do not have time to use an oven. Put frozen peas in boiling water. Turn off heat and let sit for three minutes. Pour cold milk in glass, 30 seconds. Mom and dad, this is a 15 to 20 minute meal!

So you are thinking, my kid doesn't like salmon. Some kids don't, especially when it is not fresh. Substitute salmon with a thin 3-ounce piece of chicken breast. Quickly marinate it in lemon, garlic and olive oil, cover, and bake for maybe 15 minutes at 350 degrees Fahrenheit. The total of caloric fuel it provides adds up to just a few more calories than the salmon; all of them are good for your son or daughter.

Which kid do you think has a better chance of concentrating in school and performing without fatiguing throughout his or her swim meet? The burger, fries, and soda kid, or, the fish (chicken), potato, peas, and milk kid? Which kid's body will be better fueled producing productive caloric energy for healthy growth?

Fuel As Needed: Important

Fuel your kids as their bodies and minds require it. This reality is especially true for kids with fine-tuned metabolisms.

> The human digestive tract is especially well adapted to snack-type eating rather than three major meals a day. As long as what we're eating is low in percentage of calories from fat, low in salt, and not totally without fiber as a result of ultra refining, nibbling throughout the day is no problem. The problem is that many nibble-type foods are high in fat, high in salt, and low in fiber. Potato chips, corn chips (even 'health food store' chips), granola bars, trail mix, crackers, cookies, doughnuts, cupcakes, Twinkies, ice cream, peanut butter and jelly, soda, Kool Aid, Hi-C, milk shakes, salted nuts, and a variety of candy bars are examples.[4]

When your kids are running on empty, their body must get fuel from somewhere. The message is sent, "Go to the most available source." Then the body turns to its fat supply. Once that's gone, it will go to the tissues. Yes, the body will actually eat itself. For the overweight child, initially, this may not be a problem. For the fit athlete who is active all day, it can become a real problem. For underweight undernourished kids, the problems become serious. Eating at mealtimes and timely snacking is good.

Children with empty food reserves may experience a low blood-sugar condition. This causes fatigue, irritability, loss of focus and concentration, and low energy. Children who do not eat lunch and still face academic, performing art, and/or PE classes can count on reduced mental and physical energy. Choosing to, or not to, eat a nourishing lunch can influence your son and daughter's ability to recall facts for the 1:30 P.M. science test.

Good after school snacks help them to be reenergized for after school activities, be it playing with friends, studying ballet, working out on a soccer field, or doing homework. Kids who use up their fuel need to replace it in order to be productive.

Snacking Is a Good Habit Unless the Snack Is Bad

Throw out the Snickers bar. Replace it with fresh fruit. In an empty stomach, fruit can be metabolized to produce good caloric energy in your kid's system within 20 minutes. Bananas take longer, 30 minutes. Try to choose low-sugar fruits such as berries in order to reduce the glucose spiking that may occur, or mix fruit with a protein or healthy fat. For instance, spread 100 percent peanut or almond butter on a banana. It will satisfy your son or daughter's hunger while creating a balanced energy reserve. For more sustained energy, add foods with fiber. Go for the quality, whole foods for the best results.

Better Choice Snacks

Below are some suggestions for wholesome caloric energy producing foods that most kids like!

- Fresh fruit
- Fruit salad
- Popcorn, very lightly salted and buttered
- Smoothies ... see CD-ROM recipes
- Nut butters (100 percent) with celery and carrots
- Raw or slightly steamed veggies with low-fat dip (onion) or dressing (ranch)
- Chicken or turkey wrapped in whole-grain tortilla (with ketchup)
- Rice cakes with low-fat cottage cheese/cream cheese, or PB and J
- Whole-grain cereal with 1%, skim or rice milk
- Whole-grained toast with nut butter and/or jelly
- Low-fat yogurt with fruit, topped with sunflower or sesame seeds
- Applesauce mixed with berry sauces (no sugar added)
- Hummus on whole grain or nut crackers
- Tuna fish on rice crackers
- Celery stuffed with low-fat organic cream cheese or goat cheese
- Protein shake made with rice or soy milk, frozen organic fruit, a spoonful of "no-sugar added" jam and a low-carbohydrate protein powder. Add a frozen banana!
- Hard-boiled eggs (deviled eggs using canola mayonnaise)
- Rolled-up additive-free turkey slices
- Raw or naturally roasted nuts and seeds, if not allergic
- Pita bread pockets stuffed with chicken, tomatoes, romaine lettuce, low-fat cheese
- Organic cheese cubes and a small handful of grapes (frozen!)

Short and to the point: calories in foods are the measure of energy that different foods can produce. Feed your kids quality foods that will produce high-performance caloric energy on a timely basis.

Your kids do not want to be caught running on empty.

4

Meet the Anti-Fuels

Chapter Quick Facts

- Anti-fuels are foods that sabotage the anatomical systems of the human body. On average, they represent around 70 to 80 percent of what kids eat daily.
- *Sugar* creates free radicals, stuns the immune system, turns to fat when unused, stimulates nervous and emotional imbalance, and causes disease such as Type 2 diabetes. Monthly, many kids eat about 15 pounds.
- *Sodium* (salt) can also be a public enemy. Many kids are consuming five to ten times the recommended amount.
- *Fat.* Kids consume about 30 percent of their caloric energy from fat. The bad hydrogenated and trans fatty acids are in most processed foods.
- *Dairy.* Additive-treated cow's milk is a questionable source of calcium.
- *Caffeine* stimulates repeated consumption use. It is known to deplete your kids of nutrients, especially calcium.
- *Additives*: pesticides, herbicides, fungicides, preservatives, flavorings, bleaches, dyes, and more. Many people, including kids, consume around 150 pounds a year.
- Anti-Fuels keep your kids running on empty. Replace these junk foods with foods and drinks filled with life-supporting nutrients!

ANTI-FUELS ARE NOT YOUR KID'S FRIENDS *

Every time your son or daughter has a birthday, it is a reminder of how fast they are growing up! As parents, this is a time when we usually reflect on the importance and challenges of providing him or her the tools needed to be healthy, productive, and happy. We want the best for our children. Fueling their precious minds and bodies with naturally occurring foods and drinks is key to giving our kids the best odds. Unfortunately, kids are consuming more and more anti-fuels, counter productive anti-fuels.

Anti-fuels are foods and drinks with ingredients that may sabotage the workings of the anatomical systems found in the human body. Some are chemically altered versions of whole foods. Others have little or no whole-food origin and are primarily made of chemicals created in the laboratory. Excess consumption of both versions work to undermine your kids. They can impair or weaken the digestive, circulatory, nervous, immune, and skeletal systems. They also can rob your kid's body of key nutrients and leave him or her vulnerable to the negative impact of viruses and bacteria. Over an extended period of time, an imbalance of anti-fuel consumption may zap your son or daughter of energy, cause dehydration, constipation, headaches, and weaken his or her defense mechanisms.

To date, most packaged lunches and snacks found in refrigerated sections of stores are almost an all-in-one anti-fuel product. "*Lunchables* contain thirteen teaspoons of sugar (fifty-two grams of carbohydrates altogether) enough to send your child's blood sugar soaring. This marketing nightmare contains seven different forms of sugar, seven types of sodium, nineteen different chemical additives, and hydrogenated fats to clog up his or her arteries."[1] On average in a single serving package you may find one or more tablespoons of fat and around 1200 to 1600 milligrams of sodium. Unreal! In addition, almost all this sugar, sodium, and fat hail from undesirable food sources. Imagine how this massive infusion of chem-

* **WARNING:** This chapter may negatively arouse your emotions, make you feel frustrated, irritable, and mad, tax your mind, give you an information overload headache, and take too long to read. If you are experiencing any of the above and want to skip it, stick to the Quick Facts and simply turn to Chapter Fourteen to use the Better Choices Grocery List. You and your kids may be glad you did!

icals impacts your kids during a school day. Fortunately, in August of 2003, Kraft, manufacturer of *Lunchables*, announced it "will form a 10-member advisory team of nutrition, behavior, health and communications experts to review the nutritional value of its products."[2] Hopefully this committee will recommend a healthier recipe for Lunchables. This is only one of hundreds of processed foods laden with anti-fuels.

Anti-Fuels: Sugar, Sodium, Hydrogentated and Trans Fats, Dairy, Caffeine, Artificial Additives

On average, these anti-fuels represent approximately 70 to 80 percent of what kids consume daily. Most kids devour these foods and drinks in excessive amounts. Every time we, as parents, cave in to demands for sugar, salt, fat, caffeine, and dairy found in processed, refined, and fast foods, we set our kids up for disappointments, a future of possible allergies, illnesses, and poor mental and physical performance.

Okay. You are probably thinking; "You have got to be crazy if you think my kids will give up sweets, French fries, sodas, or orange cheese." Good news! There are good-tasting alternatives. Lots of Better Choices food and drinks found at your neighborhood grocery stores have passed the taste-test taken by kids known as the Kid Kritics. (Please see Chapter Fourteen.) We have found that when kids experience the positive taste and nutritional result of eating Better Choices foods, they like how it feels. Over time, after adding these foods to your daily routine, the desire by your kids and the demands of their bodies for junk food becomes reduced. In time, junk foods can be saved as weekend treats. Gradually, these changes usually reap academic, athletic, and social rewards and motivate kids to make better choices. You will learn how it can be done. This is easier than you think! The benefits are enormous and have a lifelong impact!

It is important for you to know the true facts about these anti-fuels. Share them with your kids. They want to know some of these facts, too.

Sugar: The Number-One Anti-Fuel

Buy a 10-pound bag of sugar, put it on the kitchen table and show it to your kids. Point out that according to national averages, this is about the amount they eat monthly. Many eat more! Your kids will be astounded and in denial of this fact. So will you.

The bottom line is that kids are eating way too much sugar and are challenged by the consequences. If you doubt this, read on.

Sugar Is Like Quicksand

Once it sucks you in, it is hard to get out. In time, it can significantly alter your son or daughter's mind and body. Sugar may start out as a fiber-based natural plant such as sugar cane, sugar beets, or corn. However, manufacturers refine these plants so the extract may be sold as sweet, easy-to-use, sugar. During the refining process, the life source is tossed out. What is left is a concentrated molecular sugar product. When consumed these molecules quickly flood the bloodstream, shock the stomach and pancreas, creating acidic conditions. In response, the body searches for alkaline cells to counterbalance the onslaught of acid. The brain reacts by sending instructions to leach alkaline calcium from the bones. Over time, this may result in weakened bone structure. In addition, excessive acid conditions in the stomach impair the digestion and absorption of vitamins and minerals. Immune systems are stunned. Diseases find an easy entry. Blood sugar levels spike and fall. Emotions become uneven. The more sugar kids have the more they want. They become caught in the vicious sugar cycle.

> ...In large amounts sugar leads to obesity, hypoglycemia, diabetes, high blood pressure, heart disease, anemia, immune deficiency, tooth decay, and bone loss. It contributes to herpes, yeast infections, cancer, premenstrual syndrome, menstrual problems, and male impotence...It weakens the mind, causing loss of memory and concentration, nervousness, shyness, violence, excessive or no talking, negative thought, paranoia, emotional upsets such as self-pity, arguments, irritability, and the desire for only sweet things in life.[3]

Sugar Robs Peter To Pay Paul

Just for a minute, focus on the fact that minerals such as magnesium, chromium, zinc, copper, cobalt, and manganese are required for the digestion of refined sugar. Because these minerals have been stripped from the sugar cane or beet during the refining process, your son's and daughter's resourceful brains have to search and source their bodies for these minerals. Consequently, when sugar is consumed in excess, the body's process of leaching minerals can deplete young bodies of the very minerals that are designated to keep nervous, skeletal and other systems in balance and strong. While all this is happening, simultaneously, young bodies are also trying to grow healthy brains, bones, muscles, blood vessels, and any number of the many trillions of cells. (This cell count depends on the body size.) Ultimately, one or more bodily functions sacrifice productive functions when a young body consumes too much sugar. Refined sugar works against a growing body.

Too Much Sugar Suppresses the Immune System

Really, it does. The good guys (white blood cells) that fight the bad guys (viruses and bacteria) are deactivated.

> According to Kenneth Bock, M.D., an expert in nutritional and environmental health, with practices in Rhinebeck and Albany, N.Y., two cans of soda (which together typically contain 20 to 24 teaspoons of sugar) reduce the efficiency of white blood cells by 92 percent – an effect that lasts up to five hours.[4]

Five hours! In addition, while the good guys are stunned, the bad guys (free radicals) zoom around freely multiplying in numbers, thereby opening the door to mental and physical degenerative diseases, and bacterial and viral illnesses.

Sugar and Hormone Stress

Eating sugar stimulates the release of hormones, primarily insulin. Here begins a chain reaction resulting in excessive elevated levels of other hormones such as cortisone and epinephrine. This leads to the rapid release of glycogen that is stored glucose (blood sugar). Glycogen is supposed to be released slowly by the liver to fuel the muscles. When the glycogen is released too fast, this fuel may be used up more quickly. If this happens when your son or daughter is taking a test, or running a race, he or she will be running on empty. Repetition of this process brings on exhaustion and possible physical injury. Young athletes who eat sugar before a competition face a double-dilemma. Both their minds and bodies become stressed. You can make it a triple-dilemma when you add the fact that while performing mental and physical feats, their young bodies are trying to grow.

Sugar Messes with the Body and Mind

Statistics are identifying the disturbing increase of obesity, diabetes, immune-deficiency illness, and behavioral disorders among children and young adults. Furthermore, diseases and illnesses traditionally identified with older adults are showing up in greater numbers among adults in their twenties and thirties. Type 2 (Adult Onset) diabetes is a good example. Yes, there are other contributing factors to the development of these health conditions. But, you would be foolish to deny the relationship that exists between the contributing factors of sugar and these health problems.

Type 2 Diabetes: "Increasingly, health care providers are finding more and more children and teens with Type 2 diabetes, a disease usually seen in people over the age of 40."[5]

"Today, 25 percent of all new cases of adult-onset diabetes are occurring in people under the age of twenty. Dr. Gerald Bernstein, president of the American Diabetes Association, comments: 'What we are learning, unfortunately, is this is now a disease of children. Type 2 diabetes is making alarming gains among youth ... '"[6]

Dr. Lori Laffel, head of the pediatric unit at Boston's Joslin Diabetes Center, says, "Over the years, we always saw an occasional child with Type 2. It was a handful a year. Now there is an epidemic of Type 2 diabetes in youth, absolutely."...During the early 90s, Joslin's totals increased five times. Since then, they have doubled again.[7]

One in three American children born in the year 2000 will go on to develop diabetes, the US Centers for Disease Control and Prevention reported here Saturday (August, 2, 2003). The majority of these cases will be adult onset, or Type 2 diabetes, which is strongly associated with obesity and a lack of exercise.[8]

Diabetes in children has reached epidemic proportions, especially in overweight children, say scientists ...at the meeting of the American Diabetes Association.[9]

Diabetes is disruptive to the every day lives of kids unfortunate to have contracted it. Often it leads to a nervous disorder, blindness, or amputations. This is scary.

Obesity: To be obese, you have to be about 30 percent or more over your ideal weight. Researchers have noted that millions of Americans, including children, are obese. Since one in five kids are obese, odds are that maybe every fifth parent who is reading this book is related to an obese child. Can you believe it? That is a lot. Too much fat on a body is usually an indicator that the child is not eating nutrient-filled food. In addition, most are eating too many anti-fuels such as sugar. Ten to twenty pounds of sugar a month is a huge amount of caloric energy that must be burned through use in order not to be stored as fat. It will certainly over-stimulate digestive and nervous systems as well. In addition, other organs and bodily functions become challenged. A diet of too much sugar can result in obesity, lead to cardiovascular disease, diabetes, immune disorders, and emotional challenges.

Behavioral Risks: The pancreas' job is to control the amount of sugar that enters the bloodstream. When a lot of sugar is eaten, the hormone, insulin is called on to bring a high blood sugar level down to normal. When too much sugar is eaten, the pancreas is stimulated to produce too much insulin, too often. This creates a low-blood sugar level condition, also known as hypoglycemia. Low-blood sugar can lead to cellular starvation. Most importantly, brain cells also become starved. Here is the behavioral connection: "As the blood sugar drops, the cerebrum — the area of the brain responsible for thought, learning, and moral and social behavior — starts to shut down, and the brain diverts its dwindling energy resources to the brain stem, which controls the more primitive responses: the drives for food, sex, aggressive/defensive instincts."[10] Yes, there is a correlation between a low-blood sugar level and an increase in food binging, sex drive, and violent behavior. Crime, excessive sexual activity, eating and drinking (binging) are some of the disturbing behaviors plaguing today's kids. Sugar plays a role here.

Emotional Roller Coaster: You have probably witnessed kids expressing emotional highs and lows after eating a large dose of sugar. "It (sugar) triggers the opiates in the brain, which makes you feel good."[11] Because the feel good feeling does not last, an emotional and energy dive follows. Fatigue and irritability take over until there is more stimulation with more sugar. Some compare this sugar roller coaster behavior with emotional drug behavior.

Sugar and Fat: A Double-Negative

Unused sugar turns to fat. Unused fat turns to fat. Excess fat leads to overweight and obese kids. This puts them on the road to heart and degenerative disease, diabetes, as well as a myriad of emotional dysfunctions. Research has found that sugar and fat supply three out of every five calories produced by foods eaten by the average American. Chances are, this ratio is higher for kids as they eat little else. The more knowledge you have on this subject, the more you are able to prevent potential health problems for your kids. Please read on.

Sugar Has Over 75 Names: It is Confusing

Many sugars are man-made. The few that are made by mother nature are rarely used in their original form. Here are some of the commonly used versions. Are you ready?

> Acesulfame K (Sunette and Sweet One), Aspartame (NutraSweet and Equal), Barley Malt, Brown Rice Syrup, Fructose or Levulose, Glucose, Honey, Lactose, Maltose, Rice Syrup, Saccharin, Sorbitol, Mannitol, Xylitol, Sorghum, Sucanat Evaporated Cane Juice, Sucrose, Beet Sugar, Blackstrap Molasses, Brown Sugar, Cane Sugar, Carmel, Corn Fructose, Corn Sweetner, Corn Syrup, Date Sugar, Demerar Sugar, Dextrin, Dextrose, Fruit Fructose, Grape Sugar, Grape Sweetener, Herbal Sweetener, High Fructose Corn Syrup, Invert Sugar, Molasses, Ploydextrose, Raw Sugar, Sugar and Turbinado.[12] Also Stevia, "Granulated Sugar, Powdered Sugar, Specialty Sugars, Liquid Sugars, Maple Sugar, Sucralose Sucraryl, Syrup Blend, Allose, Altrose, Arabinose, Erythrose, Galactose, Gulose, Idose, Lyxose, Mannose, Psicose, Rhamnose, Ribose, Saccharose, Sorbose, Tagatose, Talose, Threose, Xylose, Sylulose."[13]

New additions to this list are Splenda and maltitol crystals. Watch for the terms "natural flavors." This last one is the sneakiest secret ingredient. We have no way of knowing what they are. If you do not want to memorize the unfamiliar names, just know that an ingredient word ending with the letters –ose, or –ol, is sugar. One or more of the sugars listed above is found in most processed foods.

Sugar Is Simple

Sugar is nothing more than a simple carbohydrate. All sugars are made up of simple carbohydrates. There are three versions, each made up of different number of chains of simple carbohydrates (saccharide means sugar molecule):

- Monosaccharide, Mono (one) — one sugar molecule
- Disaccharide, Di (two), — a combination of two sugar molecules.
- Polysaccharide, Poly (many) — a combination of three or more sugar molecules linking long and complex chains.

Simple carbohydrates have names, identifying their distinct properties. The following combinations of simple carbohydrates (sugars) are found in foods.

- Sucrose — common sugar made from fruit, sugar cane, tubers such as sugar beets, grains, seeds, or maple syrup. Disaccharide.
- Fructose — comes from naturally ripened produce and is highly processed. It is found in hundreds and hundreds of processed food and drinks, some of which are labeled as "no sugar added." (Watch out, diabetics!) Other names are levulose and fruit sugar. Monosaccharide.
- Glucose — is a product extracted from fruit, grains, and plants such as corn and potatoes. Also, glucose is produced in the human body through the digestion of carbohydrates coming from grains, breads, cereals, pastas, starches, milk products and some vegetables. Monosaccharide.
- Lactose — is a milk sugar, formed in the mammary glands of lactating animals. It requires the enzyme, lactase, for digestion. After two years of age, most children no longer produce lactase needed for the digestion of milk.
- Disaccharide. Galactose — is found in dairy products, derived from lactose. Monosaccharide.
- Maltose — is derived from grains, usually barley. Disaccharide.

Processed Sugars

Some sugars are more naturally processed: unrefined sugar (sugar cane), maple syrup, sorghum molasses, blackstrap molasses, rice syrup, barley malt, honey, fruit juices, fruits syrups, date sugars and amasake. These naturally sourced sweeteners may withstand less processing and thus may retain some of their original nutrients. Because they all are comprised of simple carbohydrates, they are all sugar.

Though the origin of corn syrups is corn, they are heavily processed to the point of removing any potential nutrients found in this plant. High-fructose corn syrup is created by applying high heat during the processing phase which produces a free radical-filled end product. Consumption can cause notable stress on your daughter and son's bodily systems. By adding so much high-fructose corn syrup, corn syrup, and other corn sugar derivative sweeteners to so many foods and drinks, food manufacturers have added another negative consequence to sugar consumption, food allergies. Research has determined corn to be a common allergy food among children that is known to raise havoc in the circulatory and nervous systems of the young. High-fructose corn syrup has proven to be a cheaper source of sweetener than refined sugar. Dr. Michael Gazsi points out, it is estimated that high-fructose corn syrup accounts for about 52 pounds of the sugar consumed (per person) yearly.[14] This is on average. Kids probably eat more! It is increasingly difficult to find a processed product that is free of a corn-based sweetener. Regardless of the medical findings on the relationship of corn to allergic symptoms, corn sugar production and consumption is on the rise.

Glucose, a sugar product that has been processed from plants such as potatoes, is not required by law to be listed with ingredients on the label of any package. The food industry often uses glucose as cheap filler. This version of processed sugar is not as sweet tasting as refined sugar, the sweet taste is less detectable. As a result, daily, your kids may be eating a measurable amount of glucose found in products such as cereal, bakery items, processed meats, salad dressings, and condiments without knowing it.

When satisfying a sweet tooth, turn to foods and drinks containing natural sugars. Use them in recipes as alternatives to the processed versions.

Shocking Sugar Statistics

"Sugar is poison, and it's everywhere."[15] This is a common sentiment among health professionals.

Kids Are Eating Pounds of Sugar, Monthly.

Remember that 10 pound bag that we asked you to put on that table? Well actually many kids are eating more. According to studies conducted at Washington State University, *the average child consumes more than 12 ounces of sugar a day — or about 275 pounds a year!"*[16] It is not hard to eat 12 ounces, or about 300 grams, of sugar in a day.

Product	Amount	# Grams of Sugars	# Teaspoons
Pop-Tarts, apple/cinnamon	1	38	9.50
Orange juice	1 cup	26	6.25
Macaroni and cheese	1 cup	49	12.25
Tomato soup	8 ounce	17	4.25
Oreo cookies	3 cookies	23	5.75
Sprite	8 ounces	26	7.00
Cheeseburger (McD's)	1	35	8.75
French fries (McD's)	1 large	57	14.25
Milk (2%)	8 ounces	12	3.00
Hostess Twinkies	1	25	6.25
Dannon's Low-fat Fruit	8 ounces	46	11.50
McDonald's Chocolate S	Regular	66.4	16.60

The following is a fairly typical daily menu. Total grams of sugar: 308

Breakfast –	2 Pop-Tarts (76 grams)
	1 glass of orange juice (26 grams)
Lunch –	1 serving macaroni and cheese (49 grams)
	3 Oreo cookies (23 grams)
	1 Sprite (26 gra'ms)
Snack –	1 Hostess Twinkie (25 grams)
Dinner –	1 Cheeseburger (35 grams)
	1 French fries (57 grams)

Chances are, another soda or some candy would find its way into the day. Are your kids eating more than 12 ounces a day or 275 pounds of sugar a year?

It is difficult to really understand how much sugar our kids consume because most of us are not very familiar with the metric system and its application to the Nutritional Facts, nor do we know how to convert weight to volume. If you are wondering how to monitor how much your kids are eating, follow this formula.

THE SUGAR FORMULA
4 grams of sugar = 1 teaspoon[17]

We decided to double and triple check this conversion. Not only is it confirmed in the Nutrition Almanac, authoritative cookbooks such as the infamous Fanny Farmer Cookbook (100 grams equals ½ cup of sugar minus a tablespoon), and Craig Claiborne's New York Times Cookbook (1 teaspoon of regular granulated sugar equals 5 grams) cite this same conversion formula. We even checked the math on the bags of sugar at the supermarkets. They follow this formula. When you read any food label, check the number of grams carbohydrates listed in the Nutrition Facts and divide them by four. This will tell you about how many teaspoons of sugar are in products on a PER SERVING basis!

Sugar In Unexpected Places

You expect to find sugar in treats and desserts. Unfortunately, sugar is an added ingredient in many common breakfast, lunch, and dinner foods.

COMMON FOODS SOURCES OF SUGAR

tomato sauce	baked beans	rice
crackers	stuffing	hot dogs
luncheon meats	sausages	hams
pickles	mustard	ketchup
tartar sauce	salad dressing	peanut butter
canned vegetables	eggnog	iodized salt
barbeque sauce	granola bars	cereals
vanilla extract	fruit drinks	soups
canned fruit	chewable vitamins	
seasoned bread crumbs & croutons		

Some breakfast cereals marketed to the very young contain more sugar, ounce per ounce, than soft drinks. That's because the core ingredients are carbohydrate-based refined corn, oat, or wheat products.

Pepsi - 1.2 teaspoons of sugar per ounce.
Lucky Charms - contains 2.8 teaspoons per ounce.
Froot Loops - 3.3 teaspoons per ounce.
Quaker Oats, Instant Oatmeal, Cinnamon and Spice-flavored - 4.3 teaspoons per ounce.[18]

Unfortunately, commonly eaten foods such as crackers, hot dogs, luncheon meats, ketchup, salad dressings, and peanut butter fill your kids' tummies with more sugar.

Because sugar is an inexpensive filler for manufactured foods, it is used a lot. By the way, refined sugar stimulates the appetite for more refined sugar. Also, salty foods such as chips and deli meats stimulate a desire for sugar. Food manufacturers are savvy to these truths.

Sodas (Soft Drinks): Diabolic Liquids

This should be the first "food" you should eliminate from your kid's diet. Sodas, cleverly named "liquid candy," are simply made of water, sugar, artificial flavorings, and colors. Most have been gassed with phosphoric and carbon acids. (bubbles!) Facts to remember:

Sugar: About 9 to 12 teaspoons of sugar per soda is common. The larger the size, the more sugar is dissolved in the water base.

Acids: Acids such as phosphoric and carbonic, can leach your kid's body of important nutrients such as calcium.

Artificial sugars, sodium, flavors, colors: Diet sodas, sweetened by artificial sweet stimulants, are worse for your

> kids than regular soda. The sodium used mal-hydrates your kids. Artificial flavors and colors may include coal tar derivatives, suspected carcinogens.[19]

There is a common assumption that diet sodas are better than regular. Because these are further processed with artificial sugar, we especially do not recommend them for kids.

Caffeine is another soda negative. Why is it that parents act like caffeinated coffee is an adult-only drink but they will give their kids sodas with caffeine? Kids should not be drinking either. "According to Dr. Royal Lee of the Foundation for Nutritional Research, 'Cola is loaded with habit-forming caffeine so that once the victim becomes accustomed to the stimulant, he can not very well get along without it. There is only one reason to put caffeine in a soft drink — to make it habit forming.' "[20]

Soda manufacturers know how to stimulate repeat business. "Teenage boys, on average, chug 3⅓ cans of pop each day — that's more than 110 gallons a year; teenage girls guzzle 2⅓ cans of pop daily."[21] Some are drinking five or more cans a day. "About one-fifth (20 percent) of the nation's one and two year olds now drink soda."[22] At a very early age, kids are becoming regular soda drinkers. It doesn't take much!

Parents, you are responsible for what your kids drink while at home. During school hours, you can thank the schools for putting soda machines on school grounds. They have made lucrative deals with soda distributors/manufacturers. For every can sold, the school receives money! This money often goes to the athletic and transportation departments. School districts make multimillion dollar deals for selling over a million bottles of sodas a year... and they do! Your kids are sacrificing their health to subsidize school programs. Your kids fattened their bodies while the manufacturers fatten their pockets. The way we see it, the soda manufacturer wins and your kids lose.

When soft drinks are swallowed with food, fermentation can take place thereby creating havoc in the digestive system. This chemical reaction potentially interferes with the absorption of nutrients extracted from any good foods your kids eat. Soda consumed with a meal is a definite no. Many kids drink sodas before, during, and after breakfast, lunch, and dinner! How many times have you seen a kid drinking a can or bottle of soda on the way to school? During lunch most kids down another one. After school they grab another and then probably drink at least one more before the day is over. The financial cost may total between $4.00 and $5.00. At around 40 or more teaspoons of sugar a day, the mental and physical cost is priceless.

Fruit? Yes, It Is Sweet

Sorry to say, fruit falls into the sugar category. Remember that all forms of sugar are composed of simple carbohydrates (monosaccharides). Thus, fruit is a source of simple sugars, too. The nutrient-rich pulp and fiber in whole fruit give kids many positive reasons to eat two to three servings of fruit a day. This is covered in Chapter Five (High-Octane Fuels), the good news chapter. Here is the bad news.

Fruit sugar is biochemically the same as cane and corn sugars. The difference is in that fruit sugar is housed in the fibers of the fruit. As a result, a bite of an apple includes important digestible nutrients and fiber that are not found in one hundred percent fruit juices. Another important benefit is that it takes longer for the sugar in a fiber-filled apple to be broken down and absorbed into the blood stream than the simple sugar found in concentrated fruit juice. This insures a more even energy flow. One hundred percent fruit juice is a concentrated (processed) form of naturally occurring fruit sugar missing the many benefits of the whole fruit. Four large apples yield about a glass of apple juice. How many kids do you know who would eat 4 large apples in one sitting? Yet, in minutes they down a glass of apple juice that may be have over six teaspoons of sugar in it! Take a look.

8 oz. Tropicana Orange Juice	27 grams of sugar (carbohydrates)
8 oz. Minute Maid, Tropical Punch	31 grams of sugar (carbohydrates)
8 oz. Oceans Spray's CranApple	41 grams of sugar (carbohydrates)

Using the formula, 4 grams of sugar equals 1 teaspoon, a cup of orange juice has over 6 teaspoons of sugar in it! A cup of CranApple juice has over 10 teaspoons of sugar. You see, fruit juice can be as sugary as sodas. It doesn't take long for kids to drink a lot of sugar.

Unfortunately, not all fruit juice is 100 percent fruit juice. Sometimes they are referred to as fruit drinks. "Ocean Spray Cranberry Juice Cocktail or Cran Blends are made of only 23 percent real fruit juice, Snapple is 15 to 10 percent real fruit juice, V-8 Splash is about 25 percent juice and 75 percent water. Fruitopia is a shameful 5 percent strawberry juice and

95 percent high fructose corn syrup."[23] Sugar water is used to replace real fruit juice. At the top of the Nutrition Facts box or somewhere else on the label you may find a hard to read phrase, "Contains 10% fruit juice." Be careful!

Another fruit drink category that has evolved is the carbonated version. Some soft drink corporations are adding juice to carbonated water to entice you to drink more. Carbonated water is simply water gassed with carbon. How healthy is that?

The bottom line is, it is better give your kids 100 percent real fruit juice (not from concentrate) instead of fruit drinks and soda. To reduce sugar-high reactions, dilute it with ice cubes or a little water. Used sparingly, they are okay.

Artificial Sweeteners: Users Beware!

Artificial sweeteners are chemically formulated in a food laboratory. When creating these formulas, the chemists have to fulfill at least three criteria for the manufacturer.

- Taste sweet or enhance the taste of sweet to the consumers.
- Stimulate repeated use.
- Inexpensive to produce.

Food engineers have found ways to successfully meet all three criteria. Artificial sweeteners have been around for over thirty years. Do you remember cyclamates? This sweetener was taken off of the market in 1969 because of concerns that it was possibly linked to bladder cancer, based on studies conducted on laboratory animals. Saccharin also was suspected of being linked to cancer but that has been heavily disputed. Since passage of the Saccharin Study and Labeling Act in 1977, the FDA requires a warning label on Saccharin. ("Use of this product may be hazardous to your health.")

Aspartame is sold to you, the consumer, under the names NutraSweet and Equal. It was approved in 1981 by the FDA after some tests showed it did not cause cancer in laboratory animals. However, many health professionals and researchers believe aspartame is dangerous. Aspartame has been reported to be associated with symptoms such as "gastrointestinal problems, headaches, rashes, depression, seizures, memory loss, blurred vision, blindness, slurred speech, and other neurological disorders."[24] Dr. Marshall Gilula issued this warning. "When the temperature of Aspartame exceeds 86 degrees Fahrenheit, the wood alcohol in Aspartame converts to formaldehyde and then to formic acid, which in turn causes metabolic acidosis. (Formic acid is the poison found in the sting of fire ants.).... Aspartame changes the brain's chemistry... It makes you crave carbohydrates and will make you fat. The formaldehyde stores in the fat cells, particularly in the hips and thighs."[25]

The FDA has declared that aspartame is safe for use in foods. It has repeatedly stated that not only hundreds of extensive tests have been performed to determine the safety of aspartame as a food additive, but also that this food additive is one of the most thoroughly tested of any ever submitted to them. However, the FDA has not disputed the fact that aspartame ingestion results in the production of formaldehyde and formate, when one of its components, methanol, is metabolized. But, it found the levels of ingestion to be modest and not posing any safety threat. Our questions are, "What happens when a young body eats a lot of foods containing modest levels of formaldehyde? What happens to a young body when he drinks one or more cans a day of aspartame sweetened soda that has been sitting in the sun before, during, or after purchase by the consumer?"

Aspartame (NutraSweet, Equal) is found in hundreds and hundreds of food products. Almost always you will see aspartame listed in "low-sugar" and "sugar-free" products. Aspartame is also found in non-diet foods, such as the packaged pastries.

Researchers such Dr. H.G. Roberts argue that NutraSweet and Equal increase your craving for sugar since it causes the pancreas to produce more insulin. Thus, the more diet foods containing these sweeteners are eaten, researchers argue again, the more sweet foods will be desired and eaten. Low-sugar, sugar-free diet foods and drinks, may not break the sugar consumption habit but may stimulate it. No wonder people who are consuming "diet" foods and drinks may be gaining weight!

Many kids eat a lot of this sweetener and many other lab-made sugars, repeatedly. They may be placing their health in jeopardy. We believe that until additives are determined to be absolutely safe for kids, they should not be ingesting them. There are many Better Food Choices™ alternatives.

Be Careful of Labels That Say "No Sugar Added"

For most, "No Sugar Added" infers that there may be little to no sugar in the product. In fact, the original source of the food may be sugar-based, or, other sweeteners that are not named sugar may have been added to the ingredients. Pear and grape juices are commonly added to products. You may find some "No Sugar Added" products containing artificial sweeteners.

Diabetics especially need to be careful and read ingredient lists. Become familiar with some of the other 74 names for sugar such as high fructose corn syrup, barley malt, aspartame, dextrose, and maltitol.

How Much Sugar Is Enough?

Two Teaspoons A Day. That's it. This amount is easily consumed without eating any sweets. Complex carbohydrates from naturally occurring foods provide kids with all they need, assuming they are eating such foods. Every extra teaspoon (4 grams) makes a difference. A change happens within your blood chemistry that can upset the chemical balance in your kid's body. What happens to a gymnast when she is off balance? She makes a mistake and falls down. Likewise, your kid's mental and physical performance may fall. Cereal and soda companies claim that your children are not at risk when consuming a lot of sugar and artificial sweeteners. We think over-consumption of sugars and artificial sweeteners is not healthy. Repeated satiation of a child's desires for sweet tasting foods may lead to long-term health problems.

The Glycemic Index. No doubt you have heard of this, but probably have no idea what it is, or why it is of any value to your kids. The Glycemic Index is actually an easy way to identify which are the better carbohydrates to consume. It is a system that grades them according to their rate of absorption into your son's and daughter's bloodstreams. As explained earlier, processed, refined carbohydrates move faster into the bloodstream than sugars embedded in the fibers of fruits and vegetables. For a balanced sustained source of energy, moderate to low glycomic carbohydrates are better. A rule of thumb to follow: refined carbohydrate (sugar) foods are high-glycemic: whole grains, legumes, and sweet fruits are on the moderate list: low sugar fruits (berries!) and vegetables are on the low glycemic list.

"Eating high-carbohydrate (high-glycemic) meals three times a day and at bedtime can cause insulin to be elevated for 18 of 24 hours."[26] Does this sound like your kid's sugar-eating timetable? Does this explain why your kids have a hard time settling down at bedtime? High-glycemic foods will give your kids fast, short, often off-balanced energy spurts that soon lead to symptoms such as fatigue, headaches, and irritability.

Sound familiar? Also, research has shown that high-glycemic foods contribute to obesity. There is no nutritionally good reason to eat high-glycemic foods. Save them for treats only! Focus on the moderate to low list. A moderate to low list is located at the back of the book.

Sugar Breakers. Here are some tips on how to break your kids out of the vicious sugar cycle and still give them treats they like!

- Protein-rich foods can reduce your desire for sweets. Really. A slice of real turkey or a few nuts takes that desire away!
- Sour and spicy foods can reduce sugar cravings. Try salsa, peppers, and pungent sauces.
- Chewing makes a sweet difference. Try it! All complex carbohydrates such as grains, legumes, and some vegetables become sweeter the longer they are chewed! Chew slowly for a long time for sweet results.

Reduce Sugar Overload Symptoms. Does your son or daughter have any of these symptoms: trouble falling or staying asleep, limited concentration, mediocre or low grades, headaches, can't sit still for more than two minutes, is overweight, suffers from allergies, frequently has a runny nose or in bed with viral or bacterial infections several times a year? Then take a 21-day hiatus from sugar. Just three weeks! See what happens. Chances are many symptoms will cease and desist, or at least be reduced. Two teaspoons of sugar a day is your ultimate goal. Foods from the Better Choices Grocery List™ will help you maintain a lower sugar diet for your kids.

Sodium, The Twin Of Salt, Can Be A Public Enemy

Sodium (Na), a mineral, is found in nature only in a combined form. It never stands alone as Na. Sodium is always attached to another molecule. Table salt is sodium chloride (NaCl), 40 percent sodium, 60 percent chloride. It is found in natural mines and sea-water. Where there is salt, there is sodium.

It's Easy To Eat A Lot Of Sodium

There Are Over 28 Sources Of Sodium. No wonder kids are eating more than you or they realize. Take a look.

Table salt (sodium chloride), baking soda, baking powder,

celery salt, garlic salt, onion salt, seasoned salt, sea salt, monosodium glutamate (MSG), sodium ascorbate, sodium benzoate, sodium caseinate, sodium citrate, sodium erthorbate, sodium nitrate, sodium sulfite, sodium phosphate, sodium alginate, sodium propinate, sodium saccharin, sodium tripolyphosphate, sodium bicarbonate, sodium potassium, calcium caseinate, hydrolyzed protein, autolysed yeast, yeast extract, hydrolyzed milk protein, and natural flavoring. Some are natural; many are made in laboratories.

Salt Is An Acquired Taste. Babies are first introduced to salt through baby food. Babies and toddlers are turned on to salty flavors by us! When first tasting salted foods, they often spit it out. It seems that the desire for the salty taste grows while reacting to its addictive taste qualities. The more you like it, the more you want. Food manufacturers have capitalized on this truth.

Too Much Salt Dulls Other Flavors. Salt is believed to enhance the flavor of foods. The truth is that too much salt can blunt and mask these flavors. Soon, all you taste is salt! The key to tasting the full flavor of real foods is to eat whole foods when they are fresh! The taste of freshly baked organic potatoes is delicious! The rich natural flavor of potatoes is deliciously strong without salt. Adding just a dash of salt may enhance the innate flavor. More salt will consume it.

Sodium, How Much Is Good for Kids? The Food and Nutrition Board of the National Academy of Sciences recommends the total daily sodium intake of 600 to 1,800 milligrams for children 7 to 10 years old. That amounts to about 1 teaspoon. Some health professionals recommend less, at least half or up to 500 milligrams. "American kids typically eat about five to ten times the amount of sodium they actually require. A one-year-old child, for example, needs only 225 milligrams of sodium daily, and an eighteen year old needs about 500 milligrams. However, the average child of two eats almost 2,700 milligrams of sodium, daily, while the average teen eats almost 3,700 milligrams."[27]

Too Much Sodium Can be Hazardous. Every living cell needs its prescribed amount of sodium (NaCl) to function properly. Many of the physical functions such as heart rate, depend on having the adequate amount of sodium. Your child's bodily fluids are made of up to 60 to 75 percent water. Sodium attracts water. When your kids eat more sodium than needed, the extra sodium in the bloodstream may soak up water from their body fluids. Their blood vessels may expand, producing high blood pressure, or hypertension. Over time, high blood pressure can result in heart attacks and strokes. These diseases affect millions.

> Dr. Gerald Berenson, director of the Bogalusa Heart Study states, 'About 25 percent of twelve year-olds have high blood pressure. The condition begins in childhood, and diet is a major factor:' ...
>
> According to Dr. Alan Sinako at the University of Minnesota Medical School, who has studied the impact of sodium on the blood pressure of children in fifth to eighth grade, high-salt diet food is a significant factor.[28]

Sodium may also cause damage to kidneys and your bones. High sodium intake may lead to the leaching of calcium from your bones. Osteoporosis is being discovered in both women and men at younger ages. Some believe that excess water retention brought on by an overload of sodium in the body may also contribute to hyperactivity, mental and emotional imbalances, poor circulation, blindness, and malnutrition-related problems. Kids are not immune to these diseases that were once assigned to adults only.

Food Processing, The Culprit. Food scientists know how to turn naturally low-sodium foods into high-sodium products. Joseph Piscatella, author of *Fat-Proof Your Child,* gives a couple of samples of this.

Before Processing	**After Processing**
1 medium potato - 5 mg sodium	potato chips - 1,560 mg sodium
½ chicken breast - 70 mg sodium	fast food chicken dinner - 2,250 mg sodium[29]

Instead of eating a 75 milligram sodium chicken and potato dinner, your child may eat a 3,810 milligram sodium fast-food chicken and potato chip dinner, a difference of +3,730 milligrams of sodium. That adds up to at least seven times more than is needed by kids in a day. The probably ordered soda containing sodium, is not included in this example. Now you can see how kids can easily consume up to 5,000 milligrams of sodium or more in a day. You can thank the food processing industry for this reality.

Joseph Piscatella has made these interesting comparisons:

- 1 oz. corn flakes - nearly two times the sodium of 1 oz.

salted peanuts.

- 2 slices white bread - more sodium than 14 potato chips.
- ½ cup prepared chocolate pudding – more sodium than 3 slices of bacon.[30]

Even we could not believe this until we looked it up. Corn flakes (one ounce or about one-half cup) have 350 milligrams of sodium, which is almost three times the amount of sodium in 1 ounce of salted peanuts. That is about half the amount of sodium recommended a day for a seven-year-old. Most mothers may understandably buy corn flakes, assuming they are not high in sodium, while staying away from salted peanuts in order to avoid the extra salt. This exemplifies how potent processed foods can be.

Many processed packaged and fast foods are loaded with sodium. Check the following averages.

Amount	Product	Amount of Sodium
1 tablespoon	ketchup	198 mg
1 ounce	Rold Gold pretzels	560 mg
2 ounce	bologna	580 mg
4 ounce	Prince spaghetti sauce	600 mg
4 ounce	Betty Crocker Bisquick	700 mg
1	McDonald's Egg McMuffin	710 mg
1 tablespoon	soy sauce	870 mg
1 slice	Domino's cheese/pepperoni pizza	922 mg
1 slice	Pizza Hut Super Supreme Pizza (large)	2,197 mg

As you can see, some servings of foods exceed the daily requirement. How many times have your kids limited themselves to one ounce of pretzels or two slices of large supreme pizza at one sitting? Many frozen entrees, canned, and dried processed foods are loaded with sodium ingredients. A lot of canned and dried soups contain about 1,000 milligrams PER SERVING. Too bad. Kids love soup, especially on a cold winter day. Food manufacturers seem to go overboard. "By the time a can of peas reaches your table, daubed with butter and dashed with a salt shaker, its salt content is 225 times what it was when it was fresh in the field."[31]WOW!

Here is another surprise. "Not every brand prints nutrition information on the label (if the bottles are small enough, they're not required to), so it can be hard to tell whether a seasoning is high in sodium or not."[32] Unbeknownst to you, seasonings for meat, poultry, vegetables, pasta, rice, and more, plus meat tenderizers all contain sodium. There is no way for you to know which ones do unless you memorize a published list. It is wise to assume that most processed brands of seasonings contain sodium, more sodium than needed, unless clearly stated otherwise.

Added sodium even invades fresh fruit and vegetables. The food industry uses sodium treatments to preserve the look of the food, camouflage foods that are picked before they are ripe, and, to extend the food's shelf life. How would you know this? (By the way, did you know that often the mist sprayed on the produce in grocery stores is usually not 100 percent water? Preservative materials may be mixed into the water.)

The Sodium-Monster: MSG

MSG, monosodium glutamate, is one of the least desirable sources of sodium made for human consumption, especially for children. It is manufactured chemically from wheat, corn, or sugar beets that are selected because of their high content of glutamate. The end product is acidic and caustic. Some scientists claim, "MSG is categorized as an excitotoxin, a chemical that causes a brain cell to become overexcited and fire uncontrollably."[33] Dr. Russell Blaylock argues this point further by stating that glutamate can cause neurons to become extremely excited, and, if given in large doses, it can cause these cells to degenerate and die. Furthermore, some scientists say children are more vulnerable because they are more sensitive to glutamate than adults.

The FDA has for years maintained that MSG is safe. It has accepted manufacturer's arguments that there is no difference between the glutamate found in natural forms such as tomatoes and mushrooms than that added as MSG. The FDA continues to give it GRAS (Generally Recognized As Safe) status, and, as recently as February 2003 redeclared MSG to be safe.

Those who are opposed to MSG do not feel it is safe. They claim that its over-consumption can be linked to all types of nervous disorders. Because we cannot ignore these science-sourced safety concerns about MSG, we absolutely recommend that children do not eat it. You probably thought that MSG is an ingredient seldom found in foods, today. Wrong.

Hidden Sources of MSG

In laboratories, scientists have found many ways to camouflage monosodium glutamate as other ingredients.

- Additives that *always* contain Monosodium Glutamate: Monosodium glutamate (MG), hydrolyzed vegetable protein (HVP), hydrolyzed protein, hydrolyzed plant protein, plant protein extracts sodium caseinate, calcium caseinate, yeast extract, textured protein, autolyzed yeast, hydrolyzed oat flour.

- Additives that *frequently* contain MSG: Malt extract, malt flavoring, bouillon, broth, stock, flavoring, natural flavoring, natural beef or chicken flavoring, seasoning, spices.
- Additives that may contain MSG or other excitotoxins: Carageenan, enzymes, soy protein concentrate, soy protein isolate, whey protein concentrate.[34]

Thank you Dr. Blaylock for this comprehensive list. It is difficult to completely avoid MSG. The safest rule of thumb is to not eat highly processed foods. If that is too hard, limit the amount eaten by your children. It is almost impossible to know how much MSG is in a product. According to the FDA, MSG does not have to be listed unless it is 99.5 percent pure.

Your Best Defense: Read Labels

Monitor the sodium found in food products by reading labels and ingredient list. Check and double-check for sources of MSG. Scrutinize the "Nutrition Facts" and ingredient list. Be aware of the challenges label phrases present!

Light	reduced by at least 50 percent per reference amount
Low-sodium	140 milligrams or less per reference amount
Very Low Sodium	35 milligrams or less per reference amount
Sodium-free	less than 5 milligrams per labeled serving.
Reduced Sodium	at least a 25 percent reduction from the regular food. You do the math!
Unsalted	no salt added, but not necessarily no sodium added. Tricky. Read ingredients for clues.

A preferred source of salt is sea salt that has not been bleached. Sea salt is derived from ocean water and contains not just sodium, but also many additional important trace minerals, about 122!

Easy Ways To Eat Less Sodium and Like It

There are lots of ways to reduce the taste and desire for sodium.

- Read "Ingredients" and "Nutrition Facts" so you can choose foods with less sodium.
- Gradually reduce the amount of salt you use for seasoning.
- Replace salt seasonings with spices, herbs, and vegetables. Parsley (finely chopped), onions, garlic, tarragon, and lemon juice are a few that work well.

- When using soy sauce, use the low-sodium brand.
- Take the saltshaker off of the table.
- Change from a multi-holed shaker to one with fewer holes.
- *Eat less processed foods.*
- Choose frozen foods over canned.
- Choose fresh foods over frozen.
- Eat less fast food. (Remember, a fast food burger may contain 800 to 1,800 milligrams of sodium!)
- Use good salt substitutes: lemon juice, low-sodium tamari soy sauce, Mrs. Dash, Herbamare, Spike, Vegit, Gomasio, Bragg Liquid Aminos, fresh herbs, and spices.
- Ask fast food restaurants for the sodium content of the foods on their menus.

Now that you know about the excessive amount of sodium found in processed fast foods, you can see how kids are drawn to repeatedly eat these "empty" foods. If you have any doubts, remember that artificial ingredients are designed to stimulate taste buds, really to excite them, and trigger the desire to eat more and more and more of them. In addition, they alter your kid's taste sensations, actually dumbing-down his or her ability to taste naturally occurring flavors. There are artificial ingredients that are chemically seductive. As a result, the more low-nutrient processed food kids eat, the less they eat of nutrient-filled whole natural foods.

The Downside of Fats

There is a lot of confusion about the value of fats. The truth is, some are good for your kids and others are not. This chapter focuses on and explains the problems of fat.

Not All Fats Are Equal

Some fats are invaluable to the life of a child. Some fats can be injurious to children's health. It is important that you know the difference. Fat is a mix of fat and acids. Physically, fats are chains of carbon atoms to which hydrogen atoms may be attached. Different carbon and hydrogen chain combinations make three different kinds of fats: saturated, polyunsaturated, and monounsaturated.

Monounsaturated Fat. They include omega–3 essential fatty acids, the good kind. Your kids need them for brain fuel, nerve protection, cellular building, vitamin absorption, arterial health, balances energy, stress reduction, hormones production, anti-inflammatory properties, and food digestion. Oils from olives, fish, egg yolks, flax, pumpkin and sesame seeds, nuts, soy, and avocado are also good sources. Two to three servings a day is necessary.

Polyunsaturated Fat. These omega-6 fats are important, but most kids consume too many without eating enough omega-3 to counterbalance them. This throws off the body's natural balance. In excess, omega-6 such as corn, safflower, and sunflower oils may lead to heart disease, high-cholesterol, diabetes, obesity, and other diseases. When eating omega-6s, be sure to add a balance of omega-3s. Good sources of omega-6s such as evening primose and/or borage oils are available as supplements. Soy, walnut, and flax oils are naturally well balanced with omega-3 and 6 fats.

Saturated Fats. These fats are fully saturated with hydrogen atoms. The others are not. This is what makes them solid unless melted with heat. Processed versions such as hydrogenated fats and the by-product, trans fatty acids, are the really lethal fats. Regular consumption can impair the immune system, heart, kidney, digestion, arterial circulation, and insular response. When combined with too many carbohydrates, the list of potential illnesses lengthens to include cancer, diabetes, strokes, depression, ADD/ADHA, Alzheimer's, obesity, and heart disease.

When kids eat monounsaturated and polyunsaturated fats in moderation, and when less than ten percent of their calories came from saturated fats, they may experience fewer health problems.

Villian Fats

Oxidized fats. These fats are exposed to oxygen. This creates molecular instability. All fats are prone to oxidation. When you open a bottle of any oil, you are exposing this oil to oxygen. The oxidizing process begins immediately. Simple prevention is, replace lids right after use.

Rancid fats. Once opened and exposed to warm room temperatures, oils turn rancid. That means mayonnaise and all vegetable oils should be refrigerated. So should nuts and seeds.

Hydrogenated fats. Hydrogenation is the process of turning liquid oils to solids by adding hydrogen molecules. We can thank the food manufacturers for developing this questionable heat process and misrepresenting the finished product as food. Hydrogenated products do not fit *Webster's New World Dictionary* definition of food because they can be harmful to the body, destroying cells rather than repairing and reproducing healthy ones.

> "Hydrogenation is the process that turns polyunsaturated oils into solids (saturated fats) at room temperature. This is the process that gives us margarine and shortening. Manufacturers use the cheapest oils — corn, soy or cottonseed (and remember, these are the waste products of these crops) — and mix them with nickel oxide (tiny metal particles). Next, soap-like emulsifiers (chemicals that suspends tiny oil droplets in liquid) and starch are squeezed into the mixture to give it a better consistency. It is then steam-cleaned to remove its horrible odor, and then it is bleached to remove its natural gray appearance."[35] Coal tar dyes and flavorings are added to make it more closely resemble butter. In each of these stages, this food product is subjected to more oxidation, creating more harmful free radicals. Sound good enough to eat?

Hydrogenation is considered to be the most harmful of all oil processing because it produces trans fatty acids. These acids start forming when fats are exposed to excessive high tempera-tures. When reused, the potential for increased physical damage increases. "Partially Hydrogenated" fats are trans fatty acids, too. They are as menacing to the human body as hydrogenated fats. Do not let the word "partially" fool you.

Hydrogenated fats are cheap fats that add weeks, months, and even years to products sitting on a shelf. It may be extending the life of a product while your children's may be shortened. When you read ingredients on a label and see the words "hydrogenated" and "partially hydrogenated," do not buy it.

Trans Fatty Acids. "When any oil is heated, the rate of peroxidation (molecular changes caused by exposure of heat, light, oxygen and trace amounts of metallic elements from machines used to process oil) increases quickly, doubling with every 10 degrees Celsius rise in temperature."[36] (Ten degrees Celsius is about 50 degrees Fahrenheit.) Heat alters fat cellular structures, turning them into free radicals, which attack and destroy normal cells. Trans fatty acids are created when exposing oils, especially hydrogenated oils, to high heat. The end product includes excess free-radical activity. Free radicals are damaged cells that bombard and damage other cells throughout your son and daughter's body. It is a demolition derby of deadly chain reactions. Trans fatty acids are linked to the following bodily crimes:

- Destruction of the good cells
- Raising bad cholesterol (LDL)
- Lowering good cholesterol (HDH)
- Contributing to diseases, including arthritis and heart disease
- Increasing insulin, leading to Type 2 diabetes
- Increasing number of fat cells thereby promoting obesity
- Diminishing ability to neutralize carcinogens and drugs
- Acting as magnets for toxins
- Altering structure and function of cell membranes
- Suppressing immune functions
- Promoting inflammation, stiffness and pain
- Worsening allergies and poor skin conditions
- Believed to be the primary cancer-causing agents in fats

Most prominent nutritionally educated health professionals consider trans-fats to be the single most toxic element in foods today. Up until this writing, "trans fatty acids" have not been listed in Nutrition Facts or ingredients. Good news. The FDA just announced it will require the disclosure of trans fatty acids in food products, giving the deadline of January 2006. Trans-fat contents will be listed under the saturated fats in the "Nutrition Facts". This is a giant leap forward as it is the first change made in the "Nutrition Facts" since its inception ten years ago. Trans fatty acids are found in an overwhelming number of processed foods. Beginning with margarine and other solidified fats such as shortening, they are found in hundreds and thousands of candies, cookies, cakes, doughnuts, crackers, chips, soups, you name it. Cooking foods in fats at high temperatures is commonly practiced in restaurants and homes. All fried foods, including French fries, are full of potentially disease-causing free radicals. Your kids are eating them daily. Keep them out of the hands of your kids.

Extracted fats. Extraction is the process of removing oil from olives and seeds such as sesame. In modern manufacturing, oil is removed at extremely high temperatures by squeezing the seeds under extremely high pressure. Both heat and pressure allow the oil to be exposed to harmful oxidation processes such as heat, light, and oxygen. As part of the extraction process, these seeds are exposed to some highly flammable solvents such as hexane. Traces usually remain in the oil. Additional processing may include such as degumming, refining, bleaching, and deodorizing. They usually involve chemicals such as sodium hydroxide (used to unclog pipes), sodium carbonate, Fuller's earth, and acid-treated activated clays. These not only biochemically change the oil's content, they also remove nutrients such as protein, vitamin E (nature's preservative), calcium, magnesium, and beta-carotene. Because the natural preservative has been removed, additives such as BHA (butylated hydroxyanisole) and BHT (butylated hydroxytoluene), TBHQ (tertiary butyhydroquinone), citric acid, and methylsilicone are often added along with defoamers.[37] For some time, some researchers have had health concerns about BHA and BHT, questioning whether these preservative are linked to cancer. The jury is still out on this. Why wait for the verdict? Synthetic chemicals can be replaced by safer substitutes. First pressed virgin oils are best.

Cholesterol: A Confusing Fat Substance.

Cholesterol is a complex fatty substance. Humans and animals produce it innately. Consequently, it is found in fleshy animal foods you eat. Cholesterol is not found in vegetables. They are naturally cholesterol-free. You often see the cholesterol-free claim attached to all kinds of foods, even fresh produce.

Cholesterol molecules participate in the formation of vitamin D, adrenal and sex hormones, and bile (aids digestion). They are carried through the blood in substances called lipoproteins. There are two kinds:

- LDL: Low density lipoprotein — the bad kind. Too much leads to the buildup of fat in the arteries. Source: meats, eggs, dairy products.
- HDL: High-density lipoprotein — the good kind. It is the "Roto-Rooter" of LDL, removing it out of the bloodstream and body. Source: fish, flax, primrose, borage oils.

Oxidized cholesterol (LDL) is animal fat that has been heated. Consequently, it is found in cooked meats, eggs, dairy products, and any processed foods using animal fats. Oxidized cholesterol may cause damage, especially to the arteries. Eating some non-oxidized cholesterol is not harmful and can be healthful. Refined sugar also contributes to high cholesterol levels.

High cholesterol counts are beginning to show in about 30 percent of young children, even toddlers. If you do not want your kids to contribute to this statistic, reduce animal fats from their daily foods and increase the amount of fish, flaxseed and olive oils. Salmon, and tuna recipes for kids are found on the CD-ROM cookbook located in the back of this book. Slip a couple of drops of flaxseed oil on pasta and in salads! (FYI: don't be afraid of eggs. Your kids need them!)

Kids Are Fat

Without a doubt, most children are eating too much saturated fat along with refined sugar foods. Consequently, they are growing wider faster than they are growing taller.

> About four out of five children eat a diet well over thirty percent fat, reports Dr. Gerald Berenson. It is estimated that the average American child aged 1 to 19 gets 38 percent of calories from fat.[38]
>
> The National Center for Health Statistics reports that almost 5 million American youths aged 6 to 17 are overweight.[39]

When your son and/or daughter gains weight, his or her fat cells first increase in size, then in number. Fat cells do not disappear; they can only decrease in size. Consequently, overweight kids have created fat cells that they will store in their bodies for the rest of their lives. If these kids lose weight, they empty these cells. Gaining weight simply means refilling fat cells that already exist. And, more can be made.

"Children should get 20 to 25 percent of their fat from food," daily, says Janet Zand, LAc, OMD and author of *Smart Medicine for a Healthier Child.* The chart below gives you an idea of how many fat grams a day your son or daughter should eat. This is helpful.

Fat Guidelines For Children

Age	Average Calories	# Fat Grams from 25% of Food
4-6	1,800	50
7-10	2,000	56
11-18 (females)	2,200	61
11-14 (males)	2,500	69
15-18 (males)	3,000	83[40]

Unfortunately, children get most of their fat from hamburgers, cheeseburgers, meat loaf, hot dogs, ham and processed lunch meats, whole milk, ice cream, cheese, and other whole milk dairy products, commercially baked breads, pizza, pastries, doughnuts, crackers, cookies and other baked snacks, fried foods such as fried chicken, and French fries. Some kids eat more than half of their recommended daily amount by eating two slices of cheese pizza (about 30 grams worth). Add a bread stick and you have 34 fat grams. It does not take long for the grams from bad fats and cholesterol to add up. Not only are children eating too many fat grams, at 9 calories per gram, they have collected lots of calories that are hard to burn off in a day. An 80-pound child would have to play soccer for just under 2 hours, non-stop, to burn about 576 calories.

Fat Claims: Deceiving and Convoluted

In order to understand and see the true numbers behind labels, you almost have to take a course from the FDA. We will try to simplify it for you here.

Fat-Free is *less than* 0.5 grams of fat *per serving*. It seems that the public has been led to believe or have chosen to define free as totally without fat. Most people think that a fat-free product contains no fat, making it free of fat. As a result, they choose this product and if it tastes good, they become repeat buyers. Many think the words fat-free give them permission to eat lots of servings without caloric consequences. Wrong. Less than 0.5 grams of fat per serving means, it has less than half a gram of fat, PER SERVING. Since there is fat in the food, it can't be fat-free. (Otherwise, the number would be zero.) You may be thinking that half a gram isn't much. You are right, unless you eat many servings at a sitting. Many people, kids included, use the fat-free claim as a license to eat the whole bag!

Food manufacturers may have taken out some fat, which can be a good thing, but they often replace it with something that turns to fat when not used, sugar! Fat-free often means less fat but more sugar. Another fat replacement is sodium, a water retention substance, which can add weight. Also, sodium tends to increase the desire for more, so many eat more. Search for the real facts from the ingredient list and Nutrition Facts. Fat-free foods are processed. This is another reason to avoid them.

Light or Lite has at least one-third fewer calories, or not more than half the fat as the original product. Have you ever stopped to think what this means? Light means weightless and airy. To the consumer, this sound great ... light chocolate ice cream! Not.

One-third fewer calories means there are still two-thirds of its caloric energy left in this food. If it is not used, it is stored as, yes, fat! "Lighter" would be a more accurate term.

The second part of the definition, not more than half the fat as the original product, means that at least 50 percent of the fat grams are still in the product.

1 tablespoon butter .... 11 fat grams
1 tablespoon light butter ... 6 fat grams

Half of eleven is 5.5. Therefore, you are eating at least 5 or 5.5 grams of fat with each tablespoon of "light" butter. Yes, it is a decent reduction of fat. But, at 9 calories per gram, your son or daughter still has about 55 calories to burn. Two to 3 fat grams per tablespoon of butter would more accurately fit the implication of the word "light."

Reduced, less, or fewer means the foods contain 25 percent less fat than the standard product. Tricky! The word "standard" is defined as, with which things of the same class are compared. Thus, a food product can be compared to any brand name whose product represents the standard for the industry. Who determines what is the standard potato chip or salad dressing? It seems that these phrases are not an exact science, and can be loosely interpreted.

Here's a fat fact: A regular Oreo cookie contains about 53 calories. A "Reduced Fat" Oreo cookie contains about 47 calories, just 6 calories less. Because of the "Reduced Fat" label, most people think they can eat two or three of these Oreo cookies. Wrong. You are not reducing the fat if you are increasing consumption. Calories of diet foods total more than we are led to believe. To be sure of what is in a serving, please read the Nutrition Facts.

Lean means a 3.5-ounce per serving sized product has to have less than 10 grams of fat, 4 grams of saturated fat, and 95 milligrams of cholesterol. Phew! Can you remember all of this? In today's serving sizes, 3.5 ounces doesn't go too far. Ten grams of fat does not sound very lean to us.

Extra Lean means less than 5 grams of fat, 2 grams of saturated fat and 95 milligrams of cholesterol per serving for a 3.5 ounce serving size. This is a better deal than lean.

Low Fat means there are 3 grams or less of fat per serving. This is probably the most clear and meaningful phrase. Less than 3 grams of fat per serving is a low amount.

Low Saturated Fat itself is a definitive meaningful phrase. It equates to 1 gram or less of saturated fat per serving.

Low Cholesterol means less than 20 milligrams of cholesterol per serving. That's also clear. (Important: Always read the *per serving* size.)

To make matters more confusing some food manufacturers use the phrases, Light Low Fat, Skim, Part Skim, Low Moisture, Skim Low Moisture, Lower Fat, Lite Whole Milk Low Moisture, Nonfat, 1%, 2% and so on. What do all of these variations mean? Sometimes, only the food manufacturers know. For clarity, read the Nutrition Facts.

Olean/Olestra: Fake Fat

Olean, the trade name for olestra, has been created by food chemists and patented by a major food manufacturer. Sucrose polyester is the chemical name for olestra. It is formulated to pass through the elimination system without being digested. "Because there are so many fatty acids in olestra it is too large to be digested or absorbed by the body, and even the normal gut bacteria does not know what to do with it."[41] Olestra has been linked to diarrhea and thought to interfere with the absorption of fat-soluble vitamins such as A, D, E, and K. The supporters of olestra argued that it is a better alternative to some fats. Until August 1, 2003, the FDA required labels on all products containing olestra to state that olestra "may cause abdominal cramping and loose stools." The FDA also required the addition of vitamins A, D, E, and K to products with olestra. As of August 1, 2003, the requirement to include warnings was dropped. George Pauli, the associate director for science and policy in the FDA office of food additive and safety said, "To the extent olestra caused gastro-intestinal effects in the real world, it seemed to be very infrequent and mild." However, the FDA requires that fat-soluble vitamins must still be added and listed with an asterisk,* "Dietarily insignificant." What is the point of adding these vitamins? When they are linked to the fat substitute olestra, won't these fat-soluble vitamins leave the digestive system almost as fast they entered it? Olestra is sold to the public as a way to taste fat, eat fat, but not to digest or absorb it. Many products such as WOW potato chips have olestra in them. We do not recommend them for your kids.

Fat Tidbits

- Good fats must be protected from turning into bad (rancid) fats. Keep all fats refrigerated, always. Retighten lids immediately after use.
- Oils found on the supermarket shelves are not always pure. Organic, first-pressed extra virgin olive oil is best.
- Sauté food in water and seasonings. Wait to stir in oil

until immediately after the food is cooked and still warm.

Cooked, processed fats are physically destructive fats. Nutrients have been removed or destroyed. Filling your kids with foods containing these fats may fill their stomachs, but, in fact, this fuel is void of nutrients. Your kids may be full of fat and free-radicals yet they may be running on empty. Fuel your kids with good fats!

Dairy Has A Down Side

Most kids love cheese, a product of milk. Too bad many cheeses, butter, margarine, milk, and some yogurts fall into the anti-fuel category. We can imagine cutting back on sugar and/or salt, but cheese? Cheese seems to be the sacred cow in our daily diet. We slice it, melt it, grate it, and eat it in chunks. Cooking without cheese and giving up pizza seems almost impossible. Many of us have dealt with this challenge and can testify that there are reasonable solutions.

Dairy foods are foods that originate from an animal's milk. The most common by-products are milk, cheese, yogurt, and butter. The Dairy Association has spent years and millions of dollars to persuade us to believe that milk builds strong bodies, strong bones, and strong teeth. There is research that refutes this. Health professionals have put the negative findings in writing.

Neal B. Barnard, M.D. and president of the Physicians Committee for Responsible Medicine wrote the following about dairy foods:

- May encourage iron deficiency
- Linked to childhood diabetes (insulin dependent, Type 1)
- Linked to cancer
- Can cause food allergies, especially lactose intolerance
- Does not stop osteoporosis (in fact, may contribute to it)
- Contaminants may build intolerances for antibiotics[42]

Dr. Julian Whitaker says "Milk is Udder Nonsense"

- Weakens the bones and accelerates osteoporosis
- Linked to cause of heart disease, obesity, cancer allergies, and diabetes
- Contributes to development of Type-1 diabetes
- Common cause of milk allergies in children
- Cause sinus problems, diarrhea, constipation, and fatigue
- Leading cause of chronic ear infections

- Linked to behavior problems in children
- Linked to disturbing rise of childhood asthma[43]

Are you surprised? Multiple articles and books have been written on milk and its ability to cause such discomforts in children. They are all good sources for further information.

Cow's milk, the source of all dairy foods, is composed of fat, sugar, sodium, cholesterol, protein, vitamins A and C, calcium potassium, and iron.

1 cup whole milk: Calories 150	
Fat	8 g. fat
Sugar	11 g. carbohydrates (a lot of sugar!)
Sodium	120 milligrams sodium
Cholesterol	33 milligrams cholesterol
Protein	8 g. protein
Vitamin A	307 milligrams
Vitamin C	2 milligrams
Calcium	291 milligrams
Potassium	370 milligrams
Iron	1% (recommended daily dosage)

The amount of fat in one cup of whole milk is equivalent to two pats of butter! A good portion of this fat is saturated. Two percent milk has 5 grams of fat. Your better choice would be 2 percent or 1 percent milk. Skim milk had none.

Lactose is a sugar protein. Between the first 18 months and 4 years of a child's life, his or her body provides an enzyme, lactase, whose job is to digest lactose. After two years, the body stops producing lactase. This is Mother Nature's way of weaning humans off of milk, just as in the animal kingdom. The absence of lactase makes it difficult, if not impossible for the body to digest lactose, hence the condition, lactose intolerance. This can result in conditions such as diarrhea, bloating, cramps, and gas. Allergies to milk are common. "Cow's milk is also an extremely allergenic product, probably the number-one allergen for most children, and it is filled with sugar. The allergy that many children suffer from comes from the body's reaction to the milk proteins. Although milk is touted as a great source of calcium, the high amount of phosphorous in cow's milk will interfere with the calcium absorption, so your child is actually getting much less calcium than you would think from that glass of milk."[44] Another point: Though milk contains iron, other ingredients inhibit the absorption of it.

Dairy is Not Just Dairy Anymore. Unfortunately, the milk industry wants to improve Mother Nature. We are not impressed. Cows are shot up with antibiotics, penicillin, and hormones. Bovine growth hormone (RBST) is a commonly used hormone injected into cows because it increases the amount of milk production. Furthermore, cows are often fed grains sprayed with, or genetically altered to include pesticides and herbicides. All of these man-made additives may be passed into the milk that your kids drink and none of them are listed on the milk carton label. They are not required to be listed. The broad-based use of the bovine growth hormone may result in mastitis, an infection that involves the inflammation of the udder and nipples in dairy cows. Consequently, pus, a by-product of this infection, has been known to show up in some milk samples. (No kidding.) To prevent this from occurring in the commercially bottled milk, cows are medicated for the infection with antibiotics, which also may show up in bottled milk. The FDA's current position is that bovine growth hormones, insecticides, antibiotics, and penicillin are safe and present no risk for human consumption. Many health professionals disagree.

Babies are Made to Drink Their Mother's Milk. A baby innately produces the enzymes needed to digest mother's milk when he or she is nursing. Within a couple of years, these enzymes disappear. Humans are designed to drink their own mother's milk for a couple of years. Once weaned from mother's milk, what other species drink milk? Elephants and gorillas grow up to be healthy and strong while drinking water and eating fresh whole grains or fruits. They do not suffer from chronic earaches or osteoporosis. Human milk is innately formulated for humans, as cow's milk is for cows.

For those of us with kids who drink milk, we think it is better to buy them organic low-fat milk. Organic milks are not filled with pesticides, herbicides, hormones, and antibiotics.

Better Choices include low-fat organic milks and non-dairy products, such as calcium fortified soy and rice milks. Try and limit consumption of cow's milk to dinner or just before bedtime for a good night's sleep!

Dairy Slows You Down! All dairy products use a lot of caloric energy for digestion consequently channeling caloric energy away from muscular activity. Whole milk is rich, heavy (9 calories per fat gram), and difficult for your body to digest. Marilyn and Harvey Diamond, authors of *Fit for Life*, suggest that the next time you dust your house, first smear some milk over your shelves. Then see how easy it is to dust. They say that mucous producing dairy products (including cheese) do the same to the inside of your body. Nothing moves easily, including the transfer of energy. Think of how this affects your son or daughter when they are playing sports.

Cheese, Butter, and Yogurt Are Processed Milk

According to the Center for Science In the Public Interest, cheese is the nation's biggest source of saturated fat. The average American eats 30 pounds of cheese a year. "Americans are eating far too much fatty cheese. Unfortunately, it's everywhere: on sandwiches, on lean chicken, on salads, and even on fries. And it's doing even more damage to our hearts than beef or butter.... Many people think of calcium-rich cheese as healthful, but it's a dangerous trap. People would be better off getting their calcium from foods like fat-free (skim) or 1% milk, low-fat yogurt, low-fat cheese, or calcium-fortified orange juice."[45] In addition, it is reported that about 70 percent of cheese is eaten on sandwiches and burgers, as a snack, or on a pizza. Below, see how eating light can help.
(Read the labels!)

Cheese	Total Fat	Saturated Fat
Cream cheese (2 tbsp., 1 ounce)	10 grams	6 grams
Philadelphia Light (2 tbsp., 1 ounce)	5 grams	4 grams
Cheddar, regular	9 grams	6 grams
Cabot 50%, Light Cheddar	5 grams	3 grams
Cabot 75%, Light Cheddar	3 grams	2 grams
Mozzarella, regular	6 grams	4 grams
Sorrento Low Fat Mozzarella	3 grams	2 grams[46]

Usually, when cream cheese is spread onto half a bagel, it is a very generous coating, even 1 ounce. A slice of cheese pizza may have 14 or more grams of cheese on it, especially if the crust is filled with cheese. One ounce of cheese equals only 1.5 slices of processed cheese or about a 1-inch cube of hard cheese. Most kids eat more than that at a sitting. Much of the fat in cheese is saturated. Fat is where an animal stores toxins such as insecticides. Thus, when you eat animal fat, you are also ingesting the toxins from that animal. This is one reason why additive-free organic is better.

Many brands of cheese you see lined up on the shelves of grocery stores are not 100 percent cheese. By the way, do any of the cows you have ever seen produce orange milk? Then why do we have orange cheese? Dyes make cheese orange. Preservatives and other additives can be found in cheese. Plus, many cheeses are high in sodium. An ounce of American cheese has 337 milligrams of sodium. A 5-ounce jar of American cheese spread has 1,910 milligrams. And what do most kids dip into this jar? A salt-laden fattening chip! Other additives and preservatives are in cheese to give it shape and shelf life. Remember the origin of most cheese is cow's milk, milk that often already contains undesirable additives. Depressing and true. "Cheese spreads" is a catchall term for products that have no less than 51 percent cheese in it. However, the question of what is in the other 49 percent of the product remains. We especially wonder about the true contents of boxed bars of cheese that sits on the shelf, unrefrigerated, for days, weeks, and maybe months. Stay away from them.

Cheese Solutions

Kids love cheese. We love cheese. Here are some tips you can live with.

- Eat less. Gradually wean your family to accept fewer cheese meals and snacks.
- The goal to reach is to eat cheese just on weekends, like a hot gooey cheesy pizza! This way, your kids are eating lots of cheese just two out of the seven-day week. Their bodies can handle this amount of saturated fat, especially if they are active.
- Choose white, preferably organic cheeses. Organic dairy means that the cows sourced are not injected with growth hormones and are raised on unsprayed grains or grass. This is the best source of cheese. Plus it tends to be the tastiest even though they often contain less sodium. A good white cheese tastes delicious.
- Switch to lower fat cheeses for ingredients. At first, mix regular fat cheese with a lower fat cheese. Gradually lessen the amount of higher fat cheese. Over time, your kids won't notice.
- Parmesan cheese purchased in blocks from a good source is a better seasoning choice. Romano is good, too. When grated on sauces and salads, it adds a pungent taste to your meal. A little goes a long way.
- Don't overlook low-fat cottage cheese. It's an easily digested protein that can be used as a dip for raw veggies.
- Sheep and goat milk have a smaller molecular structure than cow's milk, making it easier for the human body to

digest. Try some sheep and goat cheeses! Feta and Romano. (Of the over 300 food and drinks tasted by the Kid Kritics, the Oak Knoll chocolate goat milk was the #1 pick at a taste testing!)

- Use alternative cheeses that are soy and rice based. Some are better than others. Try a few.

Butter: Another Enigma

Should you or shouldn't you serve it to your kids? Is margarine better? No. Yes, butter is high in saturated fat and contains cholesterol but it is less processed and is the real thing! Go easy on it. Nonorganic butter contains pesticides and antibiotics, but at least it has less hydrogenated, trans fatty acids than margarine. Margarine is a flat out no. Light versions of butter have less fat than regular butters. Again, organic unsalted butter is best. Serve sparingly.

Low-Fat Yogurt, Best In Dairy

The better yogurt brands are made from organic milk and have been made under conditions that keep the good bacteria, acidophilus, alive. Those with added fruits, that have not had sugar or any other additives added, can be a good source of vitamins and minerals. Some of the saturated fat hazards may be eliminated with low-fat yogurts.

Unfortunately, most of the packaged yogurts contain *a lot* of added sugar, artificial sweeteners such as aspartame, some dyes, and other additives. Also, sometimes heat is used during the process, killing the acidophilus. Frozen yogurts are particularly questionable in their representation of real cultured yogurt. Some are merely given a sour flavoring to adjust the taste. Others are nothing more than ice cream or ice milk to which yogurt cultures have been added. High amounts of fat and sugar can still be present. It seems that the more sugar added, the less calcium can be found in the product. Read the facts and ingredients, carefully. Toppings for yogurt and frozen yogurt add mountains of no-nos; sugar, fake sugars, dyes, chemicals, fat, fake fat, you name it. They are fun for a treat, but not often.

Enjoy Some Dairy: Careful, Not Too Much

Save fatty dairy for treats. Use low-fat clean organic, or soy and rice alternatives when preparing foods. For kids who are athletes, dancers, musicians or are otherwise active, explain how the benefits of cutting back on dairy can outweigh their anxiety of missing lots of fat cheese or sweetened yogurts. Over time, they will feel the positive performance difference ... it is a winning difference.

Caffeine Is A Drug

Caffeine is found naturally in coffee and cocoa beans, tea leaves, and cola nuts. Though it is already present in beans and nuts, additional caffeine is often added to products such as sodas. Once it gets hold of you, it will not let go without a fight. Is anyone in your family hooked on caffeine? "Caffeine is the number one psychoactive drug."[47]

> Caffeine is an addictive substance, no less so than nicotine. In addition, it is a neurostimulant, meaning that it acts in the body like amphetamine; it can cause jitteriness, anxiety, weight loss, and insomnia – all of which can lead to poor school performance. Caffeine can wreak havoc on blood sugar metabolism and insulin regulation (hello, diabetes!), and it is a drug to which your child should never become addicted.[48]

Caffeine seems to stimulate the nervous system, similar to cocaine. Marilyn and Harvey Diamond point this out in their book, *Fit For Life*. They continue to say, it is "... addictive, causing painful withdrawal symptoms when discontinued as it induces both psychological and physical dependence."[49] As you can imagine, children's smaller bodies are more prone to responding to the addictive and stimulating qualities of caffeine. Hyperactivity and irritability are two recognizable symptoms.

Caffeinated sodas deplete your kids of nutrients, especially calcium. What point is there to feeding your kids nutritious foods if they are going to drink caffeinated sodas on the same day? "Caffeine is a diuretic and depletes stores of magnesium, calcium, zinc and other trace minerals."[50] Add potassium and sodium to this list. The potential amount of calcium loss is considerable for kids drinking one, two or more cans a day of soda containing caffeine. "Drinking just one can of a caffeinated soft drink can cause a child to lose as much as 120 milligrams of calcium."[51] For kids who are drinking two or more cans a day, this amounts to a significant loss of calcium. The daily loss of other minerals is also disconcerting. Most kids are not replacing any of these minerals as fast as they are losing them with their current eating habits. Unfortunately, many kids drink caffeinated sodas for breakfast, lunch, snacks, and dinner.

Caffeine Can Last for Hours. A 12-ounce Cola usually contains around 35 milligrams of caffeine a Mountain Dew 55 milligrams. Any side effects are usually felt within an hour and take almost six hours to wear off.[52] Read that again, it usually takes almost six hours for the side effects of caffeine to wear off. Of course, within those six hours, another can of caffeinated soda may be consumed. How many milligrams of caffeine can a young body handle at a time? Not this much without consequences. Think of the teenage boys who are drinking over 110 gallons a year. Is it a surprise to anyone that they have behavioral challenges?

Caffeine is Not Listed in Ingredients. The problem is, you have no way of knowing how much caffeine is actually in a product. This fact is not required to be listed on food or drink labels. Your best move is to steer you kids away from caffeine.

Withdrawing from caffeine takes time, patience, and determination. The withdrawal symptoms include fatigue, headaches, nausea, breaking out (face), and general discomfort. Drinking a lot of water with lemon can help draw out the caffeine toxins. Again, water proves to be a helpful drink. It cleanses the body.

Artificial Additives: The Mean Machines

About 3,000 additives are allowed to be put into the foods and drinks we eat. The average American eats and drinks about 150 pounds of them a year. This works out to about 12.5 pounds a month! We have not seen a statistic on how many pounds kids consume but we suspect the number is higher. How many of these are artificial? We do not know because the contents are not listed on the label.

Additives often function as artificial appetite stimulants, flavorings, and colorings. Food chemists (engineers) and food processors have the job of creating the tastiest, most eye-appealing, and best-smelling product that will outsell any competition. They are well-versed on ways to devise additives that entice your kids to eat the whole bag! Preservatives are also additives. They infiltrate many processed foods to give them a long, cost-effective shelf life. Some food engineers are so clever that they have invented non-food foods made from an assortment of artificial additives. Sugar and cream substitutes, some candies, powdered drinks, and desserts are examples.

Kids Are Eating Thousands of Artificial Additives

Animal Drugs, Anti-caking Agents, Preservatives, Emulsifying, Gelling, Stabilizing, Thickening Agents, Food Enzymes, Firming Agents, Coloring Agents, Flavorings, Bleaching and Maturing Agents, Polishing and Glazing Agents, Sweeteners, pH Adjusting Agents, Acid Reacting Agents, Water-Correcting Agents, Sequestering Agents, Starch Modifying Agents, Yeast Foods, Carrier and Extraction Solvents, and Miscellaneous Food Additives. What do all of these have in common? They are used in the preparation and packaging of foods and drinks sold to humans for consumption.

Animals: Antibiotics and Hormones. These can be transferred into the animal products your kids eat. Antibiotics and hormones are being implanted and/or injected into animals before they are slaughtered.

> Farm animals in the United States are receiving 24.6 million pounds of antibiotics a year, The Union of Concerned Scientists noted that about 70 percent of all antibiotics are used to fatten up livestock.[53]

No doubt this number is incrcasing. Unfortunately, these antibiotics and hormones given to farm animals such as cows, pigs, and chickens, have been reported to be found in the muscle tissue of muscle foods commonly eaten by the consumer. You see, there is no practical way to extract it from the tissue before selling it to you.

> American regulators permit hormone implants on the grounds that no risk to human health has been proved, even though measurable hormone residues do turn up in the meat we eat. These contribute to the buildup of estrogenic compounds in the environment, which some scientists believe may explain falling sperm counts in boys and premature maturation in girls.[54]
>
> Based on conservative estimates, the amount of estradiol in two hamburgers eaten by an eight-year-old boy could increase his hormone levels by 10%.[55]

As you just read, some say that these ingested hormones may be contributing to the early puberty rates of girls and boys. It has been reported that young girls, as early as eight years of age, are growing pubic hair and are developing breasts. We don't know whether these additives are contributing to these facts. Again, we are concerned.

Hundreds, actually most, processed food products use meats potentially containing residues of antibiotics and hormones residues. Scientists argue that these ingested antibiotics are linked to weakened immune systems in humans. The good news is that some food product manufacturers do discriminate and choose livestock and poultry that are free of antibiotics or hormones. You will find many of these on the Better Choices Grocery List.

Chemical Plant and Soil Additives: Artificial fertilizers, pesticides, herbicides, contaminated feed, fumigants, fungicides, insecticides, rodenticides, and other soil conditioners. These often-used toxins are also found in foods, as they are absorbed into cellular structures during the growth of the animal and plant, fruit and nut trees. As sprays, toxins do not disperse or decay harmlessly. Instead, they may contaminate and pollute the earth, water, and air we eat and breathe. Any child's health will be challenged if the concentrations in the food, drinks, and air they ingest are at high enough levels. Though food manufacturers may not have actually grown and raised additive infected foods (some do), they do choose what animals and plants to buy for product ingredients. They are responsible for all their food sources.

Preservatives. These are used to help prevent chemical deterioration and microbiological spoilage. Of the many that exist, about 100 are commonly used. You can find them in lard, shortenings, chips, soup, crackers, bread, cheese, syrups, citrus fruit, fruit-fillers, and in just about every processed food.

Sequestering Agents. These agents prevent the deterioration of color, flavor, and texture. Did you know that teeny bits of metals might be present in some sodas? Manufacturers know your kids won't drink cloudy sodas so some use an acidic agent to clarify the cloudiness created during processing. Sequestering agents can also be found in dairy products in order to make them appear fresh and not sour. This method is also used in other processed foods.

pH Balancing Agents. Acid and pH adjusting agents are added to many, many foods to control the acidity and alkalinity of them. They help bread rise, preserve a flavor of butter, add flavor to drinks, plus they perform a myriad of other processing functions.

Artificial Coloring Agents. Dyes, also known as coloring agents, are used to appeal to the eye of the consumer. Foods are often colored by manufacturers in order to entice you to buy and feed them to your kids. There are about nine certified artificial colors; seven are usually used in foods. They are listed as FD and C (Food, Drug and Cosmetics) yellow, red, blue, green, and violet followed by numbers such as 1, 2, 3, and 6. Some are made from coal tar. Many are petroleum-based. Some researchers question the safety of artificial colors.

> FD and C Blue No. 2, is a dark blue powder, a coal-tar derivative, riphenylmethane; almost always contains sodium chloride or sulfate.[56]

> Tartrazine, FD and C Yellow No. 5, are suspected of having some health effects such as allergies, asthma, and hyperactivity.[57]
>
> It appears that young, developing nervous systems are particularly prone to the damage and irritation that many food colorants can cause. In an Australian study, behavioral changes associated with the intake of yellow dye included irritability, restlessness, and sleep disturbances. The more dye ingested, the longer the reaction time lasted. Younger children, aged two to six, experienced constant crying, tantrums, irritability, restlessness, and severe sleep disturbances. The older children, ages seven to fourteen, were irritable, aimlessly active, lacking in self-control, whiny and unhappy.[58]

Today, your kids may be eating green and purple ketchup, blue fries, shocking pink spreads, and foods with magically appearing colors. What's next? Food manufacturers use a few natural based colors such as annatto, carotene, saffron, and turmeric. Some are more acceptable than others. Studies have revealed that annatto may cause allergies, so watch for that one. Check your ingredients list.

Flavoring Chemicals. There are more than a couple of thousand artificial flavorings used to substitute the natural flavors of foods lost in some processing methods. Maybe 25 percent are from natural food sources. The rest are mostly synthetic. Again, the food manufacturers remove a natural part of a food and then they replace it with lab-made chemicals. Newark, New Jersey, is the manufacturing capital of flavorings in the United States. There, lots of food chemicals have been synthetically produced and patented to appeal to your kid's palate. These creative scientists can make just about anything taste and smell like just about anything and everything. It is an amazing and clever feat, one that lures your kids into eating what they want them to eat, whether it is good for them or not. "Adding methyl-2-peridylketone makes something taste like popcorn. Adding ethyl-3-hydroxybutanoate makes it taste like marshmallow."[59] Sound good?

A little bit of synthetic additives may not be hard for your kid's system to manage. Collectively, cans, bottles, boxes, and packages of artificially flavored foods can lead to additive overload.

Smellers! We call the next artificial additive group "smellers." Smellers are usually created and manufactured by the same chemical companies as those who manufacture flavorings. Studies show that you and your kid's taste buds are primarily influenced by smell. "The aroma of a food can be responsible for as much as 90 percent of its flavor."[60] The olfactory glands are considered the most influential factor in the sense of taste! Food chemists are brilliant at creating aromas that smell like the real thing. "Ethly-2-methyl butyrate smells just like an apple."[61] Hmmm.

Whiteners. You thought these were made just for your son or daughter's dirty clothes. Guess what? Bleaching and maturing agents are used extensively in breads and other baked goods. Even packaged bags of flour have been subjected to these agents. Flour, freshly ground, is yellow! When aging in natural storage it will gradually whiten. However, the geniuses of marketing decided a long time ago that the consumer should think of white flour as pure, fresh, and natural. Oxidizing agents such as chlorine and nitrogen have been used ever since to quickly whiten flour. Other products are bleached as well.

Fast Food Wonders. Fast foods depend on additives for the fast delivery of ready-to-eat foods. Additives run rampant in this industry. "A typical artificial strawberry flavor, like the kind found in a Burger King strawberry milk shake, contains the following ingredients: amyl acetate, amyl butyrate, amyl valerate, anethol, anisyl formate, benzyl acetate, benzyl isobutyrate, butyric acid, cinnamyl isobutyrate, cinnamyl valerate, cognac essential oil, diacetyl, dipropyl ketone, ethyl butyrate, ethyl cinnamate, ethyl heptanoate, ethyl heptyulate, ethyl lactate, ethyl methylphenylglycidate, ethyl nitrate, ethy propionate, ethyl valerate, heliotropin, hydroxyphrenyl-2-butanone (ten percent solution in alcohol), x-ionone, isobutyl anthranilate, isobutyl butyrate, lemon essential oil, maltol, 4-methylacetophenone. Methyl anthranilate, methyl benzoate, methyl cinnamate, methyl heptine carbonate methyl naphthyl ketone, methyl salicylate, mint essential oil, neroli essential oil, nerolin, neryl isobutyrate, orris butter, phenethyl alcohol, rose, rum ether, y-undecalactone, vanilla, and solvent."[62]

Phew. This long list is not only hard to pronounce, it is a bear to type. After reading this, if you want to order one for yourself, go ahead. Just, please, do not give one to your kids. By the way, have you ever wondered why fast food restaurants, or any restaurants, do not have to reveal or list food ingredients? We do. Seeing that the average American eats about half of his or her meals outside of the home, it seems that we have a right to know what is in the foods served at McDonald's, Burger King, Wendy's and the rest of the restaurants. At least Subway volunteers some useful ingredient information. For more information you may want to check these restaurants Websites.

Natural Flavors. Natural flavors, what are they? "The FDA says that they must be derived entirely from natural sources—from herbs, spices, fruits, vegetables, beef, chicken, yeast, bark, roots, etc...(Today) natural flavors and artificial flavors sometimes contain exactly the same chemicals, produced through different methods. Amyl acetate, for example, provides the dominant note of banana flavor. When you distill it from bananas with a solvent, amyl acetate is a natural flavor. When you produce it by mixing vinegar with amyl alcohol, adding sulfuric acid as a catalyst, amyl acetate is an artificial flavor."[63] It is impossible for us, the consumer, to tell whether a natural flavor is healthier than an artificial one. In other words, we really do not know what is in the natural flavors listed on labels. It's a company secret.

Fortifiers. One more group of additives includes the vitamins and minerals added to foods for fortification. This is a fast growing category of foods as the food manufacturers think they can drive more sales with this marketing opportunity. Added vitamins and minerals that are bioavailable are good additives. Bioavailable means they can be absorbed and used by the human body. Unfortunately, many fortified foods are fortified with non-bioavailable vitamins and minerals. Those used to replace iron are good examples. If the source of iron is ferris sulfate, it will be absorbed and used. If it is ferric orthophate or sodium iron phyrophophate, it won't be absorbed at all. Being a consumer is tough. Food chemistry majors may be able to cite the differences. The rest of us depend on reliable experts or just simply buy fresh and organic foods.

> "Food processors have in their armamentaria (arsenals) an estimated 10,000 chemicals they can add to what we eat. Some are deleterious, some are harmful, and some are beneficial. Every one of these chemicals used in food processing must serve one or more of the following purposes:
>
> - Improve nutritional value
> - Enhance quality or consumer acceptability
> - Improve the keeping quality
> - Make the food more readily available
> - Facilitate its preparation"[64]

How many food additives do you think improves the nutritional value of foods? Very few. Therefore, almost all food additives are created to give foods a better look, smell, taste, feel, and shelf life. Bottom line, their creation is bottom line driven. The cost of medical care for those affected by artificial ingredients comes out of your pocketbook.

Kids Are Less Able to Tolerate Toxins

Young bodies differ from adults in body mass. Hence, when consumed, toxins become more concentrated within their smaller structures. This makes them more vulnerable. Singularly and collectively, some additives clearly upset the mind and body's equilibrium resulting in altered physical and psychological behaviors. If your young child's reactions include: Nasal congestion, headaches, hives, edema, gastrointestinal discomforts, eczema, lethargy, drowsiness, disorientation, faintness, fatigue, insomnia, disorganized thinking, mood swings, lack of concentration, and erratic behavior. Do any sound familiar? Simply said, many additives are sickening.

> The 1989 Natural Resources Defense Council's (NRDC) report showed that, compared to adults, the average child receives 4 times more exposure to eight cancer-causing pesticides in food ... The EPA (Environmental Protection Agency) has identified 66 different carcinogenic pesticides that turn up in the average child's diet.[65]

We have decided to forgo listing the statistics of childhood illnesses that are link to these artificial chemicals. They are too depressing.

Good food alternatives, God-made foods intended for consumption, are the preferred choice. Please refer to the Better Choices Grocery List in Chapter Fourteen.

Kids Are Targeted Consumers

Starting at a very young age, kids are a delectable long-term consumer for food and drink manufacturers. Millions of dollars are spent to create, market, and sell products for kids. McDonald's was one of the first companies to capitalize on the value of kids as consumers. Young kids are a profitable target market for food and drink manufacturers. From the first time kids lay eyes on the magic of television, advertisers have an eager and captivated audience. Bright colors, happy faces, fun environments, and activities all invite kids to want the product being sold. Over time, they watch tens of thousands of food commercials, most of which are for junk food. Colored crunchy cereals are flashed before kids' faces hundreds of times. When your kids go to the stores, these cereal boxes are lined up to meet the eyes of your kids. Brightly colored packaging seals the deal. Food manufacturers are masters of behavioral science and the senses. Take your first step to protect your kids by turning off television advertising! Secondly, choose foods from the Better Choices Grocery List, Chapter Fourteen, and serve them to your kids. With the help of the Kid Kritics we are able to offer you alternatives that your kids will like.

Anti-Fuels Do Not Fill Empty Tanks

God gave humans the most complex and efficient engine known to our planet. Uncontaminated, unadulterated, fresh and naturally grown and raised foods and water were placed on this earth for human consumption. God created the tools we needed to be healthy, loving, and productive beings. For some reason, during this last century, man has decided he could improve on God's tools. Ego and greed seems to have played a part in the industrial food age. Recently, mankind has entered the biogenetic food age. Now that is really fooling with God's work.

We have stated the case that many of the foods formulated in food laboratories are empty of nutrients needed for the balanced mental and physical growth and productivity of your children. We have also explained the consequences of kids running on empty. Thank you for patiently taking the time to plow through all the anti-fuel information. The facts are overwhelming. The rest of this book is focused on giving you the information and tips on how to better fuel your kids. The first step is to move them away from junk foods.

Break The Junk Food Habit

On average, it takes about 21 days to 3 months to break a habit. It may take longer than 3 weeks to break the cycle of desiring addictive ingredients. The bit-by-bit change approach is often more successful and less stressful for kids. However, if your child is suffering from any of the reactive symptoms, cold turkey may be the best choice. (Please see your physician or health practitioner for professional guidance.)

Start in your own kitchen. Resolve to replace undesirable foods with wholesome choices. When eliminating one food, immediately replace it with a good alternative. The Better Choices Grocery List may become your best friend as it lists food replacements kids like!

Here is the list of the worst foods for kids as reported by the Center for Science in the Public Interest:

10 of the Worst Children's Foods

Soda pop
Hamburgers
Hot dogs
Ice cream
Bologna
Whole milk
American cheese
French fries
Pizza loaded with cheese and meat
Chocolate bars

The number-one worst food, soda pop, is the first to chuck. Replace it with spritzers, 100 percent grape juice (no sugar added), organic lemonade, water with lemon, *Smart* water, or just plain ice-cold bottled water. Break the soda habit; restore your kids' minds and bodies. Each month, try and remove one of these worst foods from your kid's daily menu. In ten months, your kids may be weaned from a regular diet of most of these anti-fuels! Then, both your kids and you will absolutely be rewarded with more energy, strength, and mental performance.

The rest of the chapters are full of helpful information, including solutions to make it easier to find good foods that your kids will like!

This will change your kids' lives, *positively*!

5

High-Octane Fuel!

Chapter Quick Facts

- Meet the high-octane fuels: oxygen, water, complex carbohydrates, essential fatty acids, protein, and sodium.
- All of the trillions of cells in your kid's body need to be oxygenated.
- Your kids are made of about 70 percent water! With "just 2 percent in dehydration, your performance decreases by around 20 percent"[1] Drink half your body weight in ounces.
- Complex carbohydrates, the lower glycemic foods, are efficient energy fuels. Recommendation for kids: about 50 to 60 percent of daily diet.
- All kids need Essential Fatty Acids (EFAs), which are provided by olive oil, nuts, seeds, salmon, and tuna. About 20 to 25 percent of calories should be from good fats.
- Proteins provide the building materials needed to form tissue and repair damaged cells. All living things are made of protein. Even plants! Around 15 percent of calories should be from protein.
- Good sodium is required. It is naturally found in vegetables and fruit. About 500 milligrams a day is enough.
- The right kinds and amount of high-octane fuels will keep your kids running like perfectly tuned, high-performance Porsches! Follow the Food Circles™.

High-Octane Fuels

Each one of us has great kids! They were born unto us, and we love them. Our lives are spent caring for them. We put a roof over their heads. We clothe them and send them to school. We protect them from "monsters," and we feed them!

Your kids deserve the best ... the best chance to meet their goals and realize their dreams. For this, their bodies deserve and need the best, the premium high-octane fuel. Octane is a petroleum hydrocarbon used in gas for cars. Different cars require different grades of gasoline and oils. High performance engines thrive on high-octane fuel. Your kids were born with high-performance engines. There are *trillions* of cells in the human body, anywhere from thirty to one hundred trillion, depending on the size of the body. Each and every cell has a purpose. Each and every one needs customized, precision fueling to run well. For example, cells found in skin, hair, and nails require essential fatty acids to be healthy. If your child is consuming olive oil, flaxseed oil, salmon, tuna, nuts, and avocados, they are fueling these cells with premium high-octane food. If your child is eating adulterated foods such as hydrogenated oils, no fish and nuts, he or she is not sufficiently nourishing these cells.

High-octane fuels are foods, found on this earth, which are innately designed for the consumption and absorption by humans. They grow below the ground, above the ground, hang from trees, run across the land, swim in the ocean, and fly through the sky. The sun, rain, air, and earth give them life. They, in turn, give your kids life!

Welcome the High-Octane Fuels

It is a pleasure to introduce them to you! For those who have read previous chapters, this one will feel refreshing. In Chapter One, The Food Circles were introduced and explained. They were designed to serve as your guideline of what to serve your kids daily. Since we refer to them here, for your reference, they are printed on the last page of this chapter.

Oxygen, the Most Important Fuel

Opposite of the plant life cycle, humans breathe in oxygen and exhale the waste material, carbon dioxide. Without oxygen, humans die. All of your kids' trillions of cells need to be oxygenated. Their lungs are designed to be filled with each breath. Crying babies are experts at filling each and every nook and cranny of their lungs. As children become older, the frequency and duration of crying decreases. Over time, it seems that older children and young adults take fewer and fewer deep breaths. The more active a child, the more often he or she deeply uses their lungs. When kids are playing hard and their engines are running in high gear, they find themselves gasping for oxygen. Their engines are running fast. They need more oxygen, and their bodies respond accordingly. Children's breathing patterns also change when they experience fear, anger, pain, and sadness. The breathing becomes shallower as muscles tense. During sleep, breathing slows to a pace that meets the oxygen needs of the resting mind and body. Voluntarily, your children's magical human machine provides them with oxygen fuel as needed.

Breathing Tip: Breathe Deep

This deep breathing improves the circulation that positively impacts the function of all the organs housed in your son and daughter's body. It promotes improved thinking, physical movement and sleeping patterns. It invites more calm and focused behavior. There are a lot of advantages to taking the time to go deep. For some reason, most of us tend to adopt lazy, shallow breathing habits. Encourage your kids to inhale, deeply into their lungs, daily. Clean air is preferred!

Water, Your Kids Are Made of It!

Second to oxygen, the most important source of fuel for kids covers about 75 percent of this planet, WATER! Your kid's body is made up almost 75 percent water.

Organ	% Water*
Brain	74-75
Skin	80
Blood	82-83
Lungs	90
Liver	69
Kidneys	82
Digestive Juices	86
Muscles	70-75
Bones	22-25

That's a lot of water!

(* These percentages are approximate.)

The Lungs are Saturated; 90 percent is an astonishing amount. Lungs must be moist for the intake of oxygen and excretion of carbon dioxide. Their demand for water increases with activity.

Blood is Composed of about 82% Water. Water is the key component for oxygen, nutrients, and detoxification in the body's circulatory transportation network.

Did You Realize that Your Kid's Brain is Composed of So Much Water, around 75 percent? Water, a conductor of electricity, is necessary for the transmission of nutrients and messages within the brain.

Your Kid's Muscles Depend on Water Almost as Much as His or Her Brain! There are 650 of them. Muscles must be hydrated to perform their thousands of duties.

Even Your Son or Daughter's 206 Distinct Bones are 25 Percent Water. Bones need to be sufficiently hydrated, too. Hydrated strong bones function as important scaffolding for your kid's muscular system.

Skin, the Largest Organ of the Body, Needs to Be Moist, Not Dry. Skin acts as the first line of protection for your son and daughter's body. It breathes in oxygen and releases toxins. Hydrated skin is more efficient and retains its elasticity and flexibility.

Specific Jobs of the Kidneys Require Water. Your children's kidneys need to be well supplied with water in order to filter their entire blood supply in less than an hour. A river of vital activity flows through the kidneys all day and night.

The Liver Works Hard for Your Kids. Keep It Filled with Water! With all the jobs the liver has to perform, it is not surprising that it is made of about 69 percent water. All of its life-fulfilling functions are water dependent.

Digestive Juices are 86 Percent Water. Water is the transportation element for the entire digestive process.

In total, water makes up almost 75 percent of the human body. Isn't it interesting that this planet is mostly made of water, around 75 percent, and so are we! What would happen if our earth totally lost just 3 percent of its water? Certainly, the physical balance of the earth would be altered. Land, sea, air, and man would experience devastating repercussions. In fact, earth could become uninhabitable for your kids and you. Young bodies are also significantly distressed by a water loss of just 3 percent.

The Diminishing Return of Dehydration

Have you ever thought of all ways your kid's body loses water? Water is lost during the exhalation process through the mouth and the nasal passage. When your son or daughter cries water is released through the tear ducts. (A glass of water after a good cry is a good idea!) Yawning and stinging eyes also stimulate the discharge of water through the tear ducts. Evaporation of water from the skin eliminates a small amount of moisture twenty-four hours a day, all day every day. Daily, through urination, your child loses more water. On a hot day and while playing sports, a significant amount of dehydration occurs. Warm temperatures, dry climates, physical activity, and the amount of sodium consumed all contribute to the amount of water lost daily. Even simply sitting in an air-conditioned or heated room dehydrates a young body.

When dehydrated, the human body's functions are also altered because the efficiency of every cell, organ, and bodily system depends on its water content. An inadequate water supply throws the body's biochemistry out of balance. When this happens, a "water distribution manager" receives the alert signal. Instantaneously, it then determines which organs must receive the remaining water, and which won't. Top on the priority list are the vital organs. They continue to receive the nutrients, hormones, and chemical messages through the available water highways. This innate survival system sacrifices some bodily function levels for the hydrations of others. Dehydration adversely affects your children.

> Dehydrate a muscle by only 3 percent and you can cause about a 10 percent loss of contractile strength, and an 8 percent loss of speed. Performance literally dries up.[2]
>
> When you lose 2 percent of your weight through dehydration, you lose 10 to 15 percent of your strength and endurance.[3]

It has also been noted that with a reduction of "just 2 percent in dehydration, your performance decreases by around 20 percent."[4] Loss of water can mean loss of strength, speed, endurance, memory, cognitive thinking, and even focus. All cells shrink when they are dehydrated, even the brain cells.

> "When you lose 5 percent of your water supply, your mental and physical performance declines by a hefty 30 percent. When you lose 20 percent of your water supply, you perish."[5]

Your kids have innate dehydration warning signals. Some of these you have probably experienced yourself. The obvious one is when your mouth feels dry. This may be followed by flushed skin, fatigue, weakness, headaches, and maybe dizziness. Eventually, blurred vision, shortness of breath, and rapid pulse can be experienced. With any one of these symptoms, chances are, the level of dehydration has reached three percent. Daily, through normal activity, including the exhalation process, your son or daughter may lose six 8-ounce glasses of water. This amount does not include the extra dehydration experienced during exercise or on hot days. Any and all daily loss of water must be replaced!

Water Is Cool

Overheated young bodies suffer more consequences than dehydration. It is critical to avoid a sustained condition of high body temperatures. When kids are sick, parents respond immediately. However, when young bodies become overheated by even a couple of degrees while playing games outside on a hot day, parents may not notice. Fortunately, the brain notices and responds using its resources to cool the body. The higher your kids' core temperature (98.6 degrees Fahrenheit) rises, the more their blood circulation is used for cooling. However, excess exercise can increase heat production in muscles to more than twenty times their resting rate. Even with optimum hydration and a cool environment, this heat load can raise your core temperature to 103 degrees Fahrenheit within about fifteen minutes. Young kids do not sweat significantly until their hormones kick into gear as teenagers. Thus this innate process of heat release is not as productive for them. Because it is harder for their body temperatures to cool down, it is critically important that young bodies do not become overheated in the first place.

A good air-conditioning option is to drink cold water. It acts as a cooling agent. Cold water inside the stomach helps to cool an overheated body. You may be surprised to learn that cold water is likely to be absorbed more quickly than warm water. By the way, when you add any other fluids, such as juice, to water this cooling process slows down.

Alert! When your kids are thirsty, they are already between 1 to 3 percent dehydrated. However, the human body has a built-in delayed thirst response system. As a result, if kids wait until they feel thirsty to drink fluids, it is already late! Their potential performance levels have already been diminished. Your kids need to consume water all day, every day, whether they feel thirsty or not. The way to determine if your son or daughter is dehydrated is by pinching his or her skin.

If it immediately returns to the original smooth surface, he or she is hydrated. If not, it is time for more water!

Kids Need How Much Water?

Dr. Janet Zand recommends the following:

School-age children: 2 to 2½ ounces per hour or 48 to 60 ounces in 24 hours.

Adolescents: 3 to 3¾ ounces per hour or 73 to 90 ounces in 24 hours.[6]

Add one or more glasses per hour when physically active, in 80 degrees Fahrenheit or higher temperatures, in 80 percent or more humidity, or while in dry climates. Athletes, drink half to one cup (4 to 8 gulps) every fifteen minutes, during a sports event.

Water Motto: Daily, drink half of your body weight in ounces for normal activity and conditions. Add one half cup every fifteen minutes when very active, and in heated and/or dry conditions. (Easy!)

Water Tips

Not all drinking water is simply H_2O. Not anymore. Your tap water is likely to be contaminated.

> There are about 60,000 chemical contaminants of water. Any municipal water supply is likely to harbor at least a thousand ... tap water is treated only to minimum standards, by seimentation, filtration, chemical conditioning, and disinfection with chlorine. The toxic metals, pesticides, industrial chemicals, are still in there when it comes out of your tap. So are the 50 or so chemicals used in the water treatment. So are the dead bacteria (are) killed by the chlorine, so are the carcinogenic trihalomethanes from the chlorine itself, that are known to cause liver and colorectal cancers.[7]

Unfiltered tap water may make your kids sick. Polluted water may pollute their organs, muscles, and brain. Dr. James Balch and Phyllis Balch, authors of many health and nutrition books, say that more than 700 contaminants have been found in water supplies nationwide and 200 are toxic chemicals.[8] Some are lead, mercury, aluminum, cadmium, parasites like giardia, industrial chemicals and pesticides, asbestos, radon, chlorine, and fluoride. Many of the contaminants come from the toxins we put into the air and earth. Through rain, they seep down into the lower water tables, from where we tap our water supplies. "According to the Environmental Protection Agency, more than 3.5 million pounds of toxic chemicals are released directly into the air, surface water, land and underground injection wells each year."[9] The problem is enormous. Don't drink tap water, especially if it has not been tested for impurities. Drink filtered water.

Ask Your Kids' Schools to Put Water Filters on Their Water Fountains! Many kids walk by water fountains and take sips or gulps all day long. This behavior pattern is a good thing. Unfortunately, the water coming from these fountains is usually not filtered and may have a collection of unwanted particles in it. This is not a good thing. Filters are available to attach to these fountains. Filters can make an important difference in the taste and quality of water your kids are drinking. Talk to the principal!

Safe Bottled Water. Good news: Bottled water, including imported, is regulated on three levels.

- Federal, as a food by the FDA
- State requirements. Most have their own administering body and regulators.
- BWA (International Bottled Water Association) has added a stricter set of requirements to those on the federal and state level. About 85 percent of bottled water suppliers are members of this organization and must meet its standards.

In addition, in 1974 the Safe Water Drinking Act was passed. It set the standards for maximum contaminant levels (MCL) for 84 pollutants. Pollutants fall into five categories: pathogens, metals and inorganic chemicals, synthetic organic chemicals, radioactive materials, and additives. Many believe these MCL standards need to be reassessed for safety. Bottled water is recommended over tap water.

There are several kinds of bottled water:

Artesian Well: Well water that taps the aquifer (a water-bearing underground layer of rock or sand).

Drinking: Water sold for human consumption with no additives. Most is filtered to varying degrees.

Mineral: Bottled water naturally containing minerals. No minerals may be added.

Purified: Water that has been filtered by distillation, deioniza-tion, reverse osmosis, or other permitted processes.

Sparkling: Water that contains carbon dioxide.

Innovative companies have added flavors, colors, and fortifying additives to bottled waters. Some are better than others. Carefully read the ingredient lists of these products.

Because your kids need to be drinking water throughout the day, it is better that they drink the water that is available to them than no water at all. Bottled water is a good source and it is readily available. Grocery stores shelves are full of choices.

Water is found in food. Fresh fruits and vegetables are excellent ways to add water to your son and daughter's diet. On average, they are 90 percent filled with water. Examples are:

Food	% Water Content [10]
Iceberg lettuce	95
Cucumbers	95
Celery	95
Orange	87
Banana	74

Have fresh fruit and vegetables in easy to reach places in your kitchen. A bowl of fresh fruit on the kitchen table works! Replenish it frequently.

Carbohydrates: Energy Fuel

Made of carbon, oxygen, and hydrogen, nutrient-filled carbohydrates are an important source of many nutrients and fiber for kids. All carbohydrates are sugar. All sugars are made of one or more simple carbohydrates. Complex carbohydrates consist of two or more simple carbohydrates. Good complex carbohydrates work hard for your kids. Some distinguishing factors are:

- More than one (complex) carbohydrate
- Slowly absorbed into the bloodstream
- Contains important nutrients
- Sourced from whole foods
- Unprocessed foods
- Natural sweeteners

Simple processed carbohydrates are covered in Chapter Four. This chapter focuses on complex carbohydrates that efficiently energize your kids.

Benefits Of Complex Carbohydrates

- Provide steady flow of energy to the body
- Promotes storage of muscle fuel

- Restocks muscle fuel during physical activity
- Slows down the release of glucose into the bloodstream
- Do not interfere with insulin metabolism
- Help to reduce cardiovascular disease risk factors
- High fiber beneficial to diabetics
- High fiber helps prevent the onset of some diseases of digestive tract
- High fiber helps prevent colon cancer
- Assists weight control

The Glycemic Index. This system was created to identify carbohydrates according to their rate of absorption into the body. The lower the index, the longer it takes for the sugar to enter the bloodstream after the food is eaten. This is good. The result is balanced productive energy that lasts longer. Without reading the Glycemic List, a safe rule of thumb to follow is low sugar fruits and vegetables are on the low list; whole grains, legumes (beans), and sweet fruits are on the moderate list. (Please see a more complete list in the back of this book.) Low-glycemic foods are the most efficient source of carbohydrates. When adding them to the foods found on the moderate list, you end up with a list of "Better Choices" to serve your kids.

Phytochemicals...Phytonutrients: What?

Phyto means plant in Greek. Phytochemicals and phytonutrients are plant nutrients.

Many complex carbohydrates are filled with phytochemicals. Fresh fruits, vegetables, and legumes (beans) are made of phytochemicals, vitamins, minerals, and fiber. Phytochemicals "are natural occurring compounds that plants create for their own protection and survival; they take the form of enzymes, pigments, and hormones. They give plants their color."[11] Your kids benefit from the antioxidant properties of phytochemicals because they prevent disease while boosting overall health. Every naturally occurring color offers definitive nutrients that aid in the growth, everyday productivity and repair of your son or daughter's trillions of cells. Phytochemicals are a rich source of high-octane fuel. The greater the number of different naturally occurring colored edible plants your son or daughter eats each day, the better! Yes, this is a mouthful. Please see Chapter Six, Count Colors, for more on this subject.

Vitamins, Minerals, and Fiber Filled Carbohydrates

Many are under the impression that carbohydrates are low in food value. Simple carbohydrates are, complex are not. Complex carbohydrates contain many nutrients that are needed by kids.

Fruits, vegetables, whole grains, legumes (beans), nuts, and seeds provide various combinations of the 13 organic vitamins and 17 inorganic (carbon-free) minerals that are essential for human life. Your kids' lives depend on them:

- Vitamins: A, Bs, C, D, E, K, and P
- Minerals: calcium, magnesium, phospherous, sodium, chloride, potassium, sulfur, iron, zinc, copper, iodine, manganese, flouride, molybendum, colbalt, selenium, chronium.

The quality of the planted seeds, the soil in which they are grown, and the natural nutrients provided them determine the quality of the vitamins and minerals produced in complex carbohydrates.

Fiber, a Complex Carbohydrate Component. Fiber, soluble and insoluble, helps manage the functions of digestive systems. In the age of eating soft-processed, high-fat foods, your kids are missing the fiber needed to keep things rolling. Soluble fibers are found in fresh fruits, vegetables, and legumes (beans). These fibers create a "gel" in the body that regulates the absorption of food and help to maintain healthy cholesterol and glucose (sugar) levels in the blood. Insoluble fibers taken from the husks of whole grains work as a bulking agent to create daily bowel movements thereby removing unwanted waste. Important! Most complex carbohydrates that provide rich sources of vitamins and minerals are fiber-filled. Oats, nuts, seeds, broccoli, lettuce, celery, and carrots are good examples.

How Many Servings? Doctor Janet Zand, author of *Smart Medicine for a Healthier Child,* says a child's daily total calories should 50 to 65 percent complex carbohydrates. The Food Circles recommend 4–6 servings of vegetables and 1–2 servings of fruit a day. Sad to say, many kids eat just one serving of fruit and one serving of vegetables a day. A survey of some middle school students revealed that about 80 percent ate little more than one-third of a per day recommended serving, over a three-day period. Six percent ate none at all. In this survey, fast-food French fries were not counted as vegetables since they are almost completely void of nutrients and are filled with damaging saturated and trans fatty acids. Fruit juices were only loosely counted in this survey because of their excessive concentrations of simple carbohydrates and low concentrations of nutritionally beneficial pulp. If juice had been given full credit, it would not have increased the number of fruit servings a day significantly. This survey is a snapshot of what kids across America are not eating. Many kids are running on empty. It's time to reverse this trend!

The Good Carbs. All veggies are good carbs. Go for the greens! Go for salads, colorful salads bedded with deep green lettuce. Cut up fresh raw vegetables such as carrots (baby carrots), tomatoes (cherry tomatoes), and celery. The fresher the better!

Fruit, especially those low in sugar are good carbs. Berries! Cut fruit up into bite sized pieces in the refrigerator so your kids can simply reach in and pop it into their mouths. Again, the fresher the better.

Whole grains and legumes (beans) such as whole oats and soybeans. Add them to your carb list. Good tasting with good texture whole grain products are easier to find these days. Refer to The Better Choices Grocery List™ for ones kids like to eat (Chapter Fourteen).

When choosing meals for your kids, use recipes that sneak in several colors of vegetables. In the CD-ROM, *Mom, I'm Hungry, What's for Dinner?,* located in the back of this book, you will find lots of recipes that have been taste-tested by lots of kids. We have got to do a better job of feeding our kids. Quality sources of good carbohydrates in the recommended quantity fill your kids with the high-octane, nutrient-filled foods. Well-nourished kids love to run, and run, and run!

Good, Essential Fats

Your kids need good fat. Good fats are the Essential Fatty Acids (EFAs). EFAs are essential because your kids must have them to achieve and maintain optimum health and productivity. Because your kids' bodies do not produce enough of essential fatty acids, it is essential that they eat foods rich with them. Every cell in the body needs EFAs. It is estimated that about 80 percent of Americans, and thus kids, are deficient of these important fats. For those who have read previous chapters, this will sound familiar to you. Essential fatty acids (EFAs) are monounsaturated and polyunsaturated fats: omega-3 (Alpha

Linolenic), omega-6 (Linoleic Acid), and omega-9 (Oleic Acid) fatty acids plus others that are biologically active.

Essential Fatty Acids Benefits. Enough cannot be said about the nutritional power of EFAs for kids. They serve their minds when they are standing still or running, day dreaming or taking tests, being silly or serious. The following list of benefits is impressive.

- Increase number of sending and receiving sites of neurotransmitters in brain
- Transfer vitamins A, D, E, and K through the body's system
- Help build tissues and cells
- Generate body heat
- Sooth and protect nerves
- Essential for transfer of oxygen and energy
- Keep arteries open
- Protect against stress
- Protect against inflammation
- Burn fat!
- Make good hormones
- Delay digestion of food, allowing for more efficient distribution of energy
- Give energy
- Clean arteries
- Help manage cholesterol
- Prevent insulin overproduction
- Protect and treats disease: cardiovascular, skin, nerve, and inflammatory
- Imperative for growth of hair, nails, and skin
- Have mouth appeal
- Leave full feeling!

This is a long list of positives!

How Much for Kids? We recommend about a tablespoon a day. Kids who love sugar-rich foods may need more essential fatty acids than kids who do not. Healthy fats keep glucose (sugar) and thus weight in check. Actually, it is quite simple to slip EFAs into the daily diet.

EFA Foods, Mmmm Good. Olive oil, peanuts, almonds, walnuts, macadamia nuts, filberts, pecans, pumpkin seeds, sunflower seeds, sesame seeds, flaxseeds and oils, salmon, tuna, rainbow trout, lake trout, avocado, and soy foods are key sources of EFAs. Salmon and lake trout have the most omega-3 EFA. Sardines, Atlantic mackerel, and herring top the list. Too bad they are the EFA stars. To date, we know of only two kids who like them. If yours does, you have hit the jackpot!

Serving Kids EFAs Is Easier Than You Think! Olive oil has many uses, which makes it an easy EFA food source for kids. Use olive oil in salad dressings, marinades, and stir-fries. (TIP: Stir-fry vegetables, including crushed garlic, in water and a light soy sauce or Bragg liquid aminos. When perfectly cooked, lightly coat the vegetables with olive oil, stir for a minute and serve.) Nuts and seeds are great munchies after kids have a full set of teeth and are good chewers! Tuna sandwiches are popular. Seasoned with a slightly spicy sauce, many kids really like grilled or broiled fresh salmon. (Fish that has been out of the water too long gets funky. Careful.) If your kids have fish for dinner twice a week, salads with Italian dressing made with olive oil three or four times a week, tuna sandwiches twice a week, a handful of nuts and seeds every other day, peanut butter and fruit-only jam sandwiches once or twice a week, plus any nut butter on whole-grain wheat crackers for snacks, they will be higher performers. It's okay for your kids to have a small amount of other fats in their diet as long as it is NOT hydrogenated, partially hydrogenated, or trans fatty acids. With the largest portion of their daily fats coming from EFAs, their bodies will be better balanced.

- *Oils.* We recommend olive oil, first-pressed virgin, for salads and in other recipes. Flaxseed oil ranks high and works well as an added oil. ALWAYS, we repeat always, keep oils refrigerated. Keep the lids on when not using.
- *Salad dressing.* Make your own dressing by mixing packaged seasoning by dissolving it into Balsalmic vinegar and than adding olive oil (one to three ratio). Or, make your own in large quantities so you have to prepare it less frequently.
- *Nuts and seeds.* Both are best eaten raw or dry roasted with little to no salt. Lightly salted is okay. Keep them cool. Freezing makes them super-crunchy. Kids love this! ALERT: Some kids are allergic to nuts.
- *Peanut butter! Nut butters!* Please choose 100 percent well-sealed brands, no sugar added preferably organic! Keep refrigerated! Spread some on apples, bananas, raw veggies, or whole-grain crackers.
- *Fish.* This is awesome God-made food. Choose deep cold-water fish such as dolphin-safe tuna, salmon, and halibut.

They have more EFAs because they need oil to survive in the very cold waters. Warm water fish have less. Fresh fish is key to a healthy and delicious meal.

- *Avocados.* These are super sources for nutrients, including essential fatty acids. They are densely filled with good fat. A couple of servings once or twice a week would be great!
- *Flaxseed oil.* This oil is a wonderful way to supplement several different EFAs. Flaxseed contains mostly omega-3 along with some omega-6 and omega-9! Keep refrigerated. Flaxseed oil can be used in salads or to lightly coat cooked foods JUST before serving.

Remember, because EFAs are used efficiently by the body, they are less likely to be stored in the body as fat. It is important that EFAs be eaten every day. Active children may eat more EFAs than those who are inactive. Munching a small handful of cold (frozen) raw sunflower seeds or a couple of almonds a day it an easy way to provide young bodies with healthy amounts of EFAs.

Quality fat foods eaten in the right quantity provide high-octane fuel for your kids! Keep their machine oiled with the best so they can run smoothly.

Proteins: Use It Or Lose It

All living things are made of proteins, even plants. Therefore every fruit and vegetable is made of proteins. So are whole grains and legumes (beans). When you eat them, you eat proteins. Most kids do not know this. Did you? The reason proteins are called building blocks is that they provide the materials needed to build and repair your kid's many trillions of cells. Kids need a daily dosage of protein since they are essential participants in the following functions:

- Building muscle tissue
- Manufacturing red blood cells
- Creating muscle energizing and fat burning enzymes
- Producing hair, nails, and outer layers of skin
- Building bones
- Making chemical couriers in the brain's nervous system
- Keeping the acid-alkaline pH balanced in the blood ...very important!
- Producing hormones
- Stabilizing blood glucose levels and reducing cravings for sweets
- Fighting infections

The neat thing is that when your kid's body digests protein, it turns it into amino acids. After amino acids have traveled to the cells, they are turned back into a protein source that will be "on-call," as needed, depending upon the organ and type of protein conversion demanded. What creates the demand? Action. We have emphasized that proteins are the materials used for anatomical production. They are not the builders. Active muscles are; they dictate the building action. If your kids are inactive, the protein they consume will not be used efficiently, nor will it be used to build muscles.

Proteins: Living Foods

Eggs, fish, meat, dairy, poultry, nuts, seeds, legumes (beans), fruits, vegetables, and, grains! It is comforting to know that protein is not just found in meat, though it is a potent source.

Food	Serving Size	# Protein Grams
Fruit	½ to 1 cup	averages 1
Vegetables	½ cup	between 2 to 4
Grains	½ cup	averages 6 to 7
Beans (legumes)	½ cup	ranges between 8 to 10
Nuts and seeds	½ cup	ranges between 7 to 20
Dairy	½ cup	ranges between 5 to 15
Meat	½ cup	ranges between 19 to 28
Fish	½ cup	ranges between 23 to 28

Protein Controversies

Animal and Plants Protein Sources. The difference between animal and plant proteins lies in the complexity of the protein cells. Animal sources are more complex. A few exceptions are the plant proteins that take extra energy to break their carbohydrate cellular walls (artichokes). All are useful.

Largely because of the popularity of Dr. Atkin's diet, a controversy has surfaced over the amount of protein a person needs. One reason it is that too much can adversely affect the short and long-term health of kids because protein is an acid forming food. Two to three servings a day of eggs, fish, turkey, or chicken will provide a good daily protein base. Add the little that is found in complex carbohydrates and your kids will be well fueled for growth and productivity.

In the previous chapter, we have pointed out that many commercially raised animals ingest foods that may contain herbicides and pesticides, and, may be treated with antibiotics, hormones, and other chemicals. Some of these chemicals may show up in the animal's muscle tissue, most are stored in their fat. We recommend the consumption of better sources of meat, many of which are free-range and have been fed unsprayed God-made grasses and grains. Please see our Better Choices Grocery list for brand names. Ask your supermarket store manager to order some for you!

Another biochemical factor influencing the thought that too much animal protein can be detrimental is the body's need to maintain an acid/alkaline pH balance. (More on this later!) Meat and seafood are acid-based foods. The consumption of too much animal protein can create an acid imbalance in your son and daughter's biochemical system. Use the *Food Circles* as your guide. When preparing and serving meat, choose lean additive-free/free-range meat. Stay away from large serving sizes. Choose fish over meats. Include fresh fruit, vegetables, legumes (beans), nuts, seeds, and whole grains in your protein choices.

Complete Proteins. These proteins contain adequate amounts of the essential nine amino acids that are necessary to stimulate protein production in the body. The grain, spelt is an example of a complete protein. Loaves of spelt breads are showing up in the grocery stores. Soybeans, the only complete vegetable protein, are rich with amino acids, the building blocks of protein. They are also known for their antioxidant properties, their potential for lowering cholesterol, and their possible contribution to hormonal and skeletal health. Some kids are allergic to soybeans. If you have a question about this, please consult a health professional. Food manufacturers have made it easy to weave soy products into your daily menu. Soymilks are available in original, vanilla, and chocolate. Soy burgers are commonly found in grocery stores. They look like fast-food burgers but they are nutritious. Soy and whey powders packaged in protein shakes make great smoothies. These powders can be mixed into pancake batters and baking mixes, giving both a nutritional boost. (See the Better Choices Grocery List for recommendations) Soy cheese and soy-based ice creams are showing up on grocery shelves across the nation. Try them!

The issue of complete versus incomplete proteins can be resolved with this fact. It takes the right combination of incomplete proteins to make a complete protein. Since your son and daughter's bodies innately know how to combine incomplete proteins to make complete ones, you do not need to worry about food combining as long as they are eating a variety of protein sources.

How Much Is Enough?

Rule of Thumb. Daily, most kids should fulfill their protein needs as follows:

Two-thirds of protein from legumes (beans), nuts, seeds, eggs, grains, fruit, vegetables
One-third from meat, dairy, fish

Age-Based Recommendations. Health professionals recommend that for children, 12 to 15 percent of their daily calories should come from protein.

USDA Protein Chart for Children

Age	Grams of Protein
1 to 3	23
4 to 6	30
7 to 10	34
11 to 14, boys	45
11 to 14, girls	46
15 to 18, boys	59
15 to 18, girls	44

Please note that teenage boys need more protein than girls. Also, the amount of protein needed by girls' decreases when they are 15 years old. Very active kids may need more.

Overdosing is Easy. It takes just one stop at a fast food restaurant to overload your kids with protein, usually a low quality protein.

Food	# Grams Protein
Whopper with cheese	33
French fries, medium	6
Milk (2%), 1 cup	8

Total grams of protein? Forty-seven, all in one meal. Any child, except for boys between the ages of 15 and 18, who ate this fast-food meal, has already had too much protein on this day. Once over the limit, no more protein should be eaten for the rest of the day. That means no fruits, vegetables, grains, fish, eggs, cheese, and no more meat. Choose better sources for even distribution throughout the day. Protein is a high-octane fuel only when the recommended amounts of clean nutrient-filled sources are consumed. Growing active kids need protein that thoughtfully fuels the balanced development of their entire anatomy.

Protein Solutions

Eggs. Try not to eat the same kind of proteins every day. Serve an egg dish every second or third day. Otherwise your kids will get sick of them. By the way, the lecithin present in an unbroken yolk cancels out the LDL (bad cholesterol).

Nuts and seeds. Especially really cold ones, are crunchy toppings to cereals, salads, rice and pasta. Add just before serving so they won't turn soggy. Raw nuts and seeds make great snacks when slowly roasted in a low sodium soy or tamari sauce. A small amount goes a long way. Too much goes too far.

Fish. Marinated lightly in your favorite sauce, grilled and broiled, is delicious. Tuna sandwiches made with canola mayonnaise and a dash of seasoned salt is a kid favorite!

Cheeses. Extra sharp cheddar (white, please), Romano, or Parmesan cheese grated over salads and vegetables add a great tasting protein highlight to a non-meat meal.

Seeds. Serve bagels with seeds...sesame seeds (calcium!). Spread sesame bagel halves with nut butter, or, cream cheese and smoked salmon or tuna.

Black beans and brown rice combined make a complete protein meal. Add a bit of sea salt!

Spelt bread is a great protein food because spelt is a complete protein. Some spelt breads and crackers are really good. Look for some listed in The Better Choices Grocery List.

Meat. Serve free-range, organically fed, antibiotic and hormone free meats. If your grocery store does not have them, ask them to order some. In the meantime, go to your nearest natural food stores where you should find them. Any added cost is your health insurance for the future.

All living foods, God-made foods. Fresh vegetables, fruits, whole grains, nuts, seeds, and legumes (beans) are nutrient-loaded foods containing protein. Though they have less than meat, fish, dairy, and eggs, they meaningfully contribute to your children's growth.

Protein is essential to the growth and maintenance of your kids. The right amounts of the rights kinds will serve your kids well.

Sodium Recommendations

Sodium is a mineral. It regulates the body fluids, maintaining the proper blood pH and water balance. Sodium also supports the lymph systems and is needed in the digestive, muscular, and nervous systems. The proper balance of body fluids is critical to every organ and its function in the body.

Natural Sodium

Some vegetables and most fruits are juicy because they are filled with water. The sodium found in their fibrous tissue attracts and holds the water within their skins. Without sodium, they would be dry. Vegetables and fruits are good sources of sodium. An added nutritional benefit is the potassium and magnesium duo that accompanies sodium. When combined with potassium or magnesium, larger amounts of sodium are less detrimental to the body. Most fresh fruits and vegetables contain this magic balance. Left alone, nature is in balance. Below are some good examples of natural sodium.

FOOD (one each)	#Milligrams of Sodium
Apple	1
Banana	1
Orange	2
Carrot	34
Lettuce, 1 leaf	1
Tomato	11
Broccoli, 1 cup	15
Celery, 1 stalk	50

When whole foods are eaten, your kid's body naturally ingests their sodium content and puts it to good use. Kids who are eating vegetables and fruits are providing their bodies with these much needed minerals. Natural sea salts are also valuable mineral providers (sodium choride, calcium, magnesium, phosphorus, potassium, manganese, zinc, iodine, sulphur, and copper). Ask for them at your grocery store.

Sodium Recommendations For Kids

Consuming around 500 milligrams of sodium per day is adequate for kids over five.

Yes, it is okay to add a little salt to foods. Again, the problem of over-consumption primarily stems from many processed foods eaten by kids. Keep your kids in balance by fueling them with more whole foods than processed foods.

High-Octane Fuel is a 75/25 Formula

Body's fluids have an alkaline or acidic level, measured by pH. (pH measures the concentration of hydrogen ions in the fluids.) The human body's ideal pH balance range is 6.0 — 6.8. The range is one to fourteen. Though it may vary for a few people, an ideal diet of 75 percent alkaline and 25 percent acid foods prevents a too low or too high pH level. The traditional Japanese diet follows the high-alkaline pH food formula. With little exception, the American diet follows the opposite formula, 25 percent alkaline and 75 percent acid-based foods.

Keeping a proper pH balance of 6.0 — 6.8 is a priority function of your son or daughter's body. When off balance, his or her brain will send the message, "put me back in balance", at whatever cost. This may mean that the body has to take from within if the correct ratio of acid to alkaline is not met by the foods consumed. Peter will be robbed to pay Paul. Often Peter is the alkaline calcium found in the bone. There seems to be little doubt that an overly acidic body, beginning as a child, may later lead to osteoporosis. For a while, a young body may be able to compensate for a highly acidic diet. However, over time, too much acid takes a toll. Some research suggests that common and possibly life-threatening diseases, illnesses, and social challenges engulfing our kids today may be related to an alkaline/acid pH imbalance.

Foods are measured by their alkaline and acid content. Our society bases cosmetic formulas on pH balance for hair and body products. Yet, few food manufacturers have divulged or marketed the importance of pH content of food or drinks that are swallowed into the body. How could you know that your kids are eating way too many acid-based foods? As a rule, seafood, meat/poultry, dairy, grains, legumes, nuts, and seeds, oils, and sweets are acids foods. Vegetables and fruit are alkaline based-foods. If you gradually move your kids toward consuming more fruits and vegetables than acid-based foods, other issues such as the proper amount of vitamins, minerals, proteins, carbohydrates, and fats a child should eat will be automatically resolved. Shoot for a 40 percent acid and 60 percent alkaline diet. That would be a noteworthy improvement!

You Have Got To Be Kidding!

We agree that it is hard for any of us to adjust our eating habits to eat according to this formula. In addition to offering you taste-tested vegetable recipes on the CD-ROM cookbook, *Mom, I'm Hungry, What's for Dinner?* (located at the back of this book) that kids have tested and liked, we have a trick that works! The solution lies in the magic of "superfood" powders that dissolve into liquids. If you have not heard of any, let us please introduce them to you. The best is Greens+. It consists of a combination of naturally occurring foods that are packed with alkaline nutrients. Simply stir three teaspoons in a glass of juice, or, add some to a protein shake. One tablespoon is about equal to six salad bowls of a long list of green "superfoods". Starting the day with this gives your kids a huge leap to meeting his or her alkaline and high-octane fuel needs. Gradually introduce a super food shake, with or without protein powders, to your kids by first using only a half teaspoon of the powdered greens. Over time, increase this amount until you reach the recommended three teaspoons. Disguise it in their favorite juice. At first, encourage your kids to swallow a very small portion. Hide the drink in an opaque plastic glass that has a lid with a hole for a straw. Always give your kids a straw for this drink! The fact that three teaspoons equals about six salad bowls full of many colors of vegetables is very impressive. This may be equated to six servings of vegetables!!! Explain this to your kids. They love the thought of getting their daily vegetable requirement over with in one drink. So do moms!

It pays to feed your kids real food. Fill them up with the high-octane! They deserve it. Follow the Food Circles.

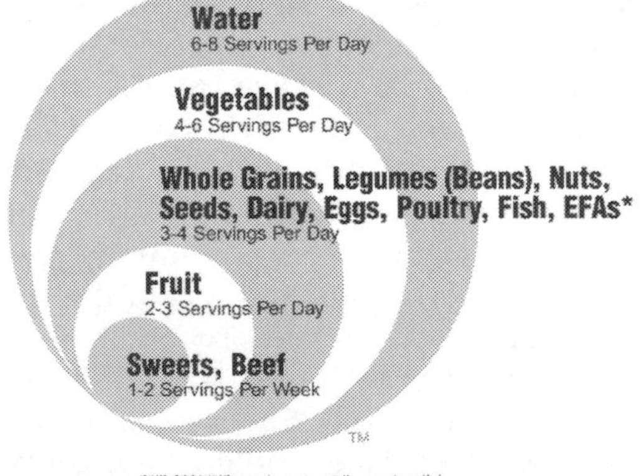

ONE SERVING equals each child's own handful.
SERVING SIZE EXCEPTIONS: Water ~ 6-8 ounces, EFAs/Seeds ~ 1 teaspoon, Eggs ~ 1, any size
*EFAs - Essential Fatty Acids (refers to oils only)

6

Count Colors!

Chapter Quick Facts

- Phytochemicals (plant nutrients) give God-made foods their colors, flavor, and scent. Thousands exist in nature.
- Phytochemicals are life-savers: Antioxidants destroy unstable disease-causing cells. Anti-inflammatory properties prevent and reduce harmful inflammation. Detoxifiers remove bad guys right out of the body.
- Only sun-ripened fruits, vegetables, herbs, grains, legumes, nuts, and seeds are fully packed with phytochemicals displaying a rainbow of colors.
- Artificial colors are found in most processed foods. Around 90 percent of artificial food colors are made from coal tar derivatives, petroleum. Kids are eating pounds a year. Studies have shown that the nervous and muscular systems of the young are at risk when consuming artificial colors.
- Eating so many artificially dyed lab-made chemicals has dulled kids' taste buds. Once weaned off dyed processed foods, naturally colorful and flavorful fresh produce will taste good!
- Introduce your kids to the concept of eating as many different colors of naturally occurring (God-made) colored foods everyday. The darker the color the better. Blueberries are tops!

Count Colors

Kids love the color blue. Green and red are the runner-ups! Of the over 214 Kid Kritics Taste Testers who answered the question of which is his or her favorite color, 54 percent said blue, 17 percent green, and 13 percent red. Purple, yellow, orange, and black all fell below 5 percent. Pink had one write-in! Gender did not seem to make a significant difference. Blue is it!

Food Colors

So, what in the world does the science of color have to do with food? All plants, including the ones we eat, are loaded with literally hundreds of colorful chemicals, called phytochemicals. They are in all plants. Phyto means plants and chemicals refer to the nutrients found in all plants, including those not meant for human consumption. Edible phytonutrient-filled plants include fruits, vegetables, herbs, grains, and legumes.

Titus Venessa, Ph.D., Sc. D., a science researcher who has devoted his career to studying food colors, states that there are two families of colors in plant foods:

> CAROTENOIDS: colors in nature that are green, yellow, and orange which turn into red, yellow, and orange colors when plant ripens. An example is a tomato that is green before it turns red. The distinguished authors of the *Color Code* report that there are over 600 different phytochemical compounds in the family of carotenoids. Fifty are in the human diet.[1]
>
> FLAVONOIDS: all colors in nature that are predominantly purple, deep reds, browns, and greens. These colors range from the chlorophyll in a new green leaf to the other end of the spectrum, the brown falling leaves of autumn. In the vegetable garden you may see a full array of flavonoid colors including green and purple lettuces and cabbage. "Eight hundred (800) have been identified to date."[2]

There are plant foods that are made of both carotenoids and flavonoids. Examples of these nutrient power-packed vegetables are broccoli, kale, Swiss chard, pink grapefruit, and kiwi.

Phytochemicals: They Work for Your Kids

Phytochemicals are God's protection invention. Their primary job is to protect plants from sunrays, pollution, and other natural and unnatural toxins. The brilliance behind God's plan is that these protective benefits are carried on into your son and daughter's body when he or she eats multiple colors of fruits and vegetables. Science is learning and confirming that phytonutrients play a significant role in protecting humans from diseases, such as cancer, and heart disease. Research is revealing that they sometimes act singularly and sometimes as a group to fight the bad guys. You probably have heard that broccoli can fight cancer. Researcher Dr. Titus Venessa explains why. The sulforaphane phytochemical found in broccoli activates a group of enzymes to quickly move a carcinogenic (cancer causing) molecule out of a cell before any harm can be done to it. Phytochemicals perform three life-saving functions.

- *Antioxidants*: Destroy destructive disease-causing unstable cells
- *Anti-inflammatories:* Prevent and reverse damaging inflammation
- *Detoxifiers:* Remove toxins, the bad guys

The power of phytochemicals lies in their potency and numbers. Your son or daughter has a strategic advantage if he or she eats more of these good guys.

Phytonutrients are also the source of a plant's scent and flavor. Kids are not only attracted to plant foods such as strawberries by their delicious red color, they are also lured by their scent and taste! Bananas taste like bananas and are pale yellow because of the caretenoids and anthyocyanins found in them. You can thank phytochemicals for the scent and flavor of onions and garlic! None of these phytonutrients are made in flavor and dye laboratories. Lucky for us, phytonutrients are not completely destroyed with heat, as are most vitamins and enzymes. Thus steamed peas or broccoli as well as vegetable soups are alive with these good guys.

Sun-ripened is best. Sun-ripened foods contain lots of phytochemicals. Unripe ones have fewer. Artificially colored fruits and vegetables contain few or no phytochemcials. Lab-made foods have absolutely none. Only sun-ripened fruits, vegetables, herbs, grains, and legumes are fully packed with phytochemicals. Sunlight activates the phytochemical production process. When this process reaches maturity, these foods are ready to harvest and eat. It is true that root vegetables such as carrots and beets, never see the sun. However, their leaves and stems serve as conduits that receive the sunlight and transform it into phytochemical nutrients. As a result, even though they grow under the soil, carrots turn orange and beets purple-red.

When fruits and vegetables are picked and boxed before being ripened by the sun, their phytochemical potency is minimized. Most commercially harvested produce is picked when green and firm in order to prevent bruising damage during transportation. Before reaching the grocery store, this produce may be gassed or dyed for coloration. Oranges are a good example. Most black olives are gassed. So are bananas. Gassing and dyeing is a common method of artificially of ripening and coloring fruits and vegetables. None of us know much about the gasses or dyes being used. This should be revealed to the consumer, especially to those with allergy concerns.

For optimum phytochemical-filled produce, buy organic or locally grown fruits and vegetables, in season! Most organic and locally farm raised produce is allowed to ripen by sunlight. In the northern hemisphere, apples are harvested in the fall and peaches in the summer. When apples appear in the stores in May, or peaches in December, you have reason to wonder when and where they were picked, how long they were stored, and whether they were gassed or dyed for the perfect ready-to-eat look. Summer and fall produce airfreighted from the southern hemisphere during our winter and spring may or may not have been treated with additives and preserving chemicals. At least they were picked in season.

Potent Phytochemicals

To avoid the overwhelming task of reading the very long list of phytochemicals found in foods along with the protective roles they play for each body part, we have simply grouped foods according to color. You can be assured that all foods listed below have some antioxidant, anti-inflammatory and/or detoxifying properties. Thus, they can play a part in preventing or potentially arresting and removing cancer, heart, and other autoimmune diseases and illnesses. Phytonutrients are high-octane fuels.

Food Color Groups

COLOR	FOOD	
WHITE	Cabbage	Cauliflower
	Garlic	Onion
	Potato, white	Turnip
YELLOW	Bell pepper, yellow	Apple
	Corn	Banana
	Potato, yellow	Grapefruit
	Squash, spaghetti, yellow	Lemon
		Pineapple
ORANGE	Bell Pepper, orange	Apricots
	Carrot	Cantaloupe
	Squash, acorn, butternut	Mango
	Pumpkin	Orange
	Sweet potato	Yam
RED	Beet	Apple
	Bell pepper, red	Cranberry
	Onion, red	Grapes, red
	Pepper, hot	Grapefruit, ruby
	Raspberry	Strawberry
	Tomato	
GREEN	Artichoke	Apple
	Asparagus	Avocado
	Broccoli	Grape, green
	Brussel sprout	Honeydew melon
	Cabbage	Kiwi
	Cucumber	Lime
	Lettuce, dark green	Kale
	Parsley	Bell pepper, green
	Spinach	Watercress
	Zucchini	
BLUE	Blackberry	Blueberry
	Plum	
PURPLE	Cabbage, purple	Grape, Concord
	Cauliflower, purple	Eggplant
	Turnip	
BROWN	Nuts, Seeds	
	Soybeans	

Phyto-blockbusters! Berries (all), cherries, sweet potatoes, spinach, broccoli, kale, red cabbage, and Concord grapes, these are loaded with protective phytonutrients. The darker the color, the better! "...vegetables that are darker not only have more antioxidant pigments — they often have more vitamins as well."[3] Authors of *Color Code* go on to quote nutritionist, Bonnie Lieberman of the Center for Science in the Public Interest, "Deep green romaine lettuce contains more B vitamins than pale iceberg. Eat a whole cup of iceberg and you get 10 percent of the U.S. RDA for well, nothing." Blue and purple foods, berries, and Concord grapes, are tops on the list. Since some work alone and some as a group, all God-made colored foods play an important role in supplying your child's body with high-octane fuel. Thus, it is best to serve your kids as many different naturally occurring colors of foods a day as possible. (Lab-made colors don't count)

Phyto-Cooking Tips

For those red and green colored foods your son or daughter resist, chop little bits up ever so finely, to make them less noticeable. Sprinkling tasteless dried parsley flakes and paprika on all prepared foods is a great way to accustom them to eating more colors. Every little bit counts! For those eagle-eyed young kids, introduce them to the sweeter versions of vegetables first. Thinly sliced yellow and red bell peppers are good choices. Your favorite dips are very helpful when it comes to introducing veggies. Another way to invite kids to eat vegetables is to grate and melt white cheese on them, lots of it at first, if necessary. Gradually reduce the cheese content. Grated Parmesan and Romano cheeses are well-received toppings. When timely, tell your kids the truth about the good guy benefits of these foods. We have found that they relate to the good guys versus bad guys analogy.

Fake Colors, Fake Foods, Consequences

Man-made color additives are usually more intense in color than natural, making them cost efficient. This is by design. A tiny drop goes a long way. In addition, artificial colors are more constant and easily blend together for predictable results. Too bad they are also questionable health additives. Artificial color ingredients placed in "foods" seem to defy the definition of food. Few will argue that they give or sustain life. Probably the most disturbing reality is that so many of the colors used have not been tested for adverse reactions. Yet, they are readily put into foods and eaten daily by kids. Some health professionals have reviewed recent artificial food coloring research and have concluded there is a real possible correlation between the consumption of synthetic coloring and hyperactive behavior. Doctor Ben Feingold's Association continues to be devoted to researching the effects food additives have on children. He "asserts that forty percent of so-called hyperkinetic or hyperactive children are really suffering from a sensitivity to certain natural food components such as salicylates and synthetic food additives, specifically artificial colors and flavors. By eliminating these elements from the diets of the children he treated, he was able to discontinue medication and improve the behavior of more than fifty percent of them. There was also a dramatic improvement in their performance at school."[4]

Coal Tar or Petroleum?

Most artificial colorings come from coal tar and petroleum-based dyes. Food chemists have discovered inexpensive ways to mimic God-made food colors using products not intended for consumption by humans and especially by kids. Some say kids are about three times more vulnerable to the biological reactions. Chances are, your kids are eating pounds of them a year. Artificial dyes are found in almost all processed foods: fruit drinks, sports drinks, sodas, processed meat (hot dogs), jellies (mint), cereals, crackers, cookies, breads (bleached, dyed flour), soups, (canned soup, broths), sauces (some sweet and sours), and salad dressings (thousand island). You name it, it's there. Watch the verbiage on the label's ingredient list. Sometimes dyes are listed specifically and some are camouflaged with words like "flavorings."

The list of man-made food dyes is long. Some have been recognized as GRAS, "Generally Recognized As Safe", by a government approval forum formed by Congress in 1958. All additives that existed in the marketplace prior to 1958 were declared exempt from premarket clearance. Since then, others have been reviewed by the authorized government agency. Ultimately, the FDA is responsible for regulating color additives. Below is a list of some of the most commonly GRAS-sanctioned used artificial food dyes.

FD & C Blue # 1 and # 2
FD & C Citrus Red # 2 FD & C Green # 3
FD & C Red # 3
FD & C Yellow # 5 and # 6
FD & C Lakes
Red Dye # 40

What the FDA and some other food safety organizations seem to overlook is the potential danger of consuming collective amounts of a number of different dyes. One serving of many kid targeted cereals includes a rainbow of different colors of dyes. Perhaps the amount in one serving alone is not initially harmful. However, add a day's worth of sodas, sport drinks, dyed candies, meats, cheese and sauces, and your son and daughter could be in dye overload. What are the mental and physical health consequences of a daily diet of dyes over time? How much is too much? Did anyone take this concern into account during the dye approval (certification) process? Who is targeted? Who ultimately pays the price for the allowance of putting so many dyes in so many foods? Your kids.

Colors Turn on Emotions

Colors stimulate emotional responses. Food engineers are paid by food manufacturers to be experts on this subject. Mega-millions have been spent researching, testing, and inventing colors that trigger irresistible appeal and positive emotional satisfaction.

When first sighting a food, your kid's eyes take mental photographs. Then his or her brain translates the different wavelengths and categorizes them according to his or her food preferences. How many times have you laid eyes on a freshly baked blueberry pie and your mouth watered? Add a scoop of vanilla ice cream and you are ready to devour it, entirely! Studies have shown that even the color of a plate on which the food is served on can alter eating habits. They say red is the winner for seconds.

Savvy marketers use color science in the packaging, advertisements, signage, and the interior décor of many fast food, convenient mini markets and major grocery stores to lure consumers and shoppers into spending more and more money. The message is, you cannot resist it, so buy it, today, now! The message to your kids is, get it for me mom. I have to have it. Don't buy into this aggressive marketing plan.

Natural Colors, A Plus or Minus

It all depends on what is meant by natural. Natural colorings extracted from natural creations may prove to be detrimental to the health of your children. Others are human-friendly. Natural means produced in nature. This does not limit the source to traditionally eaten plants. Monkeys and bugs are natural creations.

> It has been reported that some "natural" colors have been known to contain bugs and even monkey intestines.[5]

> The (carmine) colorings come in two forms: cochineal extract or carmine. Both are derived from female cochineal beetles.[6]

Maybe monkey intestines and beetles are comfortably digested by humans. Has this been tested? Why not use traditional food sourced colors instead?

Some natural colors that have been extracted for use in processed foods pose no problems. Others may be questionable since their altered molecular structure may negatively impact their natural qualities. Annatto — an extract from the seeds of the tree, Bixa orellana, is used to dye cheeses, snack foods, beverages, and cereals yellow/orange. "Studies have shown that annatto often produces allergic symptoms like skin rashes ...(It is) known to cause elevated blood sugar levels to rise precipitously, producing damage to the energy production sites in the liver and pancreas."[7] Why take this risk? Natural colors are positively healthful when they originate from God-made foods. Feed your kids white cheese!

It seems that food manufacturers are willing to push the profit envelope at the expense of your kid's health. Artificial dyes are less expensive to produce than natural colors. They extend the shelf life, and, make foods and drinks more colorful for visual appeal. These dyes are embedded in thousands of fast, fake, and nutritionally void man-made foods. One day, take a minute to count the number of color dyes used in a typical multicolored cereal. How about multicolored candies? Have you ever seen multicolored popcorn? How many cows do you know who produce orange milk? None? Then why eat orange cheese?

Choose Safe, Truly Natural Colorings

There are many safe natural occurring colors that may be used as food colors.

- The cocoa bean is brown. Hence, real chocolate fudge sauce is artificially color-free.
- Beta-carotene (carrots!) produces yellow and orange.
- Carmine from a berry, is naturally red.
- Spinach reduced to powder is a green coloring.
- Beet provides rich purple/red tones.
- Blueberries are very blue, naturally.
- Paprika, red!

There is no need to use artificial colors. Please use ingredient lists as your guide to safe food choices.

God-Made Green Foods: Low Ratings

Most of today's kids do not know the natural (God-made) delicious mouth-watering taste of fresh organic peas, and beans. Kids in Istanbul, Turkey, walk around with a fresh cucumber in their hand, munching away with satisfaction. When I first witnessed this, I could not believe my eyes. Then I tried one and understood. These cucumbers had been grown naturally, organically. They tasted sweet! When did you last have the pleasure of biting into a sun-ripened, sweet tasting, delicately skin-covered fresh green cucumber? Better yet, when did your kids ever have such a succulent experience? Instead, they are asked to eat waxed coated and sometimes color-enhanced cucumbers. Those do not taste very good. Once weaned off processed foods and onto sun-ripened foods, kids taste buds will return to their original capacity.

Do you remember when your kids were babies and ate seemingly tasteless cereal, green beans, and peas day in and day out? Babies show us that the taste for sodium is an acquired taste; they usually make sour faces. Even the taste of refined sugar, and especially artificial sugar, does not come naturally to babies. Naturally occurring sugars do. Most babies and toddlers love fruit that has not been further sweetened. Added sugar and sodium is not necessary. Artificial coloring is not either. Unfortunately, food manufacturers introduce it to them anyway.

For years, vegetables have been cooked to death and taste like mush. Some kids have no idea what a crunchy fresh, or lightly steamed green bean tastes like. Because many fruits and vegetables are grown and picked before they have ripened, the natural sun ripening sweetened process is missing. The naturally sweet flavor is never allowed to develop. Hence these fruits and vegetables taste bland. Blah! Compare the taste of a green tomato to a delicious red vine-ripened tomato.

Unfortunately, most commercial growers plant their crops in nutritionally drained, artificially “enriched” soil, which may be laden with herbicides and pesticides. This, too, affects the natural flavor, creating more bland tastes. In addition, these additives are thought to numb taste buds. No wonder kids find fruits and vegetables so tasteless. Products like French fries often do not even taste like potatoes, and are usually yellowed. What your kids are really seeing and tasting are the artificial colors, sodium, sugars, and fried fats. Yuck! Real tasty fries are made of potatoes sliced, naturally seasoned and baked. Kids love them!

Many organic fresh and frozen fruits and vegetables, served raw or cooked slightly, have won the Kid Kritics' approval. There are simple appealing ways to season and serve fresh organic or locally grown produce. Always lightly cook, preferably steam, vegetables until they are a bit crunchy. Add a dash of lemon and sesame oil. YUM!

Count Colors!

Who wants to keep track of the kinds and number of nutrients your kids are eating at each meal? Who wants to count grams of carbohydrates, fats or protein? No one we know. Kids sure don't. Do you? Count colors, instead. This is easy! Draw your kids into the fun of counting the number of naturally occurring colored foods they eat every day. When your kids eat two to three different naturally colored whole foods at each meal, they will most likely be eating many of the nutrients needed daily. Below is an example of how you can use counting colors as an indicator of the nutrient content of a meal.

Egg Salad Sandwich

Food	*Phytonutrient Colors*
Egg	white and yellow
Celery, lettuce	green
Paprika	red
Mayonnaise (canola)	white
TOTAL	4 different colors!

If the celery, lettuce, and onions are sun-ripened, this sandwich is power-packed with antioxidant nutrients that will protect your kid's body and mind. Even the paprika has a phytonutrient value. This sandwich is filled with a variety of vitamins and minerals!

Our Number-one Food Tip

Begin putting fresh or frozen berries on top of and in breakfast, lunch, and snack foods. They even taste great on top of chicken with a little lemon and honey! Mix strawberries and blueberries together for two added colors. Use parsley flakes and paprika as light toppings on dinner foods such as pasta, potatoes, rice, and chicken. In time, kids will begin to become accustomed to eating more naturally colorful foods.

Kids Like to Count Colors

Artificial colors do not count! When challenged to look for God-made foods of different colors, kids begin to allow their minds to include foods they have not traditionally eaten. In time, they will not be eating the same stuff everyday. For cooking ideas, please refer to The CD-ROM cookbook, *Mom, I'm Hungry, What's for Dinner?* located at the back of this book. It is filled with recipes that have been taste-tested by many families. Each recipe has been given a color count!

This entire chapter can be summed up in one sentence. Encourage your kids to eat many different naturally occurring (God-made) colors of foods a day.

By the way, blueberries are tops, nutritionally, and, they are blue! Kids love blue.

7

Brain Power For Academics

Chapter Quick Facts

- Hundreds of thousands of neurons, the nerve cells in the brain, communicate through over a trillion connections in microseconds! Research says that the health of neurons and quantity of their connectors can determine the level of your son and daughter's intelligence.
- Brain fuels include oxygen, water, protein, glucose, essential fatty acids, complex carbohydrates.
- The brain uses about 25 percent of the oxygen your son or daughter inhales.
- About 75 percent of the brain is composed of water. Dehydration impairs functions.
- Protein and complex carbohydrates, together, provide optimal brain performance.
- Glucose powers the "energy factories" of the brain. Too much and/or the wrong kind of sugar (refined) can seriously alter the brain's productivity.
- Essential fatty acids are the brain's ace fuels.
- Antioxidants from fruits and vegetables are free radical scavengers of unstable damaged brain cells.
- Keep your kids running on good quality and the right quantity of whole foods.

YOUR KIDS COMMAND CENTER

The brain is the command post for your children's minds and bodies. It is home of the main switchboard of their nervous system. Every function of their body depends on the messages sent and received through this communication network. The brain stores and transmits an infinite amount of information. It is responsible for thinking, feeling, hunger, behavior, memory, concentration, focus, moods, and all anatomical functions. Your kid's brain never sleeps! It works nonstop to keep all systems running 24 hours a day, using about 20 percent of the body's energy to run. The human brain is the most complicated circuitry known to mankind and it needs fuel, high-octane fuel.

"The first organ to suffer from malnutrition is the brain."[1] When not fueled properly, your son and daughter's brain chemistry will be thrown off balance. Consequently, some mental and other body functions will be compromised.

Brain Circuitry

The transmission site for information is the neuron. It looks like a fried egg with branches extending in all directions. Information is first received through its branches (dendrites). Then it moves to the egg yolk (nucleus) for processing. From there the information moves out to a thicker branch (axon) where a bud (synaptic bulb) houses and secretes chemicals called neurotransmitters. The job of these chemicals is to fire the information across the synaptic gap to a branch (dendrite) of another neuron. Thus, information is transmitted from neuron, to neuron, to more neurons. And so goes the flow of information throughout your son and daughter's brain. Jim Page from the Department of Molecular, Cellular, and Development of the University of California, Santa Cruz has pointed out that there are 100 billion neuronal cells (nerve cells) in your child's brain. Each of these cells is capable of producing 1,000 or more synaptic connections. That means about 100 trillion synaptic connections may be zooming through the young developing brains of your sons and daughters. Hundreds of thousands of neurons can communicate in microseconds. News travels *fast*!

However, when information cannot be transferred from one neuron to another because it cannot leap over the synaptic gap, it becomes useless. When information cannot be transmitted, the message becomes extinct. It has reached a dead end. For kids this could mean forgetting how to do a math word problem, not connecting with a ball, or a miscommunication with a friend. The health of the neurons, availability of neurotransmitters, and the quantity of the connectors can determine the status of your kid's intelligence, memory, emotional balance, and physical productivity.

The Brain, Digestive, and Immune Systems Are Interdependent. Let's begin with the fact that approximately 55 percent of the brain is fat, also known as lipids. Lipid fats insulate the nerve fibers and act as building blocks of the cell membranes surrounding neurons. Unfortunately, it is this fat that makes the brain vulnerable to attack by free-radical cells, which turn stable cells into unstable cells. These renegade, rebellious, and abnormal cells damage and destroy every normal cell they bump into. Then either the damaged cells die, or they become free radicals themselves. This destructive cycle of bombarding good guys, turning them into bad guys by the thousands, continues and is not stopped until antioxidant (good guy) cells outnumber them. Over time, the damage caused by free-radical cells can cause diseases such as cancer and even memory loss.

The infinite wisdom of God created antioxidants as the antidote. They destabilize, weaken and decompose those ruthless unstable cells. Your son or daughter's body innately produces some antioxidants, but not always enough to do the job. Eating foods, such as blueberries, filled with antioxidant properties, can provide the rest. As you may recall from Chapter Six, Count Colors! fruits and vegetables are loaded with phytonutrients, the power-packed antioxidant fuel.

A brain, well-nourished through the digestion of foods, is key to the full functionality of an immune system. The brain has neurotransmitters and the immune system has immunotransmitters that send messages for help when needed. Both are governed by the brain's circuitry center. Components of the immune system, such as lymphocytes (white blood cells) and macrophages (the pac man-like cells who gobble up the bad guys), rely on this communication network to direct them in the fight against viruses, bacteria, and other disease building cells. They can call up the good guys, the antioxidants, to attack and destroy the bad guys. The health of the brain's communication system impacts the health of the communication system of the immune system and vice versa. The GI track assimilates and delivers nutrients that act as essential building blocks for neurotransmitters. The brain is dependent on the efficiency of the digestive tract for delivery of nutrients it requires. Two important nutrients are the essential fatty acids (EFAs) and all the B vitamins. A deficiency of nutrients needed to build neurotransmitters and immunotransmitters can lead to diseases such as, ADD, ADHD, chronic fatigue syndrome, multiple sclerosis, Parkinson's disease, and the all too well-known, Alzheimer's disease. ADD/ADHD conditions are rampant among the young in epidemic proportions. How many kids do you know who are taking drugs such as Ritalin? Chronic fatigue syndrome was unheard of years ago. Now the numbers of young adults diagnosed with it is frightening. All of these conditions can lead to multiple sclerosis and Parkinson disease. Alzheimer's is the dreaded disease among the older population. Beware. You may see it creeping into the middle age population. It is imperative that you understand that diseases do not happen overnight. These conditions build over time. Nutrient-deprived brains open the door to such diseases. The good new is that illness is preventable and diminished through the consumption of high-octane fuel.

Better Fuel Makes Better Brains. The brain changes and grows! It is not a fixed organ. Your kids can actually increase their number of learning pathways, thereby increasing their quantity of knowledge. As you now know, the quality of your son or daughter's brain chemistry determines how well his or her brain biochemical highways work. Naturally nourishing foods, especially essential fatty acids, can actually increase the size, fluidity, and strength of brain cells. They also increase the number of information sending and receiving sites found on the network neurons, and increase the speed at which the information is transferred. Processed fake foods, the anti-fuels, will do just the opposite.

Brain Wreckers

The wrong balance of the wrong fats has the capacity of being as destructive as a ball and chain wrecker is to a building. When deficient of the good fats, and inundated with bad fats, "your cerebral tissue may become partly starved.... The outer membrane of your brain cells may stiffen and shrivel; the dendritic tentacles that reach out to form patterns of communication with other cells may become stunted; the rich chemical flood of neurotransmitters may dry up or become short-circuited, unable to gain entry to neurons and carry messages from neuron to neuron."[2] Sound bad? It is.

When Omega-6 Fats Outnumber Omega-3s. Omega-6 come from vegetable oils that often lack omega-3. The more unfriendly sources of omega-6 are oils from safflower, sunflower, and corn (found is most processed food products). The excessive imbalance of omega-6 fats to omega-3 fatty acids launches a war between the good guys and the bad guys in your kid's brain. This can also result in other learning disabilities, lack of concentration and focus, and hyperactivity. It is even said that kids with dyslexia are deficient in omega-3 fatty acids found in deep cold-water fish, flax, canola, olive, sesame, soy, and walnuts. You may be amazed to learn that dark green leafy vegetables also contain omega-3s. All can be instrumental in creating the proper balance with omega-6 oils, thereby curtailing any decline of your son or daughter's memory and thought processes.

Saturated Fats. These fats could be called the dumbing-down fats. Saturated fats stiffen cell membranes, making it difficult and sometimes impossible for information to be transferred. This negatively affects memory and learning capability. Saturated fats are known to clog blood vessels, resulting in narrowed passageways. This decreases the blood flow to the brain. Consequently, fewer nutrients reach the brain. Malnourishment follows. The accumulative effect can result in serious brain impairment.

Hydrogenated Fats, Partially Hydrogenated Fats, Trans Fatty Acids. These are fats that have been altered with the addition of hydrogen molecules, some partially, and some entirely. Trans fatty acids, the by-product of the heated hydrogenation process, are filled with free radicals; these damaged cells are known lethal enemies of brain cells. A steady diet of trans fatty acids is believed to cause short and long-term mental and physical diseases.

Sugar. Simple carbohydrates, processed sugars, artificial sugars. The brain is not spared of its damaging qualities. Save sweets for weekend treats.

Brain Fuel

There is a long list of foods that fuel the brain, foods that kids like! Though some of the following information may sound familiar to you, in this chapter we are focusing on their application to the brain.

Oxygen. The brain uses about 25 percent of all oxygen inhaled. This means that one out of every four breaths taken may be assigned to service the brain. Shallow breathers provide less oxygen to the brain than deep breathers. Take the time to remind your kids to fill their lungs! Physical activity increases the rapidity of breathing cycles. Being active in sports, performing arts, visual arts, interacting with and exploring nature, playing noncomputer outdoor games with friends, washing cars, windows and/or the dishes all can make a thoughtful difference! Turn off the TV and computer during the day and get your kids moving! Oxygenate their minds and bodies.

Water. About 75 percent of your son or daughter's brain is made of water, H_2O. Common sense tells you that if his or her brain becomes dehydrated, the brain functions will become reduced. Experts say a mere one, two, or three percent reduction of brain hydration can blur short-term memory as well as visual focus of the printed word. Plus, basic math can become confusing. Even cognitive thinking may be jeopardized. Brain cells are filled with water when hydrated. When slightly dehydrated, brain cellular functions are challenged. So are the information network of neurotransmitters. Encourage your kids to drink water before school, homework, and tests.

Glucose. Glucose, also known as blood sugar, is power fuel for brain cells. What your son and daughter eats dictates the type and amount of glucose that is fed to his or her brain. The right kind and amount affects their memory, thought process, moods, and concentration, positively. Mood swings and lower academic achievement are evidence of substandard, excessive or deficient amounts of glucose. *Young minds are especially susceptible.* If your son or daughter's daily diet is fueled with foods from the moderate to low glycemic index, his or her command center, the brain, will run smoothly and efficiently.

Essential Fatty Acids. Your son or daughter's brain is a "fat" organ. Around 55 percent of it is made of lipids fats. Water is actually trapped in these fat cells. The suppleness of brain cells is critical for its circuitry efficiency. A good balance of omega-3s, omega-6s, along with water, insures this fluidity. "Without *omega-3,* your brain cells may stiffen and wither, stifling message transmission. One fraction of fish oil (DHA) has been shown to enhance brain power, speed, efficiency, memory and learning."[3] In her book Jean Carper goes on to say "Failure to eat enough omega-3 fat is scientifically linked to an array of modern mental disorders and problems: depression, poor memory, low intelligence, learning disabilities, dyslexia, attention deficit disorder (ADD, ADHD), schizophrenia, 'senility', Alzheimer's disease, degenerative neurological diseases, multiple sclerosis, alcoholism, poor vision, irritability, hostility, inattention, lack of concentration, aggression, violence, suicide."[4] Continuing her research, she has discovered the striking new evidence that eating omega-3 fatty acids from fish can speed up brain efficiency in normal persons. It is known that the faster the transmission rate of this brain wave, the more efficiently the brain learns and remembers information.

How much is enough? Around 25–30 percent of a kid's daily caloric intake should be from good fats. When assessing how much your kids are eating, it is helpful to know that one tablespoon of omega-3 fatty acids add up to about 130 calories.

Good Food Sources

Omega-3 (DHA). Your kids' bodies cannot manufacture enough DHA to meet the daily demands. They must eat enough DHA to make up the missing difference in order to prevent brain malfunctions. The best sources are fish: salmon, trout, flounder, halibut, bluefish, and tuna. Actually sardines and herring are tops. If your son or daughter likes either, count your blessings! Most kids like tuna sandwiches. Many like fresh broiled or grilled tuna and salmon.

Lecithin. Kids need lecithin all year around, whether they are in school or not! Egg yolks and soybeans are excellent sources of lecithin.

Fruit and Veggies. The brain needs fruit and vegetables, too. A lot of them. Every color has a brain-boosting job.

- Blueberries the best! Most kids love them. Put blueberries on cereals, pancakes, waffles, and toast ... instead of maple syrup! Blueberries are also known to aid in memory improvement.

- Prunes are the warlords of the antioxidant armed forces. Berries, plums, red grapes, and raisins are also brain warriors. Cucumbers and celery pull up the rear.
- Spinach and strawberries are super antioxidants, memory boosters, and may assist in keeping the brain cell membranes supple.
- Yellow and orange fruits and vegetables! Researchers have also found that when a person's blood contains a good dosage of vitamin C and carotenoids, they are apt to score well on vocabulary, memory, and recognition. "Individuals with the highest blood carotenoids, indicating they ate the most fruits and vegetables, scored 35 to 40 percent higher on tests of logical reasoning and visual attention than those with the lowest blood levels of carotenoids."[5]

Lycopene. This is found most densely in tomatoes and tomato products such as tomato paste, plus other red colored fruits and vegetables contribute to sharper mental acuity.

Fruits and vegetables, once again, prove to be your kid's best friends.

Vitamins and Minerals. Many have brain power! Researchers have shown that nutrient deficient children, who are given vitamin and mineral filled foods, have had their nonverbal IQ scores increase. One obvious conclusion is that when children's brains are nourished, they perform better. Note that when there is an increase in IQ scores, this usually means a positive increase in brain performance. However, this does not necessarily guarantee an increase in your son or daughter's academic, physical or social performance. Every child must apply himself or herself to the task of learning!

We have grouped vitamins, minerals, and amino acids into three general brain serving functions.

Brain Fuel Suppliers

Vitamins: A, all Bs, and C.
Minerals: Zinc, Chromium, Iodine, Cobalt
Proteins: Amino Acids (L-Glutamine, L-Tyrosine, Acetyl Carnitine)
EFAs: DHA, EPA (omega-3s)

Communication Workers

Vitamins: B12

Minerals: Potassium, Calcium, Phosphorous, Copper, Magnesium, Manganese

EFAs: DHA (omega-3), PC (phosphatidyl choline), PS (phosphatidyle serine)

Immune Soldiers

Vitamins: All Bs, C, E, Pantothenic Acid

Minerals: Magnesium, Selenium, Acidophilus, Amino Acids, Chlorophyll, Fiber

EFAs: DHA, EPA (omega-3s)

These can be found in most wholesome God-made foods. Though this list focuses just on the mental benefits, these vitamins and minerals play important parts in the functions of the entire body in some way. Below is an abbreviated list of brain foods. Please see the Foods From Head To Toe Chart found in the CD-ROM, *Mom, I'm Hungry, What's for Dinner?*, located in the back of this book for a more complete list.

Brain Foods

FRUITS:	Apples	Avocados	Bananas	Blackberries
	Blueberries	Cantaloupe	Grapes, red	Grapefruit
	Lemons	Oranges	Peaches	Pineapple
	Raisins	Strawberries	Tomato	
VEGETABLES:	Beans, green	Broccoli	Cabbage	Carrots
	Cauliflower	Garlic	Kale	Lettuce, dark green
	Onions	Peas	Peppers, bell	Potatoes/skin
	Spinach	Squash, butternut		Sweet potatoes
	Yams			
LEGUMES	Black beans	Black-eyed peas	Garbanzo beans	
	Kidney beans	Pinto beans	Soybeans	
EFAs	Fish oil	Flax oil	Grape seed oil	Olive oil
GRAINS:	Barley	Brown rice	Bulgar wheat	Millet
	Oats	Rye	Whole-grained wheat	
NUTS & SEEDS	Almonds	Filberts	Peanuts/skins	
	Pumpkin	Sesame	Sunflower	Walnuts
EGGS/ DAIRY/ MEAT	Eggs	Milk, low-fat	Yogurt, low-fat	
	Beef, lean	Chicken	Turkey	
SEAFOOD	Bass, ocean	Blue Fish	Crab	Cod
	Halibut	Fillet of Sole	Salmon	Shrimp
	Trout	Tuna		

There are a lot of good foods that feed your kid's brain. There are a great variety of fruits and vegetables to choose from when planning and serving breakfast, lunch, snacks, and dinner. This is a good thing since your kids need to eat more of them per day. It just so happens that all these foods also fuel the rest of your children's anatomical systems. The more you learn the simpler the solution. Whole foods are infinitely better for your kids than processed foods.

Breakfast Alert!

Too many kids wake up empty and stay empty until lunch. They do not eat breakfast. While your kids are sleeping, their bodies are busy digesting all remaining foods and putting them to use. Growing is a key nighttime occupation of a child's body. This is one reason a good night's sleep is important. By morning, the body is usually in a fasting state. Its fuel gauge is on empty. The brain needs glucose to jump-start the mind into action. Because the brain has little to no glucose stored, it relies on a breakfast fuel to fully activate the mind. By eating breakfast your kids are firing up their brain factory for the day. Neurons are woken up from the sleep mode and put into action. When your child has revved up his or her brain, he or she is ready for school. Those who do not eat breakfast suffer from the consequences of low-blood sugar levels: diminished learning capacity, memory, and grumpy moods. Their engines are sluggish and so may be their mental and physical achievement.

> According to research by J. Michael Murphy, of the Department of Psychiatry at the Harvard Medical School, breakfast improves academic performance, psychological well-being and behavior... Non-breakfast-eaters were twice as apt to be depressed and four times as apt to have anxiety. They were also 30 percent more likely to be hyperactive and to have a variety of psychosocial problems compared with consistent breakfast eaters. When kids who rarely ate breakfast started eating breakfast consistently, their math grades on average soared a whole letter — from C to B."[6]

Better Brain Breakfast

A breakfast consisting of complex carbohydrates and protein provides optimal performance options. French toast: made from whole grain bread (nutrient-filled complex carbohydrate), coated with a scrambled organic egg (protein with a balanced number of omega-3 and omega-6 fats), buttered with a small amount of canola spread (unsaturated fat), then topped with a spoonful of blueberries (nutrient and antioxidant-filled complex carbohydrate) is a great way to start your kid's day! Given that he or she has studied for a test, answers should come more easily. That sure does make a kid feel good! A complex carbohydrate/protein combination encourages the steady flow of information. Peanut butter (100 percent, no sugar added) on whole-grain bread is another good example. By the way, toasted, peanut butter sandwiches make a great breakfast food. Add a bit of no-sugar added jam if you like.

Good IQ news! Studies reveal the brain power of vitamin C.

> Studies have shown that students with higher vitamin C levels in their blood scored better on IQ tests that those with lower vitamin C levels.[7]
>
> Jean Carper cited two studies that demonstrated that kids with the highest blood vitamin C generally had higher IQ scores by five to ten points. Also, low-C kids could raise their IQ. Further, IQ scores generally rose along with blood vitamin C concentrations.[8]

Oranges, grapefruit, lemons, and limes! Cut the oranges into sections so your kids can first make an orange smile and the bite down into the succulent fruit, sucking out the juice while chewing and swallowing the pulp and fiber. Yum!

Idea for a one-day brain menu

Refer to the CD-ROM cookbook, *Mom I'm Hungry What's for Dinner?,* located at the back of this book for some great tasting recipes kids like!)

- Breakfast: Blueberry pancakes, turkey bacon, smoothie (with greens!)
- Lunch: Egg or tuna salad sandwich with romaine lettuce
- Snack: Orange and banana slices with nuts (almonds, walnuts)
- Dinner: Fish, sweet potatoes, salad
- Lots of water!

One Last Bit Of Brain Matter

Fuel it or lose it. Well-fueled brains run well. The right foods can make the difference between a central command center that is running efficiently and one that misses some messages, or mixes them up. Stimulating your kid's brain nutritionally can lead to the creation of new neuron connectors and new brain cells, all useful for increasing the brain's functions. Now you know that this can lead to improved memory, reasoning, thinking, and learning.

Also, too many calories can cause brain damage. Surprised? This is one of many reasons why there is a lot of concern about the current epidemic of obesity among children and adults. When a body metabolizes food into caloric energy, it burns oxygen, which produces the waste material, oxidized free radicals. The more calories one eats, the more oxygen is burned for the metabolism of the food. Thus, more calories can mean more free radicals production, especially from the wrong foods. More free radicals mean more cellular damage leading to brain and other bodily disease. Fuel your kids with the recommended number of calories for their age, body style, and level of activity. Any amount above this recommendation may put their brains' health and productivity at risk.

Day in and day out, keep your kids running on good quality and the right quantity of whole foods and water. Watch them excel as students, athletes, performing artists, fine artists and good citizens of this world.

It's easy to fuel the brain.

8

Fueling Your Athlete

Chapter Quick Facts

- All athletes need oxygen! A sufficient supply improves anaerobic activity and gives athletes a higher capacity to train and compete in endurance events.
- Athletes must drink lots and lots of water all day, every day. Hydration gives athletes the competitive edge. Dehydration decreases speed, strength, and endurance. It takes 12 to 24 hours to replace fluids.
- The general fuel formula for all athletes is 60 percent carbohydrates, 15 percent protein, and 25 percent fat.
- Complex carbohydrates (vegetables, fruit, whole grains, legumes, nuts/seeds) provide the primary energy source (glucose) for the brain and muscles.
- Protein provides the materials needed to build, replace, and repair tissues. Too much causes dehydration.
- Essential fatty acids provide brainpower and energy reserves.
- "Bodily growth and repair occur ONLY during rest and sleep, never during training."[122] Eight or nine hours of sleep per night is recommended
- For the winning difference, fuel your athletes with high-octane fuels on a timely basis.

FUELING YOUR ATHLETE

Millions of kids in America, between the ages of 5 to14, are riding bikes, swimming, in-line skating, running, playing basketball, soccer, baseball, and football. More are involved in tennis, lacrosse, gymnastics, water sports, skiing, ice-skating, track and field, golf, bowling, different extreme sports, and other physical activities. This means that every day, millions of moms and dads face the challenge of fueling these active athletes. We'll bet that you are one of them. Not only must your son or daughter be fueled for the mental and physical demands of his or her sport, he or she also needs fuel for the myriad of actions and reactions required for normal growth. Young bodies are very busy at this stage of their lives. You are one of among many parents trying to figure out how to meet their nutritional needs while being overwhelmed by their schedules.

Kids today are putting in long days training hard and playing sports with the added pressure of going for the win. At the same time, they are expected to study, be attentive and involved as good students at school. In the meantime, their bodies are busy trying to grow! That's a lot of activity requiring fueling. If they are not consuming enough fuel for all the organs that are working nonstop to support all physical and mental demands, something has to give. Sooner or later, the excessive load and stress exerted on undernourished kids' bodies and minds may negatively impact their health, academic progress, athletic performance level, and social behavior. Our objective is to offer ways for you to meet the nutritional needs of your sons and daughters so they may pursue their athletic dreams and still be healthy growing kids in and out of the classroom.

THE LAW OF FUELING

Input equals output. A high-performance racing car such as a Porsche requires high-octane fuel for smooth, high precision performances? If you poured a mix of high-octane fuel and soda into a Porsche's gas tank, the engine would definitely suffer and so would its performance. Chances are that this mix of gas and soda would physically damage the engine. If you poured only soda into this Porsche's gas tank, the engine may or may not start. Maybe it would "rev up" to a sputter before quitting. For sure, some mechanisms of the motor would be damaged. Perhaps, after the proper repairs, this racing car's engine would run smoothly again. But, repairs take time, time away from practice, trial runs and races.

The human body requires proper fueling too. The human machine is the most complex, highest precision motor known to mankind. Computers pale compared to the intricacies and potential of the human body. After years of research, man still knows very little about the workings of the brain. On the average, we use about 10 percent of our brain's capacity. In fact, some researchers believe we use only 2 percent. The recent availability of MRI and brain scan radiology equipment is opening the doors to discovering the inner workings of the human body, especially the brain. The DNA code was just broken. Much is being discovered. Much is still unknown. What we do know is that the human body breaks down when it runs on substandard fuel.

Aspiring athletes push their performances to the limit, daily. Each tries to reach the top of his or her chosen field, meet goals, and in some cases break records. Anything less than high-octane fuel jeopardizes performance and usually causes mechanical breakdowns. Muscle cramps, headaches, light-headedness, heavy legs, dry mouth, inability to focus, fatigue, slowing down, feeling weak, and emotional vulnerability are some of the initial warning signals. Running on empty can mean two things. First, an athlete's fuel is void of nutrient filled calories. And secondly, an athlete's fuel tank is running out of gas. In either case, his or her body does not have the nutrients it requires to perform on demand. When your kid's engine is running on empty, regardless of his or her skills, it may lose its precision performance capability. Worse yet, it may experience a breakdown. All athletes know the cost of lost time. Smart athletes consume high-octane nutrients on a timely basis.

Fuel for Your Young Athletes

There is a lot of confusion about what and when to feed an athlete, for what sport and at what age. We are going to try and simplify these issues. For those with special needs, sports nutritionists are recommended.

Oxygen

Good breathing habits are important to athletes. Inefficient breathing patterns make it more difficult to perform optimally. A well-oxygenated mind and body support positive results. "The more oxygen you can deliver to muscles, the higher your capacity to train for anaerobic events, and the higher your capacity to both train and compete in endurance events."[1] The more an athlete conditions with good breathing habits, the more physically fit they become. This includes slow deep breathing which calms the body and mind, reducing nervous tension and aiding clear thinking. This can prove invaluable at critical times such as the beginning of a game or race.

Often, the focus of breathing is just on the inhalation of oxygen. Exhalation, the second part of breathing, is equally important. This is when waste materials are removed from the body. "The removal of carbon dioxide and other waste materials is just as important in reducing fatigue and increasing endurance as the production of energy."[2] Exercise increases the manufacturing of waste materials. They should be removed as rapidly as they are created. Tell your kids to breathe in the good and breathe out the bad.

There is a ready supply of oxygen available in the air. Clean air is best, as it does not tax the lungs with toxins.

Water

A little water can mean the difference between winning and losing. If you read Chapter Five, High-Octane Fuels, you have already learned some of the following facts. However, since they are so important to an athlete, they have been repeated below.

Water, Your Kids Are Made Of It

Organ	% of Water*
Brain	74 to 75
Skin	80
Blood	82 to 83
Lungs	90 (nearly)
Liver	69
Kidneys	82
Digestive Juice	86
Muscles	70 to 75
Bones	22 to 25

** These percentages are approximate.*

On average, water makes up almost 75 percent of your young athlete's body and he or she needs to drink water constantly. This is why:

Dehydrate a muscle by 3%: Lose about 10% of contractile strength.
Lose about 8% speed.[3]

WOW! Loss of 10 percent of contractile strength and 8 percent of speed is a measurable disadvantage for any athlete, much less a young one. Furthermore, the experts at the LGE (Sports Science) Performance Center located in Orlando, Florida note more consequential facts. Their research says that when you lose 2 percent of your weight through dehydration, you have cut your strength and endurance by 10 to 15 percent.[4] Two percent does not seem like much, but the 10 to 15 percent loss of strength and endurance can mean a lot in a meet or game. Strength, speed, and endurance are all compromised by dehydration. Wouldn't it be better for your kids and their teams to be the ones who are hydrated properly? *Hydration gives athletes the competitive edge!*

Dilemma: By the time your son or daughter feels thirsty, his or her body is already between 1 to 3 percent dehydrated. Unfortunately, the human body is wired to delay the "I need water" alert message. When your kid's mouth is feeling dry, his or her body is probably past the point of being just thirsty. It is dehydrated and his or her performance is already in jeopardy.

Young athletes have special fluid needs. Because of their size and age, kids' fluid needs are different from an adults. "Compared to adults, children produce more body heat at a given running speed, sweat less (each sweat gland produces about 40 percent less sweat than an adult sweat gland), and gain heat faster from the environment (because children have greater body surface area in respect to their body weight)."[5] When hormones enter the bodies of young athletes, their bodies have a greater ability to sweat. This is the reason why your preteen and teenage athletes' T-shirts and socks start to turn rank in middle school. "Whenever the body becomes overheated, 2 million sweat glands excrete perspiration, which is 99% water."[6] The more they sweat, the more water they need to drink.

Red Alert. Hot Athletes!

The faster and longer a motor runs, the hotter it gets. Without cooling systems, hot motors breakdown. Sweating is a cooling system, one that draws water from the body. Young bodies pay dear consequences when overheated. Of particular concern are the athletes who wear protective pads in warm temperatures. Children who play football, roller hockey, and lacrosse in warm climates, are at great risk if they are not frequently well hydrated with cold water. Helmets protect against injuries but also prevent the escape of body heat from this significant cooling site, the top of the head.

Outside the narrow range of 98-100 degree Fahrenheit, your body will always sacrifice muscle function for temperature regulation.... Heavy exercise can increase heat production in muscles to more than twenty times their resting rate. Even with optimum hydration and a cool environment, this heat load can raise your core temperature to 103 degrees Fahrenheit within fifteen minutes ... when temperature rises above 104 degrees Fahrenheit, your physiology starts to disintegrate."[7] Avoid this condition and give them the competitive edge by following hydration guidelines.

DAILY HYDRATION GUIDELINES

- Make water the first choice of drinks, day and night.
- When you first wake up, hydrate with a glass of water. Drink about eight, 8-ounce, cups of water a day. Or, use the following formula: One half of body weight equals the number of ounces of water one should drink a day.
  Example: Body weight – 128 lbs.
  One half weight – 64 lbs.
  Daily, drink 64 ounces of water, or 8 cups.
  FYI: One average mouthful of water equals about one ounce.
- Do not wait until you are thirsty before you drink water too late!
- Cold water is best. Absorbs into the body more quickly than room temperature water and it air-conditions the body.
- Add 4 glasses of water, per hour, with excessive, strenuous "sweaty" exercise.

Juice-filled fruit can be counted as it holds a lot of water. Best to limit this source to provide up to 25 percent of needed water. FYI: This source of carbohydrate, fructose, is absorbed into the bloodstream more slowly and it may cause stomach cramps. Generally, fruit juice is not a recommended fluid for immediate energy needed while playing sports. After working out, fruit juice is a good source for replacing lost energy fuel, including electrolytes.

Ways To Tell When A Body Is Hydrated:

Pinch the skin. If it immediately returns to a flat smooth surface, it is hydrated. If it doesn't this is a sign of dehydration. Pale yellow to clear-colored urine is an indicator of hydration. Dark yellow urine is a sign of dehydration. If your kids weight is the same amount before and after exercise or a sports event, they have sufficiently replaced the water lost while sweating. Smart aspiring athletes weigh themselves before and after training and events in order to monitor their hydration level.

SPORTS EVENT HYDRATION
TIMING GUIDELINE (water, only!)

Days Before – Keep hydrated (half of weight in ounces)

Couple Hours Before – 2 cups

Hour Before – 1 cup

During – ½ cup every 15 to 20 minutes. (Summer temperatures, more!)

After – 4 or more cups within first 2 hours.

(1 cup equals 8 ounces)

Because it takes about 12 to 24 hours to replace lost fluids, your kids must drink lots of water after being active in order to get ready for the next day's demands. Again, this amount depends on the weight of the child. Drinking half of their weight in ounces is an easy guideline to remember.

Coaches should take kids out of the game *every 10 to 15 minutes* to cool their bodies down, especially when playing in warm, humid weather. The game is not worth their lives. A number of football players have died from heat exhaustion. One is too many. Make sure your kid's coaches supply all the players enough water and give them lots of cool water breaks.

If the competing player does not hydrate as prescribed above, and your athlete does, then your son or daughter already has the competitive edge! If your son or daughter does not replenish lost water on a timely basis, he or she may pay the losing consequences.

Water Or Sports Drinks? It is simple. Kids need just water until they have been active for over an hour. After an hour, it's time to replenish the electrolytcs with a sports drink that does not contain fruit sugars. (Read the label!) After training or competition, it is better to first give young athletes enough water to rehydrate before they have a sports drink after training or a sports event. Even better, give them 100 percent fruit juice which contain mineral electrolytes.

Our hesitancy about sports drinks is based on the excess amount of sugar and dyes found in their ingredients. Gatorade, the original sports drink, was formulated in a laboratory for the Florida State University football team. It must be emphasized that the variables used in formulating this drink included the age, size, level, and duration of physical activity, and weather conditions (hot and humid). It was not designed for 85 pound elementary school girls or boys whose sports play is less intense over a shorter period of time than a 185 to 200 plus pound college man who is hustling for his coaches, day in and day out. The demand of replenishing fluids and electrolytes is more extensive for these big Florida football players who often play in a heat index of over 100 degrees Fahrenheit. Gatorade was made for them.

Sports drinks are made of water, simple carbohydrates (sugar), food colorings, and some nutrients. The formula is designed to go right to work in providing energy. The body uses it up immediately. For young athletes, the time for this adult drink is late in the game and after it is over. The younger the kids, the more sports drinks should be diluted because these drinks are loaded with sugar (three and a half teaspoons in one cup.) and artificial dyes such as blue and green. Sports drinks should not be used as breakfast, lunch, snack, or dinner drinks.

Water is your kid's greatest secret weapon. Fill them up! When cars run out of water, they overheat and stop running. An overheated car forfeits the race. And so it goes for young athletes. DRINK LOTS OF WATER, EVERY DAY!

Fueling Formula

In general, this formula fits most active kids' nutrient needs.

> 60 percent carbohydrates, 15 percent protein,
> 25 percent good fat ... lots of water!

Carbohydrates

Carbohydrates are sources for glucose, the primary fuel for the brain and muscles. They should mostly be from the complex group. A well-fueled brain is equally important as are well-fueled muscles. Many believe in solely focusing on training muscles to be strong, flexible, and skilled for performance.

This is a myopic view of the body's involvement in a sport. Ask Tiger Woods if that is all there is to being a winner. He knows there is much more to the game than strength. Agility, hand-eye coordination, focus, concentration, cognitive thinking, balanced moods, self-confidence, endurance, and sustained time-released energy are additional components to his game. Playing a sport well requires excellence of mind and body. Some athletes may not be well educated in schools, but they certainly are intelligent enough to be well schooled in their sports. In order to play any games, players must understand and memorize rules and strategies. Plus, they must have developed the ability to think on his or her feet. Their brains must be able to send all the messages required to swing a bat or kick a ball while keeping all other systems up and running.

As previously discussed, the Glycemic Index can be used as a carbohydrate fuel guide. It rates foods according to the speed at which the glucose enters the bloodstream. High-glycemic foods move into the bloodstream and are used faster than low glycemic foods. Foods from the medium and low groups are more long-term performance oriented than high. Below is an abbreviated version for a quick overview:

Glycemic Index of Some Foods For Athletes

HIGH		*MODERATE*		*LOW*	
Food	Rate	Food	Rate	Food	Rate
Gatorade	91	Bran muffin	60	Apple	36
Cornflakes	84	Rice, white	57	Pear	36
Pretzels	83	Rice, long white	56	Fruit yogurt, non-fat	33
Cheerios	74	Corn	55	Garbanzo beans	33
Bread, white	70	Sweet potato	54	Milk, skim	32
Grape Nuts	67	Banana, over-ripe	52	Beans, green	30
Stoned, wheat thins	67	Peas, green	48	Power Bar	30-35
Couscous	65	Beans, baked	48	Grapefruit	25
Ice cream	61	Orange	44	Soybeans	18
		Spaghetti, no sauce	41	Yogurt, plain nonfat	14
		Apple juice, 100%	40	Peanuts	12

The kinds of sport movements that benefit from the fast acting, high-glycemic, simple carbohydrates are those that require short bursts of energy such as sprint races. If a runner has to race more than once over any length of time, it is the complex carbohydrates that will bring him or her to the winning line first. The fiber-rich nutrients of complex carbohydrates cause a slower release of glucose thereby providing sustained energy. Most simple carbohydrates (refined flour and sugar) are void of nutrients and can cause energy burnout. Nutrient empty "foods" may give your kids instant energy, but are, in fact, potentially harmful energy anti-fuels. Always consider the source!

Carb-Loading. No doubt, you have heard this term bantered about. It is a scheduled method of eating carbohydrates and storing abnormal amounts of glucose in the muscles for endurance. Carb-loading may be useful to the professional marathon runner. It is not recommended for children. No athlete should attempt carbo-loading without the supervision of a health professional.

IMPORTANT: Most of the energy needed for any sports event is provided by whatever athletes have eaten during the prior week. Thus, if your athlete has been eating empty calories Monday through Friday, he or she has already compromised his athletic skills and training. A last minute loading on nutrient filled meals of complex carbohydrates is not going to sufficiently rescue the nutrient drought condition and provide the needed fuel for the following day. It is best to consistently consume the fuel needed over preceding days. Then there will be consistent sustained energy to meet athletic demands.

Protein

Just enough protein is essential for your active athlete. Contrary to popular belief, protein does not build muscles. It is only the material used to build muscles. The motion of the muscles actually builds them. Inactive muscles will not be strengthened or grow, even when they are supplied with protein. Aggressive muscular activity presents the challenge of building, breaking down, and repairing muscular tissue all at the same time. It does not take a brain scientist to figure out that a young athlete must consume adequate protein to fulfill these demands. Adequate does not mean too much! It also does not mean too little. Experts recommend that children between the ages of 6 and 10 years need to eat about 0.5 grams of protein per pound of body weight each day. According to some health professionals, a young athlete should not eat more than 0.6 grams of protein, even during intense training.

Too much protein can cause dehydration. During the metabolism of protein, the body uses more water than it does for the metabolism of carbohydrates and fat. If you recall, dehydration can cause a reduction of speed, strength, and endurance. On average a daily diet of 15 percent protein in a young athlete's diet is usually adequate. There are exceptions. Consult with a health professional for the best formula for your son or daughter.

The source and quality of protein can play a vital role in the absorption and efficiency of this protein. Timing of consumption is also critical.

Some Better Choices Protein

Animal Source	Plant Source
Egg	Almonds, raw (except for those with nut allergies)
Yogurt, low-fat	Peanut Butter (except for those with nut allergies)
Cottage cheese, low-fat	Soybeans (includes tofu)
Cheese, low-fat, white	Oat bran
Fish, cold water	Black beans
Chicken, white meat	Split peas
Turkey, white meat	Baked beans
	Protein powders, plain

Protein alternatives to 2 ounces of red meat: (Beef contains saturated fat.)

3 ounces crab meat	2 ounces canned salmon or tuna
2 ounces chicken, turkey	2 eggs
5 ounces tofu	3 tablespoons dried or canned soybeans
2 ounces fish	8 ounces sardines *[131]

Some professionals believe that about one-third of the protein in your sons or daughters diet should be sourced from animal and fish. Plants should provide the rest. Yes, vegetables, fruit, legumes (beans), and grains all contain protein. All living things contain protein. The above list of Better Choices is proof that your kids can enjoy healthy sources of protein without ingesting too much saturated fat from grain-fed beef (processed fast-food burgers). You can get a two for one deal by serving fish, which supplies essential fatty acids (brain food), and protein! Fish on the menu two times a week works wonders for a growing young athlete. Salads and fresh fruit are important sources, too!

You can stretch your food budget by reducing the amount of animal protein, especially beef. Plant proteins are less expensive than animal protein! For optimum results, combine essential fatty acids with veggies and legumes. Example: Lightly sauté garlic and finely chopped onions in olive oil and then mix with cooked seasoned black beans and rice. YUM!

Throw in some finely chopped parsley! Many kids really like black beans and rice.

Be careful about over-loading your family with protein, especially fatty animal protein. Performance is not improved with a diet of excess protein.

Good Fat

The right kinds and quantity of fats (EFAs) provide important mental and physical energy reserves for athletes. As you know, along with many other benefits, essential fatty acids are brain food. Successful athletes will tell you that sports are games of the mind. Concentration, focus, strategy, mental endurance, and execution of self-confidence all rely on the brain and its fuel for performance. So do hand-eye and physical coordination, as the brain is the body's command post. The brain's "To Do" list is long, especially when the body is working hard to win a relay race, a baseball game, or compete in any other sport. Essential fatty acids must be included in the daily diet. It is recommended that very active athletes consume enough EFAs to provide over 20 percent of their caloric needs.

Heavy consumption of saturated animal fats do not provide efficient fat sourced fuel for the muscles of your kids. When too much of this fat is ingested into your son or daughter's system, red blood cells become laden with molecules of fat that act like glue. This "fatty glue" impairs cellular activity causing an increase of free radical activity and a slow-down of metabolism. When this happens, the body has a hard time absorbing any nutrients needed to feed the tissues, muscles, bones and other body parts. A vicious cycle of impaired metabolism and nutrient assimilation kicks in when kids continue to make poor fat food choices. Their bodies will tire more quickly. Their sports performance will suffer. It is also important to know that saturated fats take a long time to metabolize, usually from two to four hours. Why would any athlete want his or her body to spend energy metabolizing animal fat foods while running down a soccer field, or leaping onto a balance beam?

When kids eat trans fatty acids, such as those found in most fast-food French fries and burgers, their young bodies must call up their good guy army to fight off these toxic enemies. Regardless of how important the event is, your son or daughter's brain will command his or her glucose and antioxidants to win this war, not the game. Better wait until long after the game to eat trans fatty acids. Better yet, keep your kids away from them.

Better Choice essential fatty acids are salmon, tuna, flaxseed oil, extra virgin olive oil, pumpkin seeds, and nuts for those who are not allergic to them. Broil, barbeque, or bake salmon or tuna with sumptuous seasonings. Mix the leftovers in rice or pasta dishes, or salads. Olive and flaxseed oils can be used to make salad dressings or at the last minute, as a very light coating for a salad. Pumpkin seeds are good toppings for salads, cereals, soups; use your imagination. Also, when combined with sunflower seeds and slowly baked in tamari or Bragg liquid aminos, they are a great snack.

Electrolytes

What are they? Do your kids lose them? "An electrolyte is an ion that is required by the body to regulate the electric charge and flow of water between the cells and the bloodstream."[9] Remember, your son and daughter are mostly made of water. His and her bodily functions depend on the flow of water throughout the systems. Without electrolytes, the fueling system becomes dysfunctional. A dysfunctional fueling system creates a dysfunctional athletic performance.

Electrolytes are minerals such as sodium, potassium, magnesium, and chloride. All are found in the nutrient-filled foods found in the grocery stores. Sodium and chloride are easily consumed because they are in salt. Natural sea salt and Celtic salt are especially rich sources. The challenge of electrolyte deficiency is attached to the duo, potassium and magnesium. Potassium is not in short supply for kids. They do eat the foods that amply provide this mineral. Examples are: oranges, orange juice, bananas, cantaloupe, potatoes with skins, apricots, prunes, tomatoes, whole grains, legumes, fish, and meats. The problem is that potassium is dependent on magnesium. Most health professionals agree that about 9 out of 10 kids are magnesium deficient. That is 90 percent! Magnesium is abundant in most complex carbohydrates such as deep green lettuce and broccoli. This is because chlorophyll is a rich source of magnesium. In addition to green vegetables, magnesium is found in nuts, legumes (beans), whole-grain, soybeans, and seafood. Trouble is, none of these foods are on kids' top ten list. Kids are not eating magnesium-rich foods. This is more serious than it appears.

Both potassium and magnesium are important to young athlete's conditioning and performance. They act interdependently. One cause of muscle fatigue is probably not what you thought it would be. According to experts, the loss of potassium in the cells of the muscle affects the rate of muscle contraction, negatively. The muscles of your son and daughter need potassium for intercellular fluid balance, nerve transmissions, and glycogen formation. These are all related to the action of contraction. No matter how hard your child tries to keep his or her muscles moving, the loss of potassium inevitably will exhaust him or her. Endurance diminishes. Consuming potassium alone, is not enough. Magnesium, is a critical partner as it regulates the potassium levels in the muscle cells. In order for potassium to perform its functions, it must have magnesium. And there is more! The proper levels of sodium and chloride are also key players. All four minerals are mutually dependent. Unfortunately, most athletic kids are consuming way too much sodium in processed food products thereby upsetting the muscular system.

Magnesium also has many other critical jobs to perform in the body of your son or daughter. Important to an athlete is the fact that magnesium helps relax muscles. Kids who are magnesium deficient have a harder time releasing and resting their muscles. Muscle cramps are too common among the youth. So is the incidence of tight muscles that make kids prone to poorer performance and injury. Do your best to turn your young athletes on to magnesium-rich, green foods and nuts. The more colors of naturally occurring foods they eat, the better their odds.

Calories

Do you want to know how many calories your kids burn as energy while playing sports?

Sports Nutrition Guidebook written by Nancy Clark offers a guideline based on weight. Below is an abbreviated version.

Calories per hour

Activity	Per pound body weight	60 pounds	90 pounds.
Bicycling, 10 mph	2.7	162	243
Golf, walking	2.3	138	207
Hiking, hilly	3.6	216	324
Jumping rope	3.8	228	342
Running, 11 minute mile	4.7	282	423
Skating, ice	2.8	168	252
Skiing, downhill	2.6	156	234
Swimming, slow crawl	3.5	210	315
Soccer	3.7	222	333
Tennis, singles	2.9	174	261
Volleyball	2.2	132	198[133]

These are estimates. There are many variables that can alter the number of calories burned. What does this chart tell you about calories? Your kids are not burning up as many calories as you probably thought. Therefore, it is not necessary to overload your kids with calories. Choose food quality over food quantity.

Counting calories can be a tedious task. There are some specific situations that warrant the time to do so. Those who are suffering from illnesses such as obesity should be guided in calorie counting by health professionals. Priming for sports events can be another reason to count calories. A sports nutritionist is recommended for this level of athletic competition.

If your kids follow the recommended numbers of servings per day per food group (see Food Circles™), eat as many different natural colors of foods a day, drink lots of water, and stay away from the anti-fuels, your young athletes will most probably be producing the number of calories needed.

Foods From Head To Toe

Some foods are particularly useful fuels for specific parts of the body. Brain foods were covered in Chapter Seven. Muscles, nerves, bones, heart, joint, spine, lungs, ears, eyes, and skin are all important to athletes. Of course, all body parts are essential to the performance of athletes. If your aspiring athlete eats some of the following foods, he or she will reap winning benefits: beans, broccoli, carrots, lettuce (dark green), bananas, berries, grapes, pineapple, tomatoes, almonds, walnuts, sesame seeds, black beans, soybeans, brown rice, oats, olive oil, eggs, yogurt, chicken, turkey, salmon, and tuna. Serve them weekly to keep your athlete's bases covered. (Please turn to page 157 for an abbreviated Foods from Head to Toe chart.)

Digestion and Exercise Do Not Mix Well

Have you ever tried to run on a full stomach? Do you remember how awful you felt? There is an explanation for this. Exercise and the digestion process compete for lead position. Digestion always wins. It takes energy to break down foods in the digestive tract. Your brain will always assign digestion as the priority need for energy. Increasing the speed of a contraction/release of muscular movement becomes secondary. Your kid's quads, biceps, and all other muscles needed to complete a physical action will have to depend on whatever energy is left over. This can add seconds to a race. It can mean not getting to the ball fast enough. A steak, eggs, and bacon breakfast is likely to slow your swimmer down. So will a grilled cheese sandwich. In addition to the consequence of a diminished performance, the combination of the muscular demands of digestion and exercise can also make a body feel nauseous and cause vomiting. It is better to follow the eating schedule guidelines described below.

GENERAL TIME GUIDELINE FOR EATING

Before:	Eat at least 2 to 3 hours before event.
	High to moderate glycemic foods.
	Stomach empty of food, filled with water 1 hour before.
After:	Water, fruit, and fruit juice.
	Rest one hour.
	Meal of carbohydrates, protein and good fats.

Examples Of Times and Meals Per Sport

Event	*Time of Day*	*What and When to Eat*
Swim meet	Morning	Night before: complex carbohydrate-rich dinner. Water! Drink lots of water throughout next morning. Light "carb" breakfast one to two hours before (bagel, toast, or fruit).
Soccer game	Noon	Night before: complex carbohydrate-rich dinner. Water! Drink lots of water throughout morning. Breakfast: cereal, toast, pancakes (avoid animal fat), protein shake. Drink water during game. Switch to sports drink after 1½ hours.
Football game	Afternoon	Night before: complex carbohydrate-rich dinner. Water! Breakfast: cereal, toast, pancakes (avoid animal fat), protein shake. Lunch: Light, noodles or PB&J sandwich. OR: Large carbohydrate-rich brunch and small snack one hour before game.
Basketball	Night	Good breakfast with protein shake. Eat complex carbohydrates all day long. Drinks lots of water all day.

Meal Menu Examples

Dinner The night before a swim meet:
Spaghetti pasta with tomato sauce
Garlic bread
Salad
Water, a lot!

Breakfast Before the meet:
Protein shake
Bagel topped with no sugar-added jam. (no cream cheese)
Water (follow water drinking schedule)

Lunch before afternoon football game:
Pancakes with 100% maple syrup or fruit-only jam.
100% diluted grape or grapefruit juice
Banana
Water, follow water schedule

Snack One hour before game:
Power bar or a light water-based smoothie with berries
Water (follow water schedule)

CELEBRATION MEALS! After training or competing, let your athletes have whatever they want, junk included, unless they have to compete or train the next day. In that case, give them a meal of their favorite carbohydrates, protein and good fats and let them choose dessert! It is important for kids to have fun along the way. Above are simple guidelines to follow. Remember, most kids are not destined for a professional career in sports. The odds are low. When they are playing, give your kids the tools to excel. Use the guidelines as a training ground for better food decisions. Be serious about this for the right reasons, to improve their mental and physical health, and to prevent injury and illness.

Rest and Sleep

Both are critically important for a growing body, especially an active body.

All athletes ask a lot of their bodies. Consequently, their bodies endure a lot of wear and tear. For young athletes, whose bodies are trying to grow at the same time, the need to refuel, rest, and sleep is critical. Rest includes downtime. It is difficult for the body to respond to action demands, such as kicking around a ball with friends after a soccer game, while at the same time trying to repair and build a soccer player's body. There are a number of kids who play two sports a day after school. Some play two different sports games on a

Saturday. They may go from a soccer game to a basketball game. Then there are the kids who train all week and compete on Saturday and Sunday. Swimmers and tennis players fall into this category. Lack of downtime, rest, and sleep, puts the body in overdrive jeopardy.

Your young athlete's magical machine can perform miraculously, but eventually, something has got to give if it is not cared for properly. It may show up as a cold or the flu. It may show itself as a headache, lethargy, exhaustion, and irritability. Your child may become more prone to injuries. "Studies show that the neuroendocrine system becomes exhausted, altering hormone levels so that optimal performance is impossible.[11] For children, the growth of organs, bones, nervous system, or muscles may be affected. Many times you see kids who are just plain exhausted. The bottom line is that the health of mental and physical performance is at risk for these undernourished and overtired young athletes.

Many studies have revealed that every body needs sleep, and most are not getting enough. Kids need nine to twelve hours sleep a night, depending on the age and activity. You will be giving your young athletes the gift of possibilities if you set bedtimes that will nourish them with rest.

Fuel your athletes with high-octane fuels on a timely basis. Balance their energy output with rest after play, and a good night's sleep of at least nine hours a night!

DRINK LOTS OF WATER!

Foods from Head to Toe Chart (abbreviated version)*

Muscles	*Nerves*	*Bones*
Alfalfa	Leafy greens	Leafy greens
Bean	Broccoli	Brussel sprouts
Tomatoes	Pineapple	Bananas
Cranberries	Strawberries	Lemons
Almonds	Walnuts	Filberts
Sunflower seeds	Pumpkin seeds	Sesame seeds
Soybeans	Garbanzo beans	Pinto
Oats	Rice, brown	Sesame oil
Fish oil	Olive oil	Yogurt, plain
Eggs	Cheese, white	Chicken
Tuna	Turkey	Barley

Heart	*Joints*	*Spine*
Artichokes	Beans	Asparagus
Broccoli	Carrots	Cabbage
Apricots	Blueberries	Blackberries
Peaches	Plums	Grapefruit
Almonds	Pine nuts	Pecans
Flaxseeds	Pumpkin seeds	Sunflower seeds
Soybeans	Lentils	Navy
Oats	Rice, brown	Barley
Flaxseed oil	Olive oil	Grape seed oil
Eggs	Eggs	Cheese, white
Salmon	Lamb	Bass, ocean

*Please see CD Rom Cookbook, Mom, I'm Hungry, What's for Dinner? or www.betterfood chocies.com for complete chart.

9

Nurturing Your Budding Artist

Chapter Quick Facts

- The primary stimuli for creativity are the five senses: seeing, hearing, touching, smelling, and tasting. Touch is the most used for artistic expression.
- Sight, the window to the world, is an invaluable sense for artists, though Stevie Wonder would question its need for musical expression.
- Sound is useful for all. A musician really needs it for music, unless he or she is a Beethoven!
- Smell, a powerful sense, arouses emotions which spill all over canvasses of art. There are more than 10,000 known scents.
- Taste is actually integrated into the sense of smell. Chefs rely on these senses for their creations. Children have more taste buds than adults.
- The sensory organs (eyes, ears, nose, mouth, and skin) need to be well nourished to be well tuned.
- Artistic disciplines also include physical and intellectual activity. All need fueling.
- High-octane fuels (oxygen, water, vegetables, fruit, whole grains, food protein, essential fatty acids) are a young artist's best friends. Junk foods are not.
- Artists are invaluable to our society. Please nourish your budding artist well.

Nurturing Your Artist

Is your son or daughter an aspiring poet, painter, drummer, dancer, photographer, singer, actress, pianist, potter, rock star, writer, composer, sculptor, designer, cinematographer, or a visionary dreaming of creating a winning Website, never stopping to ask why not?

What is his or her creative dreams? What star is he or she reaching for?

Art is Alive!

Art is defined as the products of creative work.[1] Art is a passion aching to happen. While reaching into their minds and emotions for ideas, pictures, sounds, feelings, and inspirations, young artists' creative juices flow, spilling out onto papers, dance floors, stages, or maybe monitors. Expressions of creation are revealed through many canvasses of communication including paint, music, dance, drama, crafts, sculpture, film, poetry, keyboards, and light.

Art surrounds us daily. Leaf-covered lawns, rippling lakes, and skyscrapers are works of art. Sounds in the air, whether they originate from the wind, voices, car radios, or CDs, are expressions of art. The written word read in advertising, a magazine or newspaper articles, books or speeches are all art. Motion, be it dance, ballet, tap, mime, acting, and conducting, involve communication through body movement; all display art. Food served on a plate is a picture of art. The Japanese and French are brilliant at exhibiting how carefully crafted presentations of food art can stimulate the palate!

The youth of today are very involved in art. Music serves as a lifeline to their existence. Morning, noon and night, music dances in their heads. Movement is a major source of expression for kids. Whether they are grooving to music or acting out their feelings when communicating with their friends, rhythm undulates through their bodies. Art classes in school develop artistic expression. Yet, even those kids who are not taking art in school often doodle messages onto their books. Even then, they are drawing; they are creating their own forum for a message. This is art. The computer has opened up a whole new world of art. From icons to homepages, everything viewed on the computer screen represents some version of art. Kids actively participate by choosing or even creating their own screensaver. Art is alive and active in the lives of your kids.

Artists are driven by passion. Their visions and feelings swirling on the inside are bursting, itching to be expressed on the outside! Some artists are born with so much talent that they naturally create their own visions. Most artists benefit from lessons of gifted teachers who draw out, expand, mold, shape, and squeeze every drop of talent onto the chosen canvas of expression. Passion keeps the effort alive.

Art and Your Kids Senses Are Codependent

The five senses, seeing, hearing, touching, smelling, and tasting are the primary stimuli for creativity. Sense "is the ability of the nerves and the brain to receive and react to stimuli as light, sound, impact, constriction, etc."[2] Eyes are used for seeing the magic surrounding one's existence. Ears are instruments designed to relay pleasant and unpleasant sounds. The largest organ of the body, the skin, gives sense of touch. Taste buds, located in the mouth, receive sweet, sour, bitter, and salty sensations. The nose houses the olfactory organ where scents are translated into emotions such as desire or repulsion.

Senses fuel passion. We experience and express this daily. That concert rocked! Touching that snake gave me the shivers! That tasted disgusting! Those warm chocolate-chip cookies smelled so good I ate them all. Experiences of the senses evoke passion. Without the existence of the five senses, the existence of art is questionable. However, not all five senses are required for the expression of art. Usually more than one of the senses is involved in creativity. The most frequently used sense seems to be touch.

Touch

The sense of touch gives your young artist the ability to feel shapes and textures, temperatures and pain, spatial boundaries and different pressures such as hard/soft, all of which send messages and stir emotions. In addition, touch feedback provides the brain with more precise information than that which is gathered just from sight and hearing. Interior decorators use touch to set a mood in a room. Painters and sculptors often visually stimulate viewers with a desire to touch their masterpieces. Then they put up that frustrating sign, "Do Not Touch"! Communication is heightened by touch. For dancers and actors, touch adds an especially important dimension to their work. Your kids are continuously responding to touch. Remember when your son or daughter was very young and he or she wanted to touch everything in a store? It is instinctive to want to touch to satisfy the need to identify an object and one's feelings about it.

When the skin of your artist makes contact with another surface this is registered by the nerve fibers in the skin. From there vibrations are sent through the central nervous system to the brain for interpretation. Because skin covers the body, nerve sensors in the skin are found all over the body. Healthy skin and nervous systems positively impact your young artist's sense of touch. So does the circulatory system. Poorly nourished skin, nerves, and circulation may produce a diminished sense of touch. We have all experienced the sensation of numb feet when they have "fallen asleep."

Touch is very important to the artist who uses tools to create. Painters are sensitive to the touch of a paintbrush. Clarinet players rely on the touch of their fingertips for perfect notes. Even the touch of computer keyboards can make the difference in the flow of typing one's thoughts. Pressure, textures, sensitivity are all read through the touch of an artist's fingers.

Sight

Sight, one's windows to the world, could be listed under all artistic categories. However, Stevie Wonder would rightly argue that eyes are not needed to create music. Eyes play a critical role in the expression of most art. Your young artist depends on eyes for depth, distance, dimension, and movement. Plus eyes are sensitive to different colors and contours. Ideas, emotions, and execution of art forms are all stimulated through the eyes.

The eye is made of muscles, nerves, blood vessels, and a gland. Translation of what is seen is the result of the transfer of information via the nervous system to the brain. This translation directly affects the interpretation and artistic response. Unhealthy eyes and nervous systems make it more difficult for your young artist to perform up to his or her talent ability.

Hearing

Hearing through the human soundboard, ears, is not a sense that is needed for many art forms. Sound may inspire art, but it is not required for the execution of all art. However, for most musical artists the creation of sound primarily depends on the use of ears. However, Beethoven was deaf! Thus, it is possible for one to compose great musical works without being able to hear. Clearly, it is the extraordinary artist who can do so.

Ears have awe-inspiring powers of sensitivity and range. Instantly, they are able to receive sound waves and transfer them into electrical impulses. This information is then transmitted to the brain where it is translated into high, low, fast, slow, loud, soft, melodic, caustic, friendly, unfriendly, relaxing, energizing plus additional interpretations. Music stimulates emotions. Music stimulates art as well as being art! A healthy nervous system accompanied by healthy ear mechanisms makes it easier for your kids to be involved.

Smell

Smells rouse emotions, which often pour out as an expression of art. Most people first think of smell in relation to food. In fact, thousands of odors and aromas emanate from animate and inanimate objects. Wood, wax, wool, clay, pages of a book, paint, fur, sweat, leaves, flowers, oceans, and lakes all give off smells that stimulate messages and feelings for humans. Eager painters of all ages are swooned by the salt air scent of the sea. Poets have succeeded in capturing the scent of fresh falling snow. The smell of fresh flowers has stimulated masterpieces. Artists are very responsive to emotions. It is apparent in their work. Van Gogh stroked his feelings for the French countryside all over his canvasses.

"There are more than 10,000 known scents."[3] Smells are sweet, sour, delicious, putrid, pungent, fresh, musky, floral, oily, dry, humid, wet, old, new, clean, fresh, burning, smoky, chemical, acid, plastic, dirty, rotten, fake, real, spring, fall, and the list goes on. Most smells have an association interpretation, such as, "It smells like fall. The air smells fresh. The grass smells green." Dr. Sobel notes that, "Smells are the only sense that leads from the world directly to the brain. Odors are registered in the 'oldest' part of the brain, responsible for our most basic emotional reactions: pleasure, fear, and the 'fight or flight' response."[4] Many script writers have been influenced by the smell of danger!

Particles reach the smell-sensitive regions through the nose and the mouth. The nasal passages are lined with a mucus membrane that is supplied with blood vessels, nerves, and glands. The glands supply moisture to the sniffed air particles; they must be moist before they can reach receptors. Wetness heightens smell. A wet dog smells very different from a dry dog! From the receptors, the signals are sent to the brain via the nervous system for interpretation.

Unhealthy nasal passages dampen the sense of smell and thus the productivity of performing and fine artists. Smells are flattened. Not only do your kids feel crummy when suffering from a cold; their sense of smell and taste is muted. Breathing becomes more shallow and laborious. Mental, physical, and artistic energy wanes. Fortunately the sense of smell returns in full glory when the nasal passages are healthy, again. Smells can be powerful influences in your young artist's life.

Taste

Though taste appears to be the most useless of all the art senses, it is actually integrated into the sense of smell. This reality gives taste a better role in impacting an artist's creativity. Taste and smell are chemical senses that are triggered by the chemical content of substances. Even though the tongue is able to detect only four basic tastes, sour, sweet, bitter, and salty, combinations of these expand taste sensations slightly. The taste buds are the receptor sights, from which taste sensations are converted into nerve impulses for transmission to the brain.

Chemicals must be in liquid form in order to be tasted. Sodas offer the perfect environment to excite the tongue. Dry foods are broken down by saliva before the taste organs can recognize the taste. Dehydrated foods require water to be added before tasting and eating foods. Otherwise, everything tastes bland. How many times have your heard the expression, "Ewwww, this tastes like cardboard"? Cereal always tastes better with milk. No doubt you have discovered that tough dry meat is less tasty than tender moist meat. The brain quickly identifies salt because it is highly soluble and rapidly dissolves in water. Food manufacturers use the science of moisture's impact on taste to enhance their market position among kids.

Children have more taste buds. Additional ones are located in the lining of the roof of the mouth, cheeks, and throat. Hence, kids are very vulnerable to emotional responses to foods. Has your young artist ever contorted his or her face in horror when reacting to the smell or taste of brussels sprouts? (Kids are experts at expressing riveting emotions with the greatest of ease!) It is possible that what tastes reasonably good to you may actually taste really putrid to your son or daughter. Conversely, a mouth-watering apple may taste incredibly delicious to your kids and simply satisfying to you.

Flavors can also stimulate the temperature, pressure, and pain receptors located in the mouth. This is why peppermint gives you the sensation of coolness. Spices, such as curry and ginger, taste hot. Cayenne is famous for its ability to stimulate pain in the nerve endings. Some kids love it! In turn, flavors stimulate emotions that may influence an artist's mood as he or she is creating. It certainly gives them experiential recall for choices of words, colors, and actions.

Your young artist recreates what he or she sees, hears, touches, tastes, and smells on a canvas, with words, through a camera, on a stage, with his or her voice, through the string of a guitar or piano; the list is endless.

Physical and Mental Strength, Skills, and Endurance

Let's not forget the physical requirement for artists. Many are creative athletes.

Dancers are trained in many different styles of dance. Ballet, jazz, and modern dance include a full range of physically demanding repertoires. Power and break dancing are very popular among the young. Many kids are studying tap, clogging, flamenco, square, and other ethnic styles of dance. Ballroom dancing is gaining in popularity. Ice dancing is another artistic form of movement. Whatever kind of dance your kids are studying, they are making extensive physical demands on their muscular and skeletal systems. Musicians, especially drummers, expend a lot of energy using arms, legs, abdominal, back, and neck muscles to play their instruments. They look like an octopus exercising all of their limbs at the same time. Guitarists gyrate as they play. So do sax and trumpet players, and concert violinists too! Physical training should be a part of a musician's lesson routine. Singers, from opera to rap, put forth a tremendous amount of energy when training and performing. They use a lot of body action while doing two or more things at once. Many rock, pop, and rap stars dance a mean dance while they sing. So do Broadway musical stars! For them, well-trained vocal and breathing patterns are imperative. So are good memorization skills. Actors fall into this same skill category. Tom Cruise had to be in great physical condition to play the lead in movies such as *Mission Impossible,* II. Mime artists are isometric exercise experts. Constant and intense muscle group control involves acute concentration and muscular discipline. Both are controlled by the mind. It behooves these artists to be nutritionally and physically fit, too. Input equals output. Foods that support the mind and body enable these artists to perform to their optimum ability. Performers deserve the chance to be at their best as they are developing and displaying their skills.

Visual artists such as photographers, film directors, sculptors, potters, painters, inventors, designers of Websites, sports equipment, clothes, buildings, furniture, materials, gardens, you name it, are also dependent on their mental, physical, and sensory skills. Some skills call for more intense mental activity than physical. Writers and painters spend a lot of time pouring their minds into their work while being still. If they do not move about daily, their minds, bodies, and senses may become dulled. All visual artists benefit from physical fitness for optimum mental and creative productivity and performance.

Day in and day out, aspiring artists need nourishment to achieve their dreams. Junk food diets may hamper any artist. Low blood sugar levels, a high fat diet, and malnutrition are conditions that make one feel sluggish. Such a diet may subdue creativity. It would be a shame to squelch a young artist's passion and talent with a junk food diet. He or she deserves the chance to optimize his endeavors with a well-nourished mind and body.

Artists Need High-Octane Fuel

Young artists are challenged with the task of fueling a growing body while passionately pursuing their creative expression. Artists are usually driven by emotions, led by their five senses. The process of engaging them to fulfill the challenge of their chosen art form often overrides the nutritional attention needed by his or her mind and body.

Oxygen

Oxygen is a life force for artists! Every one of the many trillions of cells in the body needs oxygen. The brain uses about 25 percent of the oxygen the body inhales. Brain activity is compromised with a reduction of oxygen. When brain activity is compromised, so is every other function of the body. Creative, as well as physical, energy may decline.

Physically active artists benefit from increasing their anaerobic and endurance capacity for optimum performance. Conditioning, combined with efficient breathing patterns, can increase the blood flow to vital organs and muscles. Subsequently, cells become well oxygenated. The results include tap dancers complete an upbeat routine of fancy footwork more effortlessly. Long phrases or notes can then be sung in one breath by singers after years of developing efficient rhythmic breathing patterns.

Every young artist benefits from the calming affects of deep breathing. Many have deadlines for their work: be it a cartoon for the school newspaper, choreographing a dance for the school dance team, completion of a painting for a school gallery showing, or memorizing lines for a school play. Deep breathing reduces nervous tension and aids clear thinking.

Water!

All artists are filled with water. The brain, an artist's center for creative transmissions, is about 75 percent water. The sensory organs are mostly made of water. So are the other supporting body parts including the lungs which are made of about 90 percent water!

Adequate hydration is important. Those artists that are physically active especially need to retain their strength, speed and endurance. Dehydrated ballet dancers have a difficult time completing many pirouettes in succession. Drummers need fast, well hydrated, arms and hands to run through speedy rudiments such as full set drum rolls. Actors and singers, while performing under hot lights, may quickly become depleted of liquids. This condition could lead to a loss of mental clarity and endurance. All artists lose water when working in an air-conditioned or heated room, under hot lights, and when outdoors in the sun and/or wind. Remember, brain cells shrink when dehydrated. Without sufficient water, messages move through the human communication network less efficiently. Keep your young artist hydrated.

- ▶ Artists, make water the first choice of drinks, day and night.
- ▶ Hydrate when you wake up. Drink about eight cups of water a day.

The general formula is: ½ body weight = number of ounces of water to drink a day. Example: Body weight 112 lbs. ½ weight = 56 lbs. Drink 56 ounces (7 cups) of water a day.

Onc mouthful of water equals about 1 ounce.

- ▶ Do not wait until you are thirsty before drinking water. ...too late!
- ▶ Cold water is best. Keeps you cool and is absorbed quickly.

* 1 cup equals 8 ounces.

Carbohydrated, Protein, Fats

High-octane foods are an artist's best friend. Junk food is not. Garbage in, garbage out may be a scary prospect for an artist. A steady mind, steady hand, and a free-flowing mind can be crucial for an artist.

We recommend a balanced diet using the Food Circles™ as a guideline. Most carbohydrates should be complex sourced. Most fats should be the essential fatty acids. Only about one third of the protein should come from meat and poultry. Fish, legumes (beans), nuts, and seeds should provide the rest. Very active artists, such as dancers, can use the athletic fueling guidelines found in Chapter Eight. Using the five senses as a guide, below is an abbreviated list of foods that are well-suited for artists. Beans, carrots, cucumbers, garlic, spinach, sweet potatoes, bananas, berries, peaches, tomatoes, almonds, walnuts, olive oil, pumpkin seeds, whole grains, soybeans, eggs, fish, and chicken are foods that nourish one or more of the senses. Have you noticed that most of the same foods are listed for athletes and academics? A more complete list of the Foods From Head to Toe can be found on the CD-ROM located at the back of this book.

Good Food Ideas For Your Kids

- Blueberries. Add them to smoothies, cereals, breads, pancakes, muffins, and waffles.
- Eggs, scramble them. Mix in shredded white cheese, finely chopped parsley, and sprinkle with paprika!
- Olive oil is the best oil for salad dressings. Add to sautéed onions and garlic, along with seasoned salt. Use as a marinade base with lemon juice and other seasonings
- Almonds, and other nuts and seeds, are delicious when roasted in low-salt tamari sauce.
- Spinach is the wonder food. Cooked mushy spinach usually triggers sour faces, yuck! However, when sneaked into lasagna or other cheese casserole type dishes, many kids will eat it. Fresh baby spinach found in bags at the supermarket blend well into salads. A little is better than none! Spinach can be camouflaged in pureed soups. A good cream of spinach soup served with croutons or garlic French bread passed the kid's taste test. Look for more ideas and recipes on the *Mom, I'm Hungry, What's for Dinner?* CD-ROM found in the back of this book.

Artists Are Invaluable To Our Society

A well-nourished young artist adds to our social landscape, even if it is in a small private way. He or she is a treasured endowment who may fill ears with wondering sounds, fill eyes with stimulating sights, fill skin sensors with wondering touches, fill noses with stirring smells, and fill taste buds with divine tastes. Your children's minds take mental photos of art, as it impresses them. These are hung in their mind gallery. Over the short and long term, all of their mental photos impact who they are and who they will become.

Please, nourish your budding artist well as we look to them to enrich our world.

10

Kid Tips

Chapter Quick Facts

- The key to motivating your kids is to know what "turns them on." Speak to your kid's dreams. Do they want to be a fireman, physician, basketball player, musician, or dancer? Then explain how good foods fuel their dreams!
- Some foods cover most of the nutritional bases: almonds, apples, bananas, bell peppers, black beans, blueberries, brown rice, broccoli, carrots, celery, cherries, chicken, dark green lettuce, eggs, fish, garlic, grapes (red!) oats, olive oil, onions peas, pineapple, pumpkin seeds, sesame seeds, spinach, squash, strawberries, sweet potatoes, turkey, walnuts, watermelon, yams, yogurt (plain).
- Try using this chapter's Better Choices Phrases such as "Water is cool. Fish can sharpen your mind. Power up on greens. Great athletes eat real food!"
- Ideas that work: Eat together at a table (no TV), dine with candlelight. Using guidelines, assign meal planning to your kids. Eat more good foods than bad. Take time to make changes.
- Be sure and replace the foods you take away with good alternatives. Examples: orange cheese with white cheese, margarine with canola spread or real butter, sodas with carbonated fruit juice, fruit drink with 100% fruit juice.
- Teach your kids the facts. Odds are, they will make Better Choices.

Kid Tips

As moms who are eager to do what is best for our kids, we are all guilty of using words and terms that are automatic "turn-offs" to them. Some of us are repeating the words of wisdom we have heard from our mothers. Others blurt out words at a moment of frustration or anger. All words leave an impression, be it positive or negative.

When trying to encourage or cajole our kids into eating foods we know are healthy for them, we often find ourselves saying one or more of the following "turn-off" and "tune-out" phrases and sentences.

Doomsday Phrases!

How many times have you heard yourself roll these off of your tongues?

- DANGLING HEALTH CARROT
  - This is good for you.
  - This is healthy for you.
  - Vegetables are healthy for you.
  - If you eat this, you won't get sick.
  - Try it. You'll like it.

- GUILT
  - Think about all the starving people in Africa.
  - Later, when you are starving, you will wish you had eaten your breakfast.
  - When I was your age, I had to eat everything on my plate.
  - Don't blame me if you get sick. I told you to eat your vegetables.
  - You will be sorry if you don't eat your spinach.
  - Why don't you eat your greens? Believe me, one day you will regret it.
  - You liked it last week!

- BRIBERY
  - Please make me happy and eat your beans.
  - Just eat one more bite. Good, now eat one more.
  - If you eat your broccoli, you can have some ice cream for dessert.
  - If you eat some of this casserole, you can go out and play afterwards.
  - If you don't eat this, no computer games for the rest of the day.
  - I'll buy you a Barbie Doll if you eat this.

- SERGEANT MAJOR
    - Clean your plate.
    - As long as you live in this house, you will eat what I serve you.
    - I have better things to do with my time than cook for you when you refuse to eat.
    - You are not allowed to leave this table until you finish your dinner.
    - Eat your breakfast, now.
    - That's it. No more treats for you.
    - I've had it. No desserts for a week.
    - If you don't finish your dinner, you'll get the rest for breakfast, tomorrow.
    - Go to your room without any dinner.

Do any of these thoughts sound familiar? Some ring our memory bells. The truth is, we all find some of these phrases slipping out of our mouth at one time or another. None of them are effective. None of them motivate our kids to like or eat the food sitting in front of them.

Winning Ways with Kids

When a group of middle school students were asked whether they considered themselves to be an athlete, artist, and/or student of the academics, many believed themselves to be an athlete or artist. Most were hesitant to believe they were "students." When asked how their career goals related to being an athlete, artist, or academic students, most athletes and artists did not associate academic skills with their aspirations. Yet, when discussing the need to memorize football plays, scripts, or the color wheel variations while applying strategies and relative thinking processes, these kids were amazed to find how involved their minds were in utilizing academic knowledge and skills. Suddenly, being a student became important! They learned that being one does not mean you have to be brilliant. Being a student is really about gaining knowledge and skills that are then put to use in an area of interest.

The truth is that good athletes and artists are good students of their passions. Many are strong academic students and most have the potential of earning above average grades. In this survey it was clear that the kids who are dreaming of being scientists, writers, scholars, or fulfilling any other academically oriented careers, understand the need for being well educated. They had not realized how physical and artistic disciplines played an integral part in their studies. After an enlightening discussion about how academics, artistry, and athletic skills apply to a wide range of endeavors, most kids altered their evaluation of themselves. Some decided they were not just athletes but students as well. A few also assigned themselves an artist and student status. Almost all of the kids declared they were all three!

Kids are eager to discover and be in touch with the depth and breadth of their abilities. They dream that their dreams will become a reality. Trouble is, dreams are more likely to stay as dreams when kids are not fueled to be physically and mentally healthy. Healthy minds and bodies empower kids to reach for their dreams.

Speak To Your Kids' Dreams

All kids have dreams, desires, and goals. Today, some girls and boys want to be professional basketball players, firemen, or astronauts. Some want to be dancers, models, teachers, or politicians, even the president. Some kids want to be rap stars, nurses or hairstylists. Others see themselves as the future Bill Gates. Many kids change their minds weekly. Experimentation with many kids, including Kid Kritics, has verified that a positive, customized dream appeal approach works.

The key to motivating your kids to eat better foods is to know what dream "turns them on." Then you can connect the foods that fuel the body parts to how they support his or her dream. Popeye was the pioneer of this concept. His dream was to be strong enough to eliminate the bully, Bluto, and win Olive Oyl's heart. We watched as Popeye lost his battles with Bluto before eating spinach. Then, just in the nick of time, when he gulped down a can of spinach, WOW, he annihilated his nemesis and Olive Oyl swooned. It is made clear that spinach is Popeye's power food. Spinach helps build strength. Strength builds confidence. Spinach breeds winners!

The desire to grow up to be like mommy, daddy, or someone else who has impressed kids can be a powerful motivator for them. Vanity and the dream to look like a favorite star are other avenues of appeal for kids, especially preteens and teenagers. Consequently, girls tend to be very responsive to the fact that broccoli helps grow long and beautiful hair. Some preteen and teenage boys are also very responsive to skin foods. Use their sensitivity to breaking out and offer them solutions through healthy skin foods such as dark green lettuce, celery, and eggs. Though these may seem like shallow goals to some people, the condition of one's hair and skin is critically important to young girls. The good news is that broccoli and dark green lettuce also supports the nerves, bones, heart, lungs, and many other vital body parts. Young boys like to run fast, be it for a soccer ball or just a race against their friends in the backyard. Muscle food provides you a window of opportunity. "Did you know that beans help make muscles grow?" "White rice will give you some energy. If you add a little brown rice, you'll be feeding your muscles, too!"

Customize this concept to your kids. Instead of telling them that oatmeal is good for them, let them know that oats help build vital muscles, nerves, bones, hearts (one per kid!), joints, spines, ears, eyes, and skin. Even though nutritionally filled foods nourish most body parts one way or another, sight the one body part that touches your son or daughter's motivational button and connect it to the food you want to serve them. The point is that it is okay to appeal to his or her dreams and vanity. You have avoided using the word, healthy, and you have caught their attention. This works!

On the CD-ROM, *Mom I'm Hungry, What's for Dinner?*, is the Foods From Head To Toe list (located at the back of this book). Refer to it for lists of food that support different parts of the body. There are foods that support most of the mental and physical needs of academics, athletes, and artists. A steady diet of these cover most of their nutritional requirements.

SUPPORTING FOODS:

Artichokes, beets, bell peppers, broccoli, cabbage, carrots, celery, corn, cucumber, dark green lettuce, eggplant, garlic, green beans, olives, onions, parsnips, peas, potato skins, pumpkin, sea veggies, spinach, squash sweet potatoes, yams

Apples, apricots, avocado, bananas, berries, coconut, cranberries, figs, grapes (red), grapefruit, honeydew melon, kiwi, lemons, oranges, papaya, peaches, pears, pineapples, plums, strawberries, watermelon

Barley, black beans, brown rice, chickpeas, (garbanzo beans), lentils, millet, oats, rye, whole grain wheat, wild rice

All nut and seed oils, plus olive oil

Eggs, white cheese, yogurt

Bass (ocean), bluefish, haddock, halibut, salmon, sole, tuna, chicken, turkey breasts, lamb.

WATER!

God-made foods that grow out of the ground, swim in the sea, and roam the lands of this earth best fuel your kids!

What Works When You Talk To Your Kids

Below is a long list of some phrases and thoughts proven effective when guiding kids to make "Better Choices." Glance through them for ideas that may work for your kids. By the way, always refer to vegetables as veggies!

Brain Matter

- The strong survive, but it is the smart that grow! (This is always a startling truth for the young.) Be smart, make Better Choices and grow!
- Successful athletes will tell you that most of the game is mental. Fuel your brain!
- Since you're the one taking the test, you decide whether to eat for better grades.
- Smart kids don't eat fake foods.
- Well-watered brains are super productive brains.
- To help your memory, drink water while studying.
- Water your brain for better test results. Drink some before exams.
- Sugar spikes mental highs and then mental lows.
- Eat good breakfasts for good grades.
- If you want to score well on your mid-morning math test, don't eat candy cereal for breakfast. Eggs and a good protein drink will give you the mental edge!
- Fish can sharpen your mind.
- Brain food needs to be consumed by all kids, whether they are athletic, artistic, or academic students.

Brawn Matter

- You really are what you eat. Just ask Andre Agassi. (Before he paid attention to nutrition, his wins were inconsistent. After expert nutritional and physical condition training, he broke tennis records!)

- Did you know that Michael Jordan and most other star athletes have nutritionists recommending what foods to eat for optimum physical and mental performance?
- Great athletes eat real food!
- Dairy slows you down. Drink (and eat) it after training or a game.
- Timing is everything. Eat pizza after the game, instead of before.
- Soda dehydrates your muscles. Drink it and they won't work as well.
- When you sweat, you need water, not dehydrating sodas.
- If you are feeling thirsty, you are already slowing down.
- You may lose 8 percent of your running speed if your muscles are dehydrated by only 3 percent.
- When your muscles are dehydrated by only 3 percent, your muscles will be about 10 percent weaker. That's a lot.
- Keep your muscles hydrated. Drink lots of water before, during, and after playing football.
- Just think, if your opponent is dehydrated and you are not, you will have the competitive edge.
- Elephants drink lots of water and they are really strong.
- Cheetahs, the fastest running mammals on the planet, drink just plain water.
- Feel the winning difference. Drink lots of water! Water is the drink of winners!
- Well-watered muscles take longer to run out of steam.
- When your body gets too hot (over 100 degrees F), it will always sacrifice muscle function for temperature regulation. Keep cool. Drink cold water.
- Keep cool when playing hot sports! Drink cold water.
- Lungs are about 90 percent water. Well-watered lungs run well.
- On average you breathe about 22 times per minute while inactive. Multiply this number by two and three times when you are very active. Better keep your lungs hydrated. Drink lots of water.
- Gorillas don't eat hamburgers. They eat fruits and veggies, foods that provide the building supplies for their super-strong muscles and bones. Ever tried to wrestle a gorilla?
- Athletes, artists, and academics excel with sharp minds and strong muscles. Power up on greens!

Empowering Bits

- Knowledge is power. Use it wisely. Make Better Choices.
- Better Choices produce better results. It's up to you!
- Telling you the facts helps you make decisions for yourself, good or bad. Are you ready for this? I think so.
- Try a bit of everything. You don't have to eat it all.
- Water is your life force. Fuel up.
- When there is high-octane fuel in your body, your performance levels can soar.
- Would you ever pour soda into a car's gas tank? Didn't think so.
- Protein foods, such as turkey and nuts, can reduce your desire for sweets. Yeah!
- God-made food is for God-made kids. That's you!

Simple Sound Bites

- Don't judge food by its color. After all, chocolate is muddy brown.
- God-made colored foods make the winning difference. Count them!
- Not all food that looks bad tastes bad. (Chicken Chow Mein!)
- Hydrated skin is beautiful skin.
- Water is cool!
- You score with water!
- Sodas are just liquid candy.
- Veggie fats are slimming!
- Dark green veggie bones are strong bones....Just ask an elephant!
- Brain food is your best bet.
- Fish is it!
- It's simple. Eat more good guys than bad (toxic) guys.
- Better foods bring better results.

Toxic Truths

- Organic foods are really good. Foods sprayed with herbicides, pesticides, and other toxins are not.
- The insecticides or hormones eaten by or injected into cows can be passed into their milk, which becomes your milk.
- Fat is where toxins are stored in mammals. Therefore, when you eat animal fat, you may be eating their toxins, too
- Anti-fuels are loser fuels.

- Powdered sugar drinks, chips, and boxed pastries that sit on supermarket shelves for weeks on end are mostly lab-made anti-fuels. Unreal.
- Artificial, lab-made chips, cheese, and ice cream are fake foods. Get Real!
- Fake foods are sickening.
- Many fast food shakes are fake shakes loaded with artificial who knows what!
- Fake foods can hang around your gut for a long time!
- How long do you think a fast food burger that your body can't digest sits in your intestines? Longer than a day? No, usually much longer.
- Your body can handle the toxins of one bag of French fries. The problems begin when it has to handle the fries, sodas, fast food burgers, toaster pastries, colored sugared cereals, grilled cheese, chicken nuggets, and potato chips day after day after day. To these toxins, add the physical demands of your sports plus the stresses of your school. This is when your body heads into overload. There is just so much this magic body of yours can handle until it breaks downs. "Overload, overload!" Sometime and somewhere it just says, "Enough."
- Would you ever put soda into the gas tank of a car? Why not? Do you think the engine will break? Dah. Soda doesn't belong in your body either.
- It's simple. Eat more good guys than bad guys. The good guys are clean water, veggies, fruits, nuts, other legumes, grains, fish, and lean meats. The bad guys are sugar (simple carbohydrates), hydrogenated and trans fatty acid processed fake foods.
- Save junk food treats for the weekends. In the meantime, enjoy fresh foods like this juicy red apple!
- Crocodiles have lived for millions of years on freshly caught food! Hmmm.

Practical Trivia

- Soda makes you thirsty.
- How many sodas does it take to overdose on sugar in a day? On average, four ounces (½ cup). On average, teenagers drink three twelve-ounce cans (4½ cups) of soda a day. That's a recipe for diabetes.
- Huge cups of soda sold at convenient stores hold about 32 ounces and have about 25 teaspoons of sugar in each.

That equals 100 grams of sugar! If you weigh 89 pounds, you would have to run just over an hour at six miles per hour in order to burn ALL of this caloric energy.

- Caffeine in sodas drain you of valuable nutrients you have eaten today.
- Caffeine is addictive. Once it gets a hold of you, it will not let go without a tough fight.
- Have you ever known a cow that gives orange milk? Then why do you eat orange cheese?
- What other species drinks milk after being weaned from their mother at an early age?
- Have you ever heard of a baby monkey drinking lion's milk? Humans are the only species that drinks milk from another species, the cow! Drink water!
- Divide your body weight in half. That is the number of ounces of water you should drink a day. On sports or performance days, drink more.
- Your blood is made of 82 percent water. Keep it flowing. DRINK MORE WATER!
- Your 650 muscles depend on water to function, NOT sodas.
- Cold water is absorbed faster than warm water. Below 50 degrees fahrenheit is best. (Michael Colgan, Ph.D. and author, Colgan Institute)
- Sugar stuns your immune system.
- The more sugar you eat, the easier it is for you to get sick.
- Too much sugar makes you fat.
- Caloric energy that is not burned is stored as fat!
- How many fast food burgers does it take to max out on fat for the day? About one half.
- How many potato chips does it take for to you to exceed your daily limit on sodium? Less than half a regular sized bag.
- Raw nuts, seeds, and beans can be slimming. Really.
- The longer you chew beans, the sweeter they taste. Same for rice!
- When you stomach is empty, eat fruit and it will be digested, flowing in your blood, and going to work for you in just 20 minutes. (Bananas take about 30 minutes)
- High goals requiring high performance need high good guy foods! The Good Guys are veggies, fruit, nuts, olive oil, beans, whole grains, free-range poultry, fish, and water!
- When you eat better foods, you can have a few treats and still stay in balance.
- It takes about 20 to 30 minutes for your brain to tell your stomach, "Full." Don't wait for this message to stop eating.

- Man has yet to out-think God. God made food for man. So, eat God-made food, instead of lab-made food.
- God designed your body to eat God-made foods.

A Few Changes Can Make A Big Difference

As parents, we sometimes need to change some habits in order to see some changes in our kids. In haste, we forget that what we do influences the behavioral patterns of our kids. Experience has proven to us that making even small changes is worth the effort.

Ideas That Work!

One or more of the following ideas may move your kids toward making Better Food Choices™ when eating breakfast, lunch, snacks, or dinner. Take the time to try the easy ones first. We recommend starting with dining with candlelight!

Eat as a family at the dinner or kitchen table with the TV off! Dining together is a social experience, a time to listen to and talk with one another. Ask each son or daughter about the good things that happened to him or her that day. Nanci Hellmich of USA Today reported that kids who ate dinner with their families ate more vegetables and drank fewer sodas than those who ate alone.[1] "Dr. Bowden and his colleagues found that kids who ate dinner with their families at least five times per week (at home or a fast food restaurant) were the least likely to take drugs, feel depressed, or get into trouble with the law. These kids were more likely to do well in school and to have a supportive circle of friends. The more poorly adjusted teens, in contrast, ate with their parents an average of three or fewer evenings a week."[2]

Unfortunately, during many meals kids are not sitting at the dinner or kitchen tables and communicating with families when they eat.

> In February of 2001, USA Today noted that children ate 42 percent of their dinners while watching TV. It is also pointed out that overweight kids ate 50 percent of their meals in front of the TV compared with 35 percent for normal-weight kids.[3]

Enjoy being together and turn the television off during breakfast, lunch, and dinner!

Dine with candlelight! This positively affects everyone's mood.

Red plates! Try serving God-made foods on red plates. It is said that people eat more when served food on red plates than other colors. Try it. If it works when serving vegetables, great! If you load up your kid's plate with mashed potatoes and gravy, choose brown or green plates. It is said that these two colors have a negative affect on one's appetite.

Serve small portions. Large portion of foods on a plate or in a bowl overwhelms kids. Better to have them ask for seconds than throw away unwanted food.

Be creative with the presentation of foods. The Japanese are very clever in using food as art. If you are artistic, go for it. For those of us who are not, just be a little creative. Example: when serving chicken in a creamy sauce, place some over a medallion of rice. Then encircle some with a thin row of bright green peas. This layout sure beats the looks of globs of chicken, rice and peas. Many of you know about the use of cookie cutters to shape sandwiches. This particularly appeals to the young! Just do not make the mistake we made of using a narrow airplane design. It fell apart. Thick ones, such as a bell shape, hold together easily. Have a little fun being creative with your kids.

Moms, cook one menu per meal, not one menu per person per meal. The sooner a child learns that the world does not revolve around him or her, the better.

Assign menu planning to your kids. Give each child one night a week to choose what is for dinner. Require them to include protein, good fats (EFAs), and complex carbohydrates (vegetables, whole grains, legumes, fruit) in the meal. Instruct them that each meal must include two to three different God-made colored foods, or more! This accomplishes several things. It gives each child the responsibility (and power!) of deciding what the family will eat for dinner once a week. Each child will become more educated about the food group choices. Each will eat what he or she wants at least one night a week. He or she will also have the satisfaction of knowing his or her sibling will have to eat his or her chosen menu. They all figure out that they, in turn, have to eat the chosen foods of their siblings. Parents should be assigned a dinner as well so it becomes a family team. Best of all, mom does not have to plan every dinner menu!!! We guarantee you, this can work!

Have your kids count colors when you shop. Whenever your kids are with you in the grocery store, ask them to pick out the fresh fruit and vegetables, gathering as many colors as possible. Kids like to make what they perceive as adult decisions. Plus, choosing colors is fun.

5 Days On — 2 Days Off: Be good (eat better foods) from Sunday afternoon until Friday afternoon. Save the treats for weekends, unless they have a competitive event scheduled. Then wait until the event is over to treat your kids. This is easy to do!

More Good Guys than Bad Guys: The goal is to have more good guys than bad guys in your kids' bodies, so the good guys can win! Shoot for a pattern of eating 60-70 percent good guys and 40-30 percent bad guys. (80/20 is ideal.) This is achievable and the results are well worth the effort. You can do this! So can your kids.

Take your time to make changes. Gradual changes are more lasting changes. Add a new food or eating habit one month or week at a time. It is said that once an old habit is removed, and/or a new habit is introduced and adhered to for 21 days, it becomes a new habit. It takes the body and mind approximately three weeks to make the adjustment. If you think about it, you will recall that most people give up their diet declarations before three weeks is up. Most last no more than a week!

You will have successes with some changes, and some won't work for your family. Always remember, when kids start to feel better and experience improvement in their endeavors, they like how it feels.

Replacement Tactics: Imperative!

Be sure and replace what you take away with something else that tastes good! No one likes to feel deprived. Not one of us. That is why so many "diets" fail. Little messages run through our heads, "Why can't I have ... I want to have ... I deserve to have ..." and so on. Kids are no different. They want tasty foods. Since French fries are the number-one vegetable eaten by kids, let's use this as an example. There are some absolutely delicious frozen baked fries in the stores that happen to be organic. (These are listed in the Better Choices Grocery List™.) Kids love them. They simply need to be heated through. Forget deep fried or most other manufactured frozen French fries. Replace sodas with sparkling juices. Enjoy Good Health Snacks crackers in place of artificially flavored and colored versions. Have a China Cola. It's made with Chinese herbs and tastes great! Kid Kritics love it. Amy's Toasted Pops uses real apples and taste better than most toasted pastries. Eat white cheese, the real thing! Get your kids the good stuff!

The Nutrition Action Newsletter of January/February 1997 gives some excellent replacement suggestions.[4] We have added to them. All are listed below. Please refer to the Better Choices Grocery List for more specific suggestions. Gradually introduce these replacement foods. Remember, 21 days is the magic number. After not eating or drinking something for 3 weeks, especially with a good replacement, your kids will usually not miss it. The first days are the hardest. By the fourteenth day, most have forgotten about the removed food or drink. When replacing the "give-up" food with the "like-it" food, the 3 weeks will pass quickly. What is key is that you have a stick-to-it commitment. Remind your kids about their dreams. Tell them the truth about the fake, junk foods.

REMOVE	REPLACE
Meat, Poultry, Seafood	
Hamburger, meatloaf	Ground turkey breast, veggie burgers
T-bone, rib eye, prime rib, etc.	Flank, round steak, sirloin
Regular hot dog, bologna, sausage, etc.	Turkey/ chicken dogs, Boca/Shelton's sausages
Poultry with skin	Poultry without skin
Fried chicken or fish	Broiled, grilled, or roasted chicken or fish
Buffalo wings	Health is Wealth Buffalo Wings
Hormone, antibiotic, pesticide,	Organic, free-range, naturally fed, injection free herbicide filled, stalled, caged
Dairy Products	
Whole or 2% milk	1% or skim organic milk
Orange cheese	White cheese
Whole fat cheese	Reduced, low-fat cheese
Whole fat ice cream	Reduced, low-fat, ice cream or yogurt
Hormone, antibiotic, pesticide,	Free-range, naturally fed, injection free herbicide filled.
Ice cream	Ice milk, sherbets, soy, or rice ice creams
Non-organic	Organic
Bread	
White bread, fake whole wheat	Whole grain bread (wheat, rye, oat, multi-grained), clean sour dough and spelt.
Regular whole wheat	Organic whole wheat, spelt, 100% sprouted grains,
Cereals	
Sugar coated, dyed, fake	Whole grain fruit juice sweetened, organic

REMOVE	REPLACE
Pasta, Rice	
White seminola	Organic artichoke (De Boles), whole wheat, rice
White rice	Organic white basmati, brown basmati
Vegetables, Fruit	
Canned	Fresh
Frozen	Organic frozen
Toxic sprayed	Organic, locally grown, seasonal
Condiments, Oils, Butter	
Ketchup	Organic ketchup
Mustard	Organic mustard
Mayonnaise	Canola mayonnaise, organic
Olive oil	Extra Virgin, first–pressed olive oil, organic
Corn, safflower, sunflower	Extra Virgin, first-pressed olive oil
Shortening (give it the heave-ho!)	Organic shortening (Spectrum)
Butter	Organic butter
Margarine	Spread, organic, white (no yellow) butter,
Chips, Popcorn, Crackers	
Regular chips	Organic, low-fat chips
Regular popcorn	Unsalted, unbuttered (salt & butter your self with real versions)
All popcorn	
Hydrogenated, partially hydrogenated	Non-hydrogenated
Artificial ingredients	Real, God-made ingredients
Drinks	
Sodas	Carbonated fruit juices
Colas	China Cola, once in a while
Fake fruit juice	100% fruit juice (organic!)
Tap water	Bottled, filtered water
Sweet Treats	Sweet Treats
Junky versions	Real (not fake) ingredients
Seven days a week	One to two servings a week.

Kids can handle giving up Bad Choices for Better Choices. Perfection is not our goal. Reasonable and effective improvement is the reachable desired goal. We have seen this process work for many kids. Try it! Don't give up. What kids don't like today, they may like tomorrow, in a week, a month, or a year. Reintroduce foods giving them a new look, using a new recipe. One day, your kids may give you the green light!

Bottom Line: Tell kids the truth. Give them the facts. Most likely, they will make Better Food Choices on their own.

11

Always Consider the Source

Chapter Quick Facts

- God-made foods have evolved naturally over hundreds of years. They grow out of the earth, live freely in oceans, fly in expansive skies, and roam open fields and plains.
- Man-made foods involve chemical formulas used to create, produce, and preserve "foods." These chemicals include pesticides, herbicides, dyes, and more.
- Organic foods are God-made foods. Since 2002, they have been governed by the USDA Organic Food Standards and Labels laws.
- Genetically Modified Organisms (GMOs) are man-made genetically engineered (GE) foods. The DNA from one species such as viruses and bacteria are spliced into the DNA of other organisms such as corn, cottonseed, and soybeans.
- It is estimated that about 70 percent of foods in grocery stores are genetically modified.
- Labeling or testing of genetically altered and patented foods is not required. The consequences of DNA changes are unknown. Allergic reactions are a big concern.
- Irradiation is a controversial method of adding shelf-life to a product. Many foods are irradiated; the list is growing. Your kids are probably eating irradiated foods.
- Request non-GMO, non-irradiated, additive-free foods at your supermarket. Read the ingredients. Fill your kids up with unaltered God-made foods!

Always Consider the Source

Have you ever bought a purse that looked like a name brand, designer version, but wasn't? In a month or two, did the snap or strap break? Remember the supposedly high-quality cotton T-shirt you added to your wardrobe, only to find little bitty holes popping out after just a few washes. How about those leather shoes that turned out to be not 100 percent leather, so they cracked and pulled apart at the seams. Does this make you mad? After all, you spent money on products that you thought should last, be durable, and were made of 100 percent quality materials. They weren't. Instead, they were "rip-offs"!

Do you see some of these trends in food manufacturing? Are you buying products that appear to be high quality but really aren't? Some manufacturers tell us that the heavily sugared cereals you buy are good for your kids. Now you know that many brands hardly fit the definition of food. It is implied that oversized burgers and fries are nutritious fulfilling meals for your kids. Wrong. Milk is supposed to be a cornerstone source of important nutrients for all of us. This is questionable. You can even question the nutrient content of some well-sprayed commercially grown produce. The carrot you or your mother ate as a child probably had more vitamins and minerals in it than those you buy for your kids today. Nutrient-empty, additive-packed, so-called foods are filling today's grocery store shelves. The good news is that there are nutrient-filled and good tasting alternatives to the many chemically engineered malnourishing cereals, toaster pastries, oversized burgers, fries, and milk products. It is the food source that makes the difference.

The Source Counts

It's simple. There are God-made foods, and there are man-made foods. Man-made foods are those artificially altered or created from scratch in a science laboratory. They can also be called lab-made foods. God-made foods are foods that have evolved naturally over billions of years. They grow out of the ground, live freely in the ocean, fly in the expansive skies, and roam the open fields and plains. These are the foods our ancestors, your grandmothers and grandfathers, and even your parents enjoyed until the industrial revolution gave birth to processed and tampered foods. Today, these naturally grown and raised foods are called, natural, organic, and free-ranged. Funny we should have to give these naturally occurring foods labels in order to differentiate them from man-made foods.

Many people view organic foods as bizarre, and their consumers as health nuts. Guess that means your grandmother, your great grandmother, and their mothers and fathers were all health nuts! You actually are an offspring of a family tree of health nuts. Your genetic map was created from two genetic maps whose DNA (deoxyribonucleic acid, the genetic material) was influenced by what was consumed over generations. Another way to say this is that you are the offspring of a family tree nourished by God-made foods. It is reasonable to question what your family tree would look like if your ancestors had been consuming the man-made foods we are eating today. We are what we eat. Your kids are what they eat. Better yet, your kids are what they digest and utilize. Think about that!

Organic, Natural, Man-Made Foods

There are three basic categories for foods found in grocery stores: organic, natural, and man-made.

- *Organic* is defined in the dictionary as "having the characteristics of, or derived from living organisms."
- *Natural* is defined by Webster, "arising from nature; in accordance with what is found or expected in nature. Produced or existing in nature; real; not artificial or manufactured."
- *Man-made* means the idea and its implementation is created and manufactured by man. As opposed to natural and organic, man-made is artificial.

Organic! Organic foods must be grown on land that has no contaminants, has been cultivated and harvested without lab-made chemical applications, and has not been genetically altered. Organic foods can be found in the produce, refrigerated, freezer, and dry goods sections of your local supermarkets. They are cultivated for the perfection of nutrients and taste, not the looks. They have been spared of synthetic herbicides, pesticides, fungicides, fertilizers, hormones, antibiotics, ionizing radiation, and cross-species genetic mutations. You can taste the difference with your first bite!

To insure you, the consumer, of what is or is not officially organic based food, the United States Department of Agriculture (USDA) has finalized the Organic Food Standards and Labels with the date of required implementation: October 21, 2002.

- *100 percent organic* labeled products must contain only organic ingredients. This may be noted on the front of the package.
- *Organic* labeled ingredients of products must be at least 95 percent organic by weight. "Organic" may be positioned on the front of the package.
- *Made with organic ingredients* labeled processed products must contain at least 70 percent organic ingredients. As many as three of these ingredients may be listed on the front of the package.
- Processed products with less than 70 percent organic ingredients may not use the word "organic" on the front of the package. These ingredients may be listed in the information panel.

The USDA Organic Seal may only be printed on the packaging of the 100 percent organic and organic approved categories. It may not appear on the packaging of foods that fit the other categories. Now, according to a USDA regulation: one hundred percent organic foods must be free of irradiation (ionizing radiation), biotechnology (GE), sewer-sludge fertilization, artificial pesticides, herbicides, hormones, antibiotics, and additives. This means a milking cow must eat organic feed for an entire year before its milk is certified organic. No traces of growth hormones are allowed in the cow. If a cow receives antibiotics for any reason, it may not produce organic milk for another whole year. Soil for organic crops must be free of non-organic farming practices for three years before commercial use. This insures that the broccoli, carrots, lettuce, and other crops grown according to the organic standards will be filled with the nutrients (minerals!) yielded from the rich clean soil in which they were grown.

Government-approved certified inspectors have been assigned to the task of examining the farmers and handlers for their compliance to these rules. From the point of origin, the seed, to the point of consumer delivery, the retail store, they are obligated to observe organic products. The livelihood of organic food producers depends on the integrity of their own farming practices, those of other organic farmers, and the inspection and maintenance of standards. One slip up and an entire crop will lose its organic rating. The oversight procedure allows for the tracking of all certified organic foods. Organic farmers are relieved that their products are regulated giving them credibility.

More good news. All of the newly established national organic food label standards apply to all U.S. and imported foods. Since so much produce is imported today, this is meaningful.

Natural? Understandably, there is a lot of confusion over what is labeled as natural on food packaging. This is because the food manufacturing and distribution businesses have conveniently modified the definition of natural food. What may have originated from nature may have been tampered and altered with what is not traditionally found in nature. Some natural foods may have been sprayed. Example: oranges sprayed with manufactured pesticides during the growing period and after harvesting are considered natural. Yet, by definition, foods produced with artificial chemicals are not natural. Another problem occurs when products with natural origins are further treated synthetically. They may be gassed, dyed or irradiated. Sprayed dyed oranges fall into that unnatural category. Also, natural ingredients are often partnered with unnatural ones in processed foods. When 100 percent whole grains are mixed with bleached white flour, the end product has been altered. This composite is not natural. In short, natural is a term loosely used on packaging. Be careful; read the ingredient list!

Man-made. Man was never supposed to outsmart God. It is difficult to understand how humans can believe that the intricacies of the biological, ecological, and genetic systems on earth can be fully understood and manipulated by man for his or her self-interest without serious consequences. Technological advancements driven by man have led to good and not so good results. We have to thank science for successful organ transplants. But, we are very concerned about the health consequences of eating man-made foods, especially for kids.

Man-made foods are different from natural and organic (God-made) foods. The phrase "man-made" refers to the science of food engineering that significantly alters food biochemistries from the origins to processed adulterated versions. This science has expanded to making man-made foods that don't even originate from nature. Unfortunately, overzealousness and often greed have led man to create foods that are:

- Depleted of natural nutrients (sometimes entirely).
- Tainted with artificial ingredients.
- Known to have toxin residues in the products.
- Processed enough to change the molecular structure of the foods.

- Injected with questionable substances.
- Originated in test tubes, artificially.
- Cross-species bred.
- Suspected of health hazards.

Man has gone to a lot of trouble and expense to improve on God's work. From the original seed, planted in naturally mineral-rich soil, nurtured by clean rain and sun, picked when ready to eat, fruit, vegetables, grains, legumes, and nuts are potent foods designed to well nourish your son and daughter. Man-made versions can't match this nutritional perfection.

You Get More for Your Money with Organic. Organic tastes better! Guaranteed. An organic baby carrot tastes better than one that has been grown conventionally in nutrient-depleted soil. In order to compensate for nutrient-depleted soil, commercial farmers heavily fertilize their crops with chemicals. "It seems that crops grown on nitrogen fertilizer take up considerably more water, thereby diluting their nutrients, sugars and flavors."[1] In addition, a large percentage of conventionally grown produce is picked before ripening and then gassed later so it will soften and be edible. The last stage of being ripened by the sun is the time when the natural sugars are produced in fruits and vegetables, giving them their sweet flavor. Most organic produce is sun-ripened. Chances are, your kids will like organic vegetables more than the other bland versions.

Organic Foods are More Nutrient-packed, Naturally. Organic foods provide greater amounts of vitamins and especially minerals than conventionally raised foods. Virginia Worthington, Ph.D. at Johns Hopkins drew this conclusion and added that the greatest difference among all vegetables tested were in magnesium, vitamin C, and iron.

> Organically grown produce was higher in most minerals and vitamins and lower in potentially harmful nitrates, which result from nitrogen fertilizers. The greatest differences among all vegetables tested were in magnesium (organic was 29 percent higher), Vitamin C (27 percent higher), and iron (21 percent higher).... Nutritional composition of conventionally grown American food has declined during the past 60 years.[2]

Sad but true, the nutrient-content of conventionally grown American food is lower than those eaten sixty or more years ago. The depleted nutrient condition of the soils covering the vast commercial farms spread around our country is just one reason why. We wish this wasn't so, but it is. Modern mass production farming practices have robbed foods of nutrients. While this may keep the retail price low, it also lowers the food value.

Some organic products, such as cereals or bread, cost about the same as nonorganic products. Most do not. On average, organic food product prices are around 20 to 30 percent more. However, you pay a price for spending money on an apple or pasta that is missing its nutrients and is permeated with a combination of artificial ingredients, insecticides, pesticides, herbicides, fungicides, bleach, dyes, and ripening agents. Over time, the combination of diminished nutrients along with the ingestion of these toxins may lead to costly medical bills for allergic reactions, asthma, flu, colds, and eventually more serious diseases, including the dreaded cancer. On the other hand, an organic apple is filled with disease fighting antioxidants, vitamin A, B vitamins, vitamin C, minerals, trace minerals, and the much needed fiber. A conclusion is that for 20 to 30 percent more in the price of organic, you are getting 100 percent of the food value that is additive-free versus an altered version that may contain as little as 20 percent of its original nutrients and added undesirable chemicals. In order to eat enough conventionally grown apples to receive the full amount of nutrients of an organically grown apple, your son or daughter may have to eat at least two apples. This also means that your son or daughter will be eating more toxins. This becomes expensive. With organic, you actually get more value for your money. More nutrients, taste, and insurance against poor health!

Pure and Perfect. Pure and perfect is ideal and for the most part unreal. Organic is not always pure and perfect. Traces of pesticides may be found in some organic produce because of what is referred to as the pesticide drift. Winds can blow pesticide or other toxic particles from conventional farms located in the geographic area onto organic produce growing not too far away. This reality can be hard to prevent. The solution lies in the increase of organically farmed land. Due to the significant rise of consumer demand for organic foods, we are seeing an increase of organic farming.

Search for the most available untainted source of fruits, vegetables, grains, legumes, nuts, seeds, essential fatty acids, dairy, eggs, chicken, turkey, lamb, beef, and fish. First and foremost, it is important for your kids to eat from each of these food groups, even if the source is not organic. Do your best in providing the most toxic-free versions. Mix organic with nonorganic foods to keep your food bills affordable. Make sure that your kids are eating two to three different God-made colored foods at each meal.

Genetically Modified Organisms/Genetically Engineered Foods

To confuse matters, the terms genetically engineered (GE) and genetically modified organisms (GMO) foods are used interchangeably. Genetic engineering is the science used to genetically modify organisms. Henceforth, we will solely refer to genetically engineered foods as GMO foods.

The Science of GMO Foods. GMO foods are the buzzwords of the 21st century. With good intentions and great expectations, scientists have been diligently searching to solve the mystery of the cellular DNA blueprint in foods. Every individual food cell contains specific genes that control the genetic traits of that food. For instance, there is a DNA blueprint for the hot in peppers, another one for the oil in salmon, and yet a different one for the oil in olives. Once the DNA pattern of the individual traits is discovered, scientists can use this information to make designer foods by inserting genes from one food into another. Genes from a mild pepper may be inserted into those of a hot pepper to create a new kind of hot pepper. Same species cross-breeding is not new. Genetic scientists went one step further by cutting, splicing and transferring DNA genes from whatever they want to whatever species they desire. In many cases, these innovations have been be motivated by the well-intended desire for positive results: weed control, disease control, food spoilage, and shelf life control. Unfortunately, this increasingly complex practice is questionable when applied to the chemical/bacterial/viral insertion or the crossing over of different species into foods.

> What do you get when you cross corn with bacteria?
> Sick corn.

This is real. This and so much more is happening right now. Many cross-species food products such as fishy tomatoes are in the works. Odds are that your kids have eaten GMO foods. A lot of it. Over 60 percent, some say 70 percent, of the foods in the supermarkets today are GMO. You have no way of knowing which ones have been altered because GMO labeling is not required. The FDA's position is that GMO foods are safe enough to eat. However, many scientists argue that comprehensive long-term safety tests have not been conducted to determine if it is safe for your kids to eat GMO foods. There are grave concerns among some researchers over the short and long term consequences of creating what some call "Frankenfoods."

Currently, there are four categories of GMO crops.

Pesticide-resistant	This is the result of the insertion of pesticides into the DNA of a plant such as corn. The purpose is to make the injected food product unappetizing to the targeted insects. Instead, it appears to promote pesticide-resistant insects.
Herbicide-resistant	This concept is the same as the one used for pesti cides resulting in the same trend of creating herbcide-resistant insects.
Built-in vaccination	Vaccinations are injected into the DNA of plants so those eating them will become resistant to the targeted disease. Problem is, you the parent consumer, have no way of knowing how much of what vaccination your kids are eating. Scientists are concerned that there are all sorts of potential reaction problems related to this practice.
Nutrient fortified	Vitamins, such as A, are injected into the DNA of plants. Sounds good. Problem is, your kids would have to eat pounds of these GE fortified foods to satisfy their daily requirements. Also, there are unknowns yet to be addressed in this GE process

Farmlands and Supermarkets are Filled with GMO Foods. "The number of acres of transgenic crops in 1999 was 98.6 million."[3] This number has increased significantly since then. Approved GMO crops to date include "canola (rapeseed), corn (including popcorn and sweet corn — not blue corn), papaya, potatoes (Atlantic, Russet Burbank, Russet Norkatah, and Shepody), red-hearted chicory (radicchio), soybeans, squash (yellow crookneck), sugar beet, tomatoes (including cherry).[4] Not all are commercially available, yet. The four genetically altered foods most commonly found in about 70 percent of the supermarkets food inventory are corn, canola, cottonseed, and soybeans. Corn syrups are in hundreds of products such as cakes, cookies, and cereals. Wheat products are soon headed for grocery stores. It was approved for genetic modification in 2004. The list of processed GMO foods is growing quickly. Most travel into the foods we buy in the grocery stores through animal feed and processed foods.

And there's more...

> There are hundreds of GM (GMO) products in the pipeline awaiting further development, approval, or commercialization. Virtually every type of popular produce has been genetically engineered in the lab. Some of these include: wheat, rice, melons, cucumbers, strawberries,broccoli, grapes, sunflower, sugarcane, sugar beet, apples, lettuce, radicchio, carrots, coffee, cranberries, eggplant oats, onions, peas, pineapples, plums, raspberries, sweet potatoes, walnuts, and barley.[5]

Genetic engineering is a rapidly developing, well-financed science. Many more cross-combinations are being researched by biotechnologists. They include DNA insertion of a variety of viruses, fish, tobacco, or insects into vegetables fruit, grains, and legumes (beans). What's next? It is unsettling. Who wants tobacco in their food? What will happen to your kids' immune systems if they eat a steady diet of foods carrying the DNA from bacteria and viruses? No one knows. As consumers, our problem is that we don't know what is in what. None of the inserted DNA species are listed in the ingredients or anywhere else on the label.

Are Your Kids at GMO Risk? Pesticides are required to be registered with the EPA (Environmental Protection Agency). The EPA then regulates which ones farmers may spray on plants in order to kill pesky insects. To eliminate the insecticide spray process, biotechnologists have created the concept of placing pesticides or herbicides right into the plant's DNA so it innately repels or kills any bugs trying to eat it. Scientists actually cut, splice, and insert these pesticides' DNA right into DNA of foods, so that they are no longer a separate substance. As parents, we are concerned that our kids may be ingesting these pesticides.

> Despite claims that these food products are based on 'sound science,' in truth, neither manufacturers nor the government has studied the effects of these genetically altered organisms or their new proteins on people especially babies, the elderly, and the sick....As a pediatric neurologist, I especially worry about the safety of modified food when it comes to children.[6]

The potential hidden allergenic properties of some GMO foods are a foremost concern of health professionals. However, the development of genetically engineered food variations is on the increase. Genetic engineering can transform a harmless food into one containing a potentially harmful allergen in at least three different ways:

1. The level of a naturally occurring allergen might be increased.
2. A gene taken from one type of food might transfer allergenic properties when inserted into another food.
3. Unknown allergens may result from foreign genes and proteins never before part of the human food supply.[7]

When pesticides and herbicides genes from one food is inserted into another, without identification, those with allergies to these chemical or food sources may become vulnerable to reactions. Anyone who suffers from allergies knows how serious an allergy attack can be, especially a surprise one. The only way your child and you can know if their food has been genetically engineered is with a clear label identifying the engineering. Otherwise you will have no clue.

And there's more. Unless your kids are drinking and eating organic dairy products, they are most likely consuming genetically engineered milk products. Meet the bovine growth-hormone (rbGH, rBST).

> It was known as early as the 1930s that injection of dairy cows with bovine pituitary extracts increased milk yield. The practice, however, was not commercially viable until genetic engineering created a cost-efficient production method. Engineers took the cow gene that created their growth hormone, altered it, and inserted it into *E. Coli* bacteria, creating a living factory. The resulting hormone is similar, but not identical to the naturally occurring variety. When injected into a cow, it boosts the whole metabolism, including an increase in mammary cell activity. This leads to increased milk production.[8]

The FDA approved the use of these hormones against the advice of many scientists. To date, it has not required companies to label foods as genetically engineered or have rbGH added to the ingredient list. The FDA has also recommended that companies, who identify their milk as being hormone-free, should also include a disclaimer saying that there is no significant difference between the milk coming from cows treated with hormones and those who are not.

Scientists disagreeing with this FDA opinion, question whether there is a relationship between of the ingestion of hormones and early puberty in humans. The average age of puberty used to be twelve or thirteen. Now lots of girls under the age of ten are experiencing puberty changes. Just look around you. Other concerns being researched are possible linkage to breast, prostate, colon, and gastrointestinal cancer, the onset of which may begin at young ages.

Scientists opposed to the FDA's position are also concerned that cow's injected with the bovine growth hormone may have infectious reactions showing up in the form of pus (dead white blood cells). To prevent this, farmers using rbGH give their cows antibiotics, which, according to these scientists, may then show up in the cows' milk and future meat products. Your kids' immune systems are already challenged with the excessive use of antibiotics. Who is keeping track of your son or daughter's immune system and how much it may be taxed?

By the way, this exact science of DNA splicing is not an exact science. What happens to the wayward viral or bacterial cells, which has been imprecisely injected into the DNA? What happens when the intended cellular metabolism is disrupted and reorganizes into an unpredicted cellular combination?

So many variables of the GMO processes are unsettling. "They say it has been proven that the DNA of such (inactivated) viruses and bacteria, when incorporated into food, is capable of surviving passage through the digestive system from where it can find its way into the bloodstream and hence, into any of the cells in the body. The viruses can then break down cell walls of organisms already infected by other viruses, genetically combine forces, and begin to grow again. ...Scientists have linked the emergence of pathogenic (disease-causing) bacteria, antibiotic resistance and more virulent viruses to horizontal gene transfer ... between unrelated species."[9] Doesn't this make you shake in your boots?

No one knows what will happen to humans who eat genetically engineered GMO foods over a period of time. Philip J. Regal, Ph.D. stated the following in a Declaration submitted in federal district court by the Alliance for Bio-Integrity in a lawsuit against the FDA seeking mandatory testing and labeling of genetically engineered foods: "It is my professional opinion that utilizing RDNA technology in production for food-producing organisms can be very powerful biologically and very different biologically from conventional forms of breeding. It entails a set of risks to human health that are not ordinarily associated with the latter. Such use of DNA technology has the well-recognized potential to interfere with the normal activities of the engineered organism, for example so as to generate unexpected and unknown toxins, carcinogens, allergens and other anti-nutritive substances."[10] Dr. Regal is a biologist in the College of Biological Sciences, Professor of Ecology, Behavior, and Evolution at the University of Minnesota, has studied and authored the safety issues concerning the use of genetic engineering extensively.

At this writing, genetically engineered foods are NOT tested for long-term safety. So far, The Food and Drug Administration (FDA) does not demand long term labeling or testing of these altered foods. They only need the manufacturers' assurances that they are safe. The United States Department of Agriculture (USDA) and the Environmental Protection Agency (EPA) does not require comprehensive testing. Instead, the biotech companies may choose to, or not to, take the step of safety testing these foods and offer the conclusions to the FDA. We believe that GMO foods should have to meet the safety test requirements required of drugs.

> Steven M. Druker, Executive Director, Alliance for Bio-Integrity: "It is still the case that the overwhelming opinion of the FDA experts was that no GE food can be presumed safe unless it has been confirmed so through rigorous toxicological feeding studies."[11]
>
> Dr. John B. Fagan: "What makes genetic engineering particularly dangerous is that no one can predict the new toxins and allergens that will develop as a result of recombination."[12]
>
> Nearly 60 percent of scientists polled by the International Society of Chemotherapy believed maize (corn) genetically engineered for antibiotic resistance to be an unacceptable risk for consumers.[13]
>
> Without labeling, says Sheldon Krimsky, Ph.D., professor of urban and environmental policy at Tufts University, "People are being made part of an experiment for which they have not given their consent."[14]

The food manufacturers know that the public thinks unfavorably of genetically engineered foods. Some surveys notated that the negative response to GE foods is as high as 93 percent June 2001 (ABC News telephone poll[15]). That sends a powerful message; we want to know. Consequently, manufacturers are concerned that required labeling of genetically engineered ingredients could mean fewer sales of these products. Food manufacturers want their cake and to be able to eat it, too. You, the consumer, have the right to know the facts, both the good and bad.

The good news is that a Genetically Engineered Food Right to Know Act is being presented to Congress. The objective is to require that food labels identify all GMO ingredients. Maybe by the time you have read this, it will have passed.

The FDA says there is no difference between man-made GMO foods and God-made conventional foods. Yet, every transgenetic (genetically engineered) process is patented as “novel foods” because of the unique scientific quantifiable difference of these foods from natural, God-made foods. The biotech companies that have been developing transgenic processes, be it for fish in tomatoes or for bacteria in potatoes, declares the process and the product to be unique (novel) so it can be patented. This entitles them to legal ownership of this technology and everything produced by it giving them the right to all royalties of products sold. God-made foods cannot be patented. They belong to those who grow them.

Other Countries Say No to Some GMO Foods and Yes to Labeling

Genetically engineered foods are banned in many countries. Others allow them but require they be labeled accordingly. (Since the printing of this book, some countries may have changed their position.) An abbreviated list is below. Please check the Website footnote for a complete world map.)

Ban or Moritorium: United Kingdom, Ireland, Netherlands, Belgium, Denmark, Sweden, Greece, Portugal, Spain, Italy, France, Germany, Austria, New Zealand.

Proposed Ban: Poland, Brazil.

Require Labeling: China, Japan, Australia, Russia, Brazil, Chile.

Proposed Labeling: Norway, Switzerland, Poland, Hong Kong, New Zealand.[16]

As you can see, many governments of many countries are concerned about the repercussions of the genetic engineering of foods. Gene pollution is forever.

More Concerns, Irradiation

Irradiation is another controversial method used by food manufacturers to destroy insects, bacteria, yeast, molds, and parasites, or sterilize reproductive systems. Benefits to the manufacturers include longer shelf life for produce, meat and herbs. The irradiation process involves the zapping of food with gamma rays of radioactive cobalt. In small dosages, this process may become a health hazard. Look at why your kids are at risk when eating irradiated foods.

The authors of *Additive Alert* point out that one chest X-ray is equal to one rad, which is defined as a measure of radiation.

1 RAD = .01 Gy = 1 chest X-ray

(As you know, extensive protective precautions are taken when your dentist or an X-ray technician takes an X-ray of your kid's teeth or bones.) This raises the red flag for us.

The following table shows the amount of radiation permitted in some basic foods, and the equivalent amount in chest X-rays.

Potatoes & onions	15,000 RADS	= 0.15 kGy = 15,000 chest X-rays
Whole wheat flour, wheat, flour	75,000 RADS	= .075 kGy = 75,000 chest X-rays
Whole spice, ground spices & dehydrated seasoning preparations.[17]	1,000,000 RADS	= 10.00 kGy = 1,000,000 chest X-rays

WOW! How can it be safe to eat foods that have been radiated a million times more than the exposure of a chest X-ray? Now you say, the food was radiated, not the body. Well listen to this.

> The huge jolts of irradiation results in the destruction of vitamins and other essential nutrients. Researchers claim that irradiation diminishes or destroys vitamins A, C, E, K, B^1, B^2, B^3, B^6, B^{12}, carotene, and thiamine (another name for B^1).[18]
>
> Physicists at Melbourne University discovered the levels of free radicals increased between three to fifty times depending on the food that was irradiated. The human body is very sensitive to free radicals produced by gamma radiation. In fact, these free radicals are capable of causing cancer and premature aging. The effects of eating irradiated foods over a lifetime are impossible to predict. Furthermore chromosome damage may not become apparent until later generations.[19]

As with so many things, many small amounts add up to a large amount. How many times a week does your son or daughter eat irradiated potatoes, wheat, wheat flour, pork, fruit, vegetables, beef, eggs, dehydrated herbs, and other seasonings such as oregano? What about citrus fruits, strawberries, other fresh fruits and vegetables, poultry and pork? It may surprise you that black pepper is one of the most widely irradiated products found in today's foods. In 2002, the USDA approved irradiated meat for the National School Lunch Program. The FDA has long held that irradiated foods are safe for human consumption. Many disagree with this position.

At this writing, Switzerland, Great Britain, Germany, Sweden, New Zealand, Austria, Romania, Abu Dhabi, the Dominican Republic, Botswana, Ethiopia, Kenya, and Australia have banned the food irradiation process. Other countries are considering such a ban.

Labeling of irradiation is an issue among the consumer, food producer, and manufacturer, and FDA. "Foods that are irradiated have to be labeled with the international symbol for irradiation and wording such as 'irradiated', 'treated with radiation', 'treated by irradiation'. Irradiated ingredients that are then used in processed foods do not have to be labeled."[20] What is being said is that the first user of the product sees the symbol or wording. The end user, you, of processed foods may not. It is up to the food manufacturer's discretion. The FDA is in the process of reviewing irradiation label requirements.

Be Informed

Few issues are moving as rapidly through the legal and governmental processes as genetic engineering. Biotech, pharmaceutical, and food industries are working feverishly to produce the latest and greatest bioengineered products, be the first to patent them, and capture the market. Attention is riveted on the ramifications and solutions to biotechnological questions. Governing agencies are finding it difficult to keep up with the advancements. The challenges and repercussions are formidable. Safety testing for short and long-term results are lacking because no company wants to lose in the race for market share.

By the time you have read this page, some of the information in this chapter may be outdated. A way for you to keep abreast of genetic engineering is to be in touch through the following Websites:

www.centerforfoodsafety.org, www.ucsusa.org, www.organic-consumers.org, www.safe-food.org, and, www.thecampaign.org. It is worth your time to be informed. The health of your kids is at stake.

Simple Solutions

Always consider the source. Ask your local grocer for non-GMO, nonirradiated, additive-free food. Read ingredient lists. Buy organic when possible. Eat as much of God-made foods as possible! They are the cleaner naturally occurring foods, the organic foods. Man has been eating them for centuries. Why is this concept so foreign to today's generations?

> Thinking himself wise, man continues to exalt his foolish and uncontrolled pride, believing he can improve upon the unparalleled working of a flawless and all-knowing Creator.[21]

Choose Better Choices, The Good Guys

Some of the food manufacturers who are dedicated to not using genetically engineered (GMO) ingredients are Eden Foods, Barbara's Bakery, Newman's O, Dean Foods Vegetable Company, Muir Glen, Westbrae, Ben & Jerry's, Stonyfield Farm, Horizon Organic Dairy, Gerber (baby foods only), Tree of Life, Cascadian Farms, Harmony Farms, Spectrum Naturals, Arrowhead Mills, Frito-Lay, GeniSoy, Lundberg, Garden of Eatin', After the Fall, Knudson, Imagine, and The Hain Food Group. (A complete list of nongenetically altered foods can be found on www.truefoodnow.org)

Fill up your kids with the foods that were eaten by their ancestors, unadulterated nutrient-filled foods!

Food Genetic Engineering Update

June 2004 (Just prior to this book's distribution.)

The Associated Press has reported that "the European Union said it would approve human consumption of a variety of genetically modified corn." (Associated Press, May 14, 2004, www.foxnews.com.) This decision will be valid in all twenty-five European Union countries for ten years. "European Commission's spokesman, Reijo Kemppinen, said the Swiss-based company Syngenta's application to sell Bt11 sweet corn would be approved at the commission's meeting. In other countries, Bt11, an insect resistant genetically engineered corn, has previously been approved: United States, Canada,

Argentina, Austria, China, Japan, Korea, New Zealand, Philippines, Russia, South Africa, and Switzerland.

More News

Vermont has become the first state to require labeling on genetically engineered seeds. (April 29, 2004, www.thecampaign.org)

For more updates on food genetic engineering, check your news media sources or our website, www.betterfoodchioces.com.

12

Kids and Diets: What, When, and How

Chapter Quick Facts

- Good diets are sensible plans that keep kids well, optimally productive, and serve as a foundation for a lifelong lifestyle of balanced mental and physical health. Junk food diets do the opposite.
- Most commercial diets are designed for adults who weigh around 145 pounds or more, not for growing kids. For these, a health professional should be consulted.
- Vegetarian Diets (Vegan, Lacto, Lacto-Ovo, or Non-Red Meat) need extra protein supplementation. Health professional supervision is essential.
- High Protein/Low Carbohydrate Diets can deprive growing kids of the complex carbohydrates and essential fatty acids they need. Not recommended for kids.
- Low Glycemic Diets, or low sugar diets, are not practical diets for kids.
- Blood Type Diet. These diets may make sense for kids who are 10 years or older. Educate yourself on this one.
- Mediterranean Diet is the common-sense diet that can be followed easily by most kids.
- Food Circles™ Diet is the only diet that emphasizes water! It is easy to understand and follow. We recommend this as a guideline for your kids.

Kids and Diets. What, When and How?

Diet ... Does hearing this word stir up anxiety, confusion, and frustration? For most of us, diet is a four-letter word. It usually implies there is something wrong with us. Something needs to be corrected. We are too fat, too cholesterol-filled, too sugar-laden, too indulgent, or just plain too lazy. Today's media, including television, magazines, advertisers, Websites, and books remind us constantly that diets may be the answer to many of our problems. The pursuit of the perfect body is the number one selling point of packaged diets. The implications are that when you go on one of these diets, you will be happy, successful, and attractive to the opposite sex. Teenagers are particularly susceptible to this alluring message. Unfortunately, so are preteenagers.

Americans have a distorted meaning of the word, diet. The *Webster's Collegiate Dictionary* defines diet "as food and drink regularly consumed. The kind and amount of food prescribed for an animal or person for a special reason." In other words, diet is also what you eat, every day. The word diet is not necessarily related to weight loss.

Bad Diets Are Bad; Good Diets Are Good

Take your pick. Whatever you son or daughter eats is defined as a diet. Good diets are sensible diet plans that keep kids healthy and serve as a foundation for a lifelong lifestyle of balanced health. Kids' bodies readily and favorably respond to nutritious foods. They feel the results and experience the positive rewards, emotionally, mentally, and physically. The basic formula of a good diet for kids is a balanced diet of nontoxic, nutrient-filled foods with a few fun foods thrown in for good measure!

Conversely, kids' bodies readily and negatively respond to nutrient-empty, toxic junk food, and drink diets. These commonly consumed junk food diets are deficient in vitamins, minerals, fiber, and phytonutrients, and are packed with sugar, animal fat, trans fatty acids, and artificial ingredients making them sickening. Many serious health conditions, such as clogged arteries, are not detected until children become adults. However, the stage can be set for these conditions during childhood, and even infancy. Obesity, diabetes, and ADD/ADHD have not waited for adulthood to exhibit their damage. Each has reached epidemic proportions among young kids. Young bodies are more vulnerable as their growing bodies need good fuel sources to encourage proper development and provide a strong healthy foundation for their lives. From mother's milk through baby food, and into regular table food, it is important that kids are fed nourishing well-balanced meals and snacks (good diets!).

Most Marketed Diets Are Not Designed For Kids

For those who believe a change in diet is needed for their son or daughter, be careful. You may think that if you just put your son or daughter on a popular diet such as a high-protein, low-carbohydrate diet, he or she may eat his or her way back to health and improve his or her behavior, academic, and physical performance. The truth is, most commercial diets are designed for fully developed adults who weigh around 145 pounds or more! Few diet formulas are customized for individual body chemistries. They certainly are not designed for your growing kids. The bottom line is that it is not healthy to pursue most commercialized diets without the guidance of a doctor who would monitor blood pressure, cholesterol levels, and other vital signs. Popular diets such as the Atkins, Zone, and Protein Power are strict adult-oriented programs. Most diets that are very limiting in protein, complex carbohydrates, and good fats are wrong for most growing kids. Children should not be candidates for commercially packaged diets. Boys and girls who are experiencing serious health problems, including obesity, should be under the supervision of a licensed health professional.

The Fat Diet! A Number-One Diet Problem

The word fat has numerous definitions according to Webster; "plump, obese, of a meat animal: fattened for market, of food: oily and greasy, well filled out, something in excess." Sounds bad. Unfortunately, much of the processed breakfast, lunch, snack, and dinner foods eaten today are heavily endowed with bad fats such as hydrogenated, partially hydrogenated fats, and trans fatty acids.

Fat is composed of numerous compounds containing carbon, hydrogen, and oxygen. They are energy-rich foods that are not soluble in water. That doesn't sound so bad. In fact, fat from a good source such as olive oil or fish provides really important fuel for your son and daughter's body.

Many published fat reduction diets send dieters away from the bad fats as well as the good fats. For kids, eliminating the good fats may negatively impact the development of their nervous system that subsequently impacts multiple physiological and mental functions. Kids need good fats such as olive and fish oils in their daily diet.

Some diets encourage the consumption of low-fat and fat-free foods. As noted earlier in this book, manufacturers of such products usually compensate for the reduction or elimination of the fat with added generous portions of simple carbohydrates, sugar! Problem is that any and all excess and unused sugar is stored as fat. This is not a very satisfactory fat reduction diet solution.

Many kids are on fat gaining diets. Kids are fat and getting fatter. Obesity is growing in epidemic proportions. So is diabetes, a fat related disease. The Center for Disease Control and Prevention recently reported that obesity grew 61 percent in only nine years (1991-2000). Statistics vary. Some say one in three kids is overweight. Some say one in five is obese. It was reported in the September 2001 issue of Journal of the American Medical Association that from 1999 to 2000 adult onset diabetes increased 49 percent nationwide. What is particularly disturbing is the recent information revealing that about 25 percent of newly reported adult onset diabetes cases are under the age of twenty-one. But, you ask, isn't diabetes a sugar related disease? It is. Many kids are eating at least twelve pounds of sugar a month. That amounts to a lot of unused caloric energy that the body then reserves as fat.

Junk Food Diets Are Bad

Everybody knows this. Yet, most kids eat junk or no food for breakfast, a fast junk food lunch, and, often a hurry up and eat-in-the-car-burger and fries dinner. This is a diet filled with trans fatty acids, simple carbohydrates, artificial ingredients, flavorings and dyes, and, little else. Few vitamins, minerals, phytonutrients, and fiber are found in the daily diets of today's kids.

When any kid lives on excessive amounts of fat, carbohydrates, and fried foods, his or her health will be compromised. Junk food diets consist of mostly empty food: French fries, pizza, sodas, pastries, cookies, frozen dinners, fried chicken or fish, pork products, hamburgers, hot dogs, too much refined wheat, candy, excessive sweetened juice or dairy products, insufficient water, and the list goes on and on and on. You get the picture. This is bad stuff. Your son or daughter's health will suffer from a diet of junk food. Unfortunately, most kids are part of today's Junk Food Generation.

Addiction Diets

How do I look? Do I look good in these clothes? Look at how fat I am. I have gained weight! I'm craving some chocolate chip cookie dough ice cream. I have to eat just one more. I want to eat the whole thing, NOW. I want some French fries. These "I" messages run through young and younger kids' heads, non-stop. In a nutshell, kids are addicted to their looks, to self-gratification, to peer pressure, and, to addictive-type foods and drinks. These thought processes live symbiotically with their actions Even young kids, influenced by television and movie images and messages, eat for looks, pleasure, acceptance, and to win. Those who carry these issues to the extreme become addicted to one of two diets, anorexia or bulimia. Anorexia could be called the "Fear of being Fat and Denial Diet." Bulimia is the binge (I deserve) and purge (no, I don't deserve) diet. Preteen and teenagers who have low self-esteem, suffer from guilt, feel unloved, or, think they are just too fat, may experiment with these emotionally related diet programs. In order to fulfill the need to be model thin and deny themselves pleasures, anorexics starve their bodies and lose excessive amounts of weight. Bulimics gratify their needs by first eating excessive amounts of whatever they want and then retreating to the nearest bathroom in order to induce regurgitation of all the foods just eaten so they won't gain weight. Both addictive diets are very serious and must be treated by licensed health professionals.

Unfortunately, addictive eating habits do not have to be that extreme to contribute to health problems. Overconsumption of sugar, caffeine, artificial ingredients such as appetite stimulants, even the "mouth feel" of fat can invite obesity, diabetes, cardiovascular diseases, and emotional imbalance. Most kids do not know that they are chemically attracted to artificial ingredients and dyes. They think they are eating a whole bag of cookies just because they taste really good. The taste makes these cookies irresistible and the nature of ingredients may be driving excessive consumption. The way you can try to help your kids not eat the whole bag, is to replace these processed artificial foods with ones from the Better Choices Grocery List™. Choose a balance of God-made foods for a balanced diet.

Vegetarian Diets

Some kids turn to vegetarian diets for their "need to be" answers. Environmental issues such as the killing of and commercial handling of animals for food prey on the minds of some kids. They may choose not to eat meat, fish or dairy for their desire to be animal or environmental activists. Others may be concerned about toxins or just plain think it's cool to be different. There are four kinds of vegetarian diets:

- VEGAN: absolutely no animal or animal derived products. This includes honey, eggs, dairy. Foods eaten are of 100 percent plant origin; vegetables, grains, seeds, nuts and legumes.
- LACTO: Allows the addition of dairy products to the basic vegan diet.
- LACTO-OVO: Allows the addition of eggs and dairy to the basic vegan diet.
- NON RED MEAT: Allows the addition of poultry and fish to any variety of the vegetarian diets.

Depending upon the health condition of your child, a vegetarian diet can be healthful in very specific cases. Any variety of a vegetarian diet should be supplemented with protein drinks and additional supplementation such as amino acids and minerals like zinc. If you choose to allow your son or daughter to be a version of a vegetarian, we recommend that you monitor your child's health along with their energy levels, grades in school, moods, and weight. Again, please consult a health professional before restricting a food group from your son or daughter's diet.

High-Protein/Low-Carbodydrate Diets

These diets include the popular Dr. Atkins, Protein Power, Heller, South Beach, and Suzanne Sommer's programs. Their plans range from the consumption of 20 milligrams of carbohydrates per day (the most strict) up to 100 grams of carbohydrates per day (the highest allowed). With these restricted carbohydrate allowances, specified amounts of high-protein and high-fat foods are recommended. One objective is to stabilize insulin. When insulin levels are out of control, disease in the form of weight gain, diabetes, heart disease, depression, nervous disorders, or just plain unruly behavior can develop in kids. Higher protein diets may keep the insulin produced by the body at a healthier level leading to balanced normal bodily functions. Higher protein diets may also help to eliminate food cravings, mood swings, and lack of focus.

There are systemic and digestive concerns about the basic formula of high-protein diets. Designed for weight loss, diabetes, depression, and cardiovascular conditions, these low-carb/high protein diets require a lot of discipline. Unfortunately, many adults have used these diets as a license to eat lots of saturated animal fat, hydrogenated fats, and trans fatty acid foods. Many bodies are not chemically designed to handle so much protein. They may experience constipation, bad breath, indigestion, and sluggish livers. Plus, many think that when on these high-protein programs, they can eat endless amounts of cheese. Cheese is a dense fat food and should be limited. Many individuals may develop excess mucous and gas buildup with increased cheese consumption. Problems do not always stem from the diet itself but the individual's misinterpretation and misapplication of the diet plan.

Other concerns include the exclusion of many complex carbohydrate plant-based essential fatty acids (EFAs) such as olive and flaxseed oils, nuts, and seeds. These are vital fuels for kids, all kids. Also, in Chapter Five (High-Octane Fuels) we spell out the critical role complex carbohydrates play in the mental and physical development of children. High-protein/low-carbohydrate diets may deprive growing kids of these needed nutrients. Fat-reduction diets involve complicated science. Kids who need to lose weight should go to a licensed health professional for supervision.

Low-Glycemic Diets

The objective with these diets is to control a person's blood sugar. Usually, the most desired goal is to lose weight. The Zone diet advocates 40-30-30 (carbohydrates-protein-fat). The Sugar Busters diet focus on several smaller balanced portions of food daily, and relies heavily on the glycemic index for most food intake. Although the goal of these dietary programs is to keep the insulin hormone in balance, several very beneficial foods for kids are forbidden on this diet. Carrots, bananas, beets, and pineapple are banned while junk foods such as commercially refined and artificial cereals, sweeteners, and diet soda are allowed. Rigid dietary programs are very difficult for children to follow and require advance planning from the parental guardian for the child. Many kids do not have the luxury to snack throughout the day and therefore a difficult time trying to stick with this diet. Several adjustments to modify this program for kids would make sense for certain individuals suffering from certain hypoglycemic, diabetic, thyroid challenges. To follow it by the book would be unwise for most children. Consult a licensed health professional before putting kids on this diet.

Low-Fat Diets

These diets are promoted heavily by the American Heart Association and by doctor Dean Ornish. Doctor Ornish advocates that only 10 percent (20 to 25 grams) of your daily calorie intake may be from "fat." However, he has recently begun to recommend fish oil supplementation, eating more complex carbohydrates like whole grains, and limiting the consumption of refined carbohydrates. While the focus on increasing the amount of vegetables consumed is extremely important, we believe that there needs to be more emphasis on the promotion of healthy fats and the reduction of too many carbohydrates. Remember, unused ingested carbohydrates turn into fat. Moderate to low-fat diets may work with overweight children as well as for those with elevated blood pressure. A diet with too little of the good fat is a mistake, especially for growing children. Again we emphasize that you consult your licensed health professional before starting your son or daughter on any low-fat diets.

Blood-Type Diets

Is your kid a blood type A, B, A/B, or O? We are willing to bet that you do not know. Surprisingly, most parents don't have a clue about their kid's blood type. Doctors usually do not routinely test for the blood types of their patients. Some birth certificates document blood types. Your son or daughter's doctors may test for it upon request.

The introduction of blood type diets follows research as documented by Dr. D'Adamo. He claims that the benefits include more energetic life, reduction of illness, natural maintenance of ideal body weight, stress management, strengthening of mental acuity, and reduction of food cravings. Part of Doctor D'Adamo's research discusses lectins (abundant proteins found in the foods we consume) and their compatibility with the antigens (cause production of antibodies in blood) in accordance to one's blood type. When a person eats a food that contains uncompatible lectins this food is labeled an enemy invader. When these opposing lectins surround these foods, the lectins start to deposit glue-like suction cups onto the cellular wall. Accumulation of these "bad" lectins within the body may lead to metabolic and hormonal imbalances, interfere with insulin production, or lead to bloating and elimination challenges. There is a lot more research supporting this diet concept. Incompatible food choices may cause your son or daughter to become tired, lose focus in school or to gain excess weight.

There are four blood types: A, B, AB, or O. Each favors a specific food group and level of exercise.

Blood Type A (Agrarian):	Population percentage, 40 percent Lower protein and fat Higher complex carbohydrates Low impact to moderate exercise
Blood Type B (Balance):	Population percentage, 12 percent Moderate amounts of lean protein, healthy fats, fresh fruits, and vegetables. Moderate exercise.
Blood Type AB (Modern):	Population percentage, 3 percent Wide variety of selected lean meats, healthy fats, fresh fruit and vegetables Moderate exercise.
Blood Type O (Old):	Population percentage, 45 percent High protein, vegetables, and healthy fats. Moderate amounts of fresh fruits Low carbohydrates. Intense exercise.

Please refer to Dr. D'Adamo's book, *Eat Right For Your Blood Type Encyclopedia,* for specific recommendations of food, beverages and supplements. Families are usually genetically of the same one or two blood types. It would be rare for a family of four to represent each of the four blood types. Thank heavens. Meal planning would be a nightmare!

This dietary regime does make sense for kids beginning at ten years, especially those with food allergies, sinus and asthmatic conditions and those who crave sweets and carbohydrates. Gradual adaptation to this food plan is not difficult. Please consult a licensed health professional who is knowledgeable about this diet.

Mediterranean Diet

Most kids can easily follow this common-sense diet. In general, the Mediterranean lifestyle reflects a balance of healthy and fresh God-made foods. Foods on this program include fresh vegetables and fruit, fish, lean protein (chicken), reasonable amounts of complex carbohydrates, fresh herbs, few refined carbohydrates, and high amounts of healthy omega fats (olive oil!). All are to be eaten daily in balanced moderate amounts. See how this differs from the commonly eaten diets of today.

The American Diet	The Mediterranean Diet
High in saturated fat	Low in saturated fat
High in sugar	Low in sugar
High in trans fatty acids	Low in trans fatty acids
High in starchy carbohydrates and baked goods	Low in starchy carbohydrates and baked goods
Low in water consumption	High in water consumption
Low in extra-virgin olive oil	High in extra-virgin olive oil
Extremely low in omega-3 fatty acids	High in omega-3 fatty acids
High in omega-6 fatty acids	Low in omega-6 fatty acids
Extremely low in vegetables	High in vegetables[1]

Those of you who have grown up in a home of Mediterranean descent or have visited the Mediterranean area know the pleasures of their menus. Instead of serving garlic bread with animal fat butter, olive oil is commonly offered in a small dish. Dipping bread into garlic or herb-laced olive oil is fun and enjoyed by kids. (Kids love eating with their fingers.) The good news is that these kids are eating essential fatty acids (brain food!) and not margarine. In this diet, smaller amounts of meat products and larger amounts of vegetables are woven into the every day recipes. Sweets are served in smaller portions, usually as treats! A Mediterranean diet is a smarter, common sense diet that we recommend for most kids.

Food Circles Diet

A diet following the Food Circles is real simple and sensible. The largest circle, water, encircles all the food groups because it is the most essential fuel for your growing kids. The second largest circle is the vegetable circle because kids need to eat more servings of vegetables a day than any other remaining food groups. The third circle is filled with essential fatty acids (EFAs), whole grains, legumes (beans), nuts, seeds, dairy, eggs, poultry, fish, and lamb. The next sized circle is for fruit. Kids need to eat less fruit than vegetables. Red meat and sweets occupy the smallest circle, as kids are to eat them only once a week. Take a look at the Food Circles below.

Food Circles

The Food Circles are the brainchild of some Kid Kritics. With some tweaking, this graphic became a clear easy way to

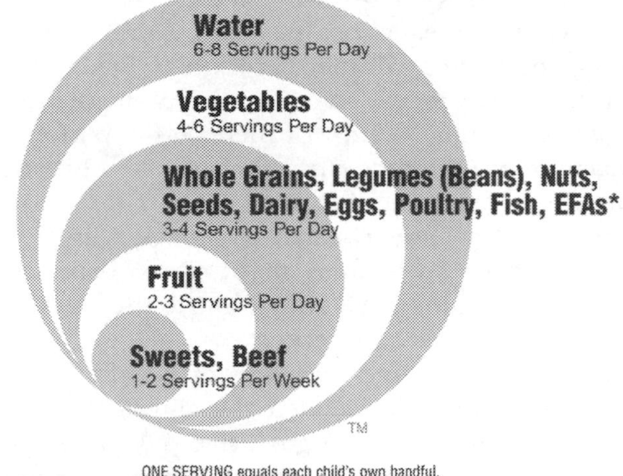

ONE SERVING equals each child's own handful.
SERVING SIZE EXCEPTIONS: Water – 6-8 ounces, EFAs/Seeds – 1 teaspoon, Eggs – 1, any size
*EFAs - Essential Fatty Acids (refers to oils only)

understand and remember a symbol. Please introduce it to your kids. Use it as a guide. With each food group, always consider the source. Instead of trying to change all eating habits at once, strive to gradually add servings of each group to your kid's daily diet. It takes time to change. Remember that serving sizes are customized to your son and daughter since one serving equals a comfortable handful for him or her. With the Food Circles as a guide, in time, you will positively adjust your shopping and cooking habits. As you may have noted, the Food Circles diagram is the only one that emphasizes the importance of water in a kid's daily diet. We highly recommend following the circles when fueling your kids!

Which One Is Best?

For most kids, we believe that the Food Circles will balance and best fuel your kids. The Mediterranean diet complements them. When you do move in this direction, the odds heavily favor the fact that you will be serving, and they will be eating and drinking Better Choices. Remember the easiest rule of thumb: eat at least two different God-made colors of food per meal. Three is better! For kids with special health imbalances, the guidance of a licensed health professional is a must. A customized well-balanced, high performance diet is your goal. Your kids can look forward to a renewed balanced energy and focus, a strengthened immune system, and an improved behavioral pattern because they are choosing the right foods for their body!

Five Days On, Two Days Off!

This is what makes a healthy diet work. Follow the Food Circles guide Sunday dinner through to Friday lunch. Friday dinner is a free-for-all! Stay clear of most junk food on Saturday but enjoy some. (Athletes and performers should stay away from junk food until their weekend events are over.) Do the same during Sunday until dinner. Then it is back on to the Food Circles plan. Launch the week with a good-tasting nutritious dinner on Sunday night. From experience, regardless of good intentions, we know that dinner menus tend to go downhill as the week progresses!

What five days on and two days off accomplishes is a combination of having experienced the physical, productive and emotional achievement of a good five days with the reward of an unrestricted, you can have whatever you want Friday night. Plus treats are still allowed on Saturday! What generally occurs over time is a reduction of desires for sweets, sodium, and junk food in general. Taste buds positively change with a regularity of a diet of Better Food Choices™. We are talking about a lifestyle change.

It is all up to you! Make better food choices. Don't always go along with whatever everyone else is eating! Feed your kids what they need to stay well fueled. When given the knowledge as to why certain foods are more productive foods than others, kids take an interest and cooperate. Tell them the facts. Eventually, they may infect their friends with the good news.

It's your kid's life. Give him or her the competitive edge. Fill your God-made son and daughter with God-made food!

13

Better Choices Grocery List

Chapter Quick Facts

- This is probably the most useful chapter for you in this book. Use this product-specific grocery list as your food bible.
- Grocery list requirements: good food sources, ingredients, nutrition, and taste.
- We read the ingredients and nutrition facts of almost all the foods and drinks found on grocery store shelves. This comprehensive grocery list is the result.
- Kid Kritics approved foods are noted by asterisks. Chances are your kids will like them.

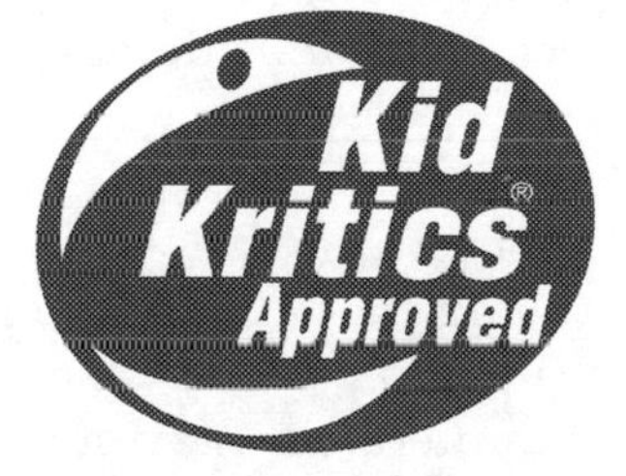

- Foods and drinks generally known to be liked by most kids are also included.
- This comprehensive list is organized by food category, such as bread, cereal, chicken, and chips. It is laid out for food identification. Organic foods are noted in bold print.
- Use the Better Choices Grocery List™ for easy to prepare and serve foods and drinks. Your kids won't be running on empty anymore!

Better Choices Grocery List

This is probably the most useful chapter in this book. The food and drinks found on the grocery list initially had to pass three assessments: ingredients, nutritional, and taste. We spend days walking up and down the aisles of several major supermarkets, natural food markets chains, and independent health food stores, reading hundreds upon hundreds, maybe thousands, of labels of the foods and drinks stocked on the shelves. This took a lot of time and was exhausting, but was necessary in order for us to evaluate the food and drinks available to you, the shopper. Painstakingly, we read the ingredient lists in search of high-octane and anti-fuels. It was important to elimi-nate the foods infused with too much bad fat, sodium, sugar, and additives. Foods with a welcomed list of reasonably healthy ingredients then had to satisfy the nutrition needs of your kids. Then we turned to the Nutrition Facts for specific data on the content of the ingredients. This provided us with a nutritional crossover checking process. The end result gave us a list of foods that we could recommend for clean and balanced nutrition, the Better Choices Grocery List.

However, as we all know, if kids do not like the taste of any foods recommended on our Better Choices Grocery List, buying them would be a waste of your hard-earned money. Cooking them would be a waste of your precious time. Thus, we turned to our Kids Kritics for their vote. Who better could tell us if kids like a specific food or drink?

Kids Kritics Approved

The Kid Kritics are an ever-growing group of boys and girls between the ages of five and fourteen. The gender split has been almost even. Lucky for us, kids love to taste test foods and they gladly give us their unadulterated, honest, and candid opinion! For each item tasted, they had to say yes or no to a series of questions. A few questions included were: Does it look good? Does it taste good? Would you want it for breakfast, lunch, snack, or dinner? (This question was adjusted per meal appropriateness.) Would you want your mom or dad to buy it? Then each food or drink was given a rating from one to five, five being the best! By the time the answers are evaluated, it became clear whether they liked it or not. The foods thus far given the Kid Kritics seal of approval were clear winners. Those that fell into a borderline rating were not included. Neither were the obvious rejections. Consequently, the odds of your kids liking foods and drinks given the Kid Kritics seal of approval are good.

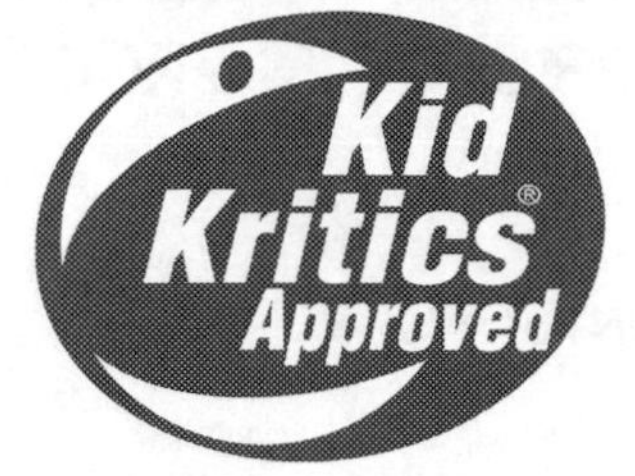

There are foods and drinks on the recommended grocery list that have not been taste-tested by the Kid Kritics. However, most are commonly known to be liked by many kids. Kid Kritics taste-testings are being continued after publication. The results will be published on our Web site, www.betterfood-choices.com. Realistically, not every kid will like every food listed. However, the use of the Better Choices Grocery List will really increase your odds of success.

Hundreds of new food and drink products are added to the grocery store inventory every year. Yearly, hundreds of foods and drinks are also removed from the shelves or altered. This fluctuation of additions and subtractions is challenging to monitor. As a service, we will attempt to keep you updated with the web page Better Choices Grocery List.

We tried to organize this grocery list by breakfast, lunch, snacks, and dinner to make your job easier. It became very confusing and unpractical. Instead the foods and drinks are listed by categories such as baking ingredients, bread, cereals, chicken, and chips. It is an easy to read comprehensive list.

All organic foods are highlighted by bolding the letters. Kid Kritics approved foods and drinks are identified with an asterisk.

BRANDS TO TRUST™ is an abbreviated grocery list that has been created for your grocery shopping convenience. It was designed and coated for you to carry in your purse. As the name implies, this is a list of food and drink brands we feel you can trust for the entire product line. Exceptions are noted with the phrase ONLY. Brands to Trust is not listed in this book but is a separate product available to you.

Following is the first generation of the Better Food Choices Grocery List. Use it when you plan. You will find this list on the easy to carry CD-ROM, *Mom, I'm Hungry, What's for Dinner?* (cookbook). Take this CD to work and logon to the recipes and grocery list when trying to figure out what you are going to cook for dinner. May this list bring you peace of mind!

BETTER CHOICES GROCERY LIST

Description	Product	Brand Name
BAKING INGREDIENTS		
BAKING POWDER	Baking Powder, aluminum-free	Bob's Red Mill, Rumford
BAKING SODA	Baking Soda	Arm & Hammer
CHOCOLATE CHIPS	Chocolate Chips	Chatfield's, Ghiradelli, Newman's Own, **Sunspire**
COCOA	Cocoa Mix	**Ah!Laska, Country Choice**
COOKIE/BROWNIE MIXES	Chocolate Chip Cookie Mix	**Arrowhead Mills**
	Oatmeal Raisin Cookie Mix	**Arrowhead Mills**
	Brownie, original	**Arrowhead Mills, No Pudge***
CORN BREAD	Cornbread Mix	**Arrowhead Mills, Upcountry**
FLOUR	Pastry	**Arrowhead Mills, Hodgson Mills**
	Spelt	**Arrowhead Mills, Bob's Red Mill Hodgson Mills**
	Yellow Cornmeal	**Arrowhead Mills, Bob's Red Mill**
	Unbleached, white	**Arrowhead Mills, Bob's Red Mill, Hodgson Mills**
	Whole Wheat	**Arrowhead Mills, Bob's Red Mill,** Gold Medal (whole grain), **Hodgson Mills**
PANCAKE FLOURS	Buttermilk Pancake Mix	**Arrowhead Mills, Upcountry Organics**
PIE CRUST	Graham Cracker	**Arrowhead Mills**
SHORTENING	Shortening	**Spectrum***
SPRINKLES	Sprinkelz, all kinds	**Let's Do Organic!***
VANILLA EXTRACT	100% Vanilla Extract	**Flavorganics**, Frontier, Mc Cormick's, **Simply Organic**
BARS (snacks)	Puffins Blueberry Yogurt	Barbara's Bakery
	Energy Bites, oatmeal raisin	Power Bar
	Manatee	Endangered Species
	Puffins, P.B. & Choc. Chip	Barbara's Bakery
BEANS (legumes)		
CANNED	Baked Beans	**Bearitos (fat-free), Eden, Westbrae**
	Black Beans	**Bearitos, Eden, Goya, Westbrae**
	Chili Beans	**Westbrae**
	Garbanzo Beans	**Eden, Westbrae**

Description	Product	Brand Name
	Great Northern White	**Eden, Westbrae**
	Kidney Beans	**Eden, Westbrae**
	Refried Kidney Beans	**Eden**
	Refried Black Beans, fat-free	**Bearitos, Eden**
	Soybeans	**Eden, Westbrae**
	White Beans, small	Goya
CHILI	Chili, black beans	Health Valley, **Bearitos**, Shelton's*
	Chili, chicken	Shelton's
	Chili	**Eden, Westbrae**
	Chili, turkey	Health Valley, Shelton's
	Chili, vegetarian	Health Valley
DRIED	Black Beans	**Arrowhead Mills**, Goya, **Tree of Life**
	Chickpeas (garbanzo)	**Arrowhead Mills**, Goya, **Tree of Life**
	Kidney, red	**Arrowhead Mills**, Goya, **Tree of Life**
	Lentils	**Arrowhead Mills**, Goya, **Tree of Life**
	Pinto	**Arrowhead Mills**, Goya, **Tree of Life**
	Soybeans	**Arrowhead Mills**, Goya, **Tree of Life**
	Split Peas	Goya
FROZEN	Burritos, bean & cheese	**Amy's**
	Burritos, bean & rice	**Amy's**
	Burritos, black bean & veggies	**Amy's**
	Edamame	**Cascadian Farms,** Sea Point Farms,
	Enchiladas, black beans	**Amy's**
	Enchiladas, cheese	**Amy's**
REFRIGERATE	Hummus, plain	Cedar's, Hannah, **Swan Gardens**

BEEF (additive-free!)

Description	Product	Brand Name
DELI	Roast Beef, slices	Applegate Farms*
	Oven Roasted, plain	Boar's Head
FRESH CUTS	Ground Beef, Flank Steak London Broil, New York Steak, Top Sirloin, Stew Cubes	Coleman, **Green Circle,** Laura's Lean Beef, Mayer Natural Angus, **Organic Valley**
REFRIGERATED/ FROZEN		
	Beef Sticks	Shelton's*
	Burgers	Coleman, **Organic Valley**
	Franks (hot dogs)	Applegate Farms, Coleman
STICKS	Beef Sticks	Applegate Farms, Shelton's

BREAD

Description	Product	Brand Name
LOAVES	Ultimate Kids Bread	**Alvarado Street Bakery***
	9-Grain	Pepperidge Farm
	8 Grain Sandwich	**Todd's**
	Crunchy Grains	Pepperidge Farm
	Multi-Grain Oat	**Rudi's**
	Multi-Grain	S. Rosen's

Description	Product	Brand Name
	Jewish Light Rye	**Rudi's**
	Spelt Bread, (wheat-free)	**Rudi's, Todd's**
	Sprouted California Bread	**Alvarado Street Bakery**
	Sprouted Soy Crunch	**Alvarado Street Bakery**
	Sprouted Wheat	**Alvarado Street Bakery, Rudi's***
	Sourdough Wheat	Pepperidge Farm, **Rustics***
	White	**Rudi's, Rustics*, Todd's**
	Whole Wheat	**Rudi's, Rustics, Todd's**
BUNS	Hamburger Buns	Alvarado Street Bakery, **Rudi's, Todd's**
	Hot Dog	Alvarado Street Bakery, **Rudi's**
	Hot Dog, flourless	Ezekiel
TORTILLAS	Tortillas	**Alvarado Street Bakery, Garden of Eatin, Rudi's,** Zapata
PASTRY SHELLS	Fillo Pastry Shells	Fillo Factory*
PIE CRUSTS, please see BAKING INGREDIENTS		
PIZZA CRUSTS	Pizza Shell, sprouted wheat	**Alvarado Street Bakery***

BUTTER/SPREADS

Description	Product	Brand Name
BUTTER, no additives (salted and unsalted)	Butter	Alta Dena, Cabot, **Horizon***, Land O'Lakes, **Organic Valley**
SPREADS, no additives	Soft Canola Spreads	Canoleo, Spectrum*

CANDY

Description	Product	Brand Name
	Gummi Bears, all kinds	**Let's Do Organic!***
	Gummy Bears/ Worms	**Planet Harmony**
	Jelly Pebbles	Woodstock Farms
	Chocolate Malt Balls	Sunspire
	Sun Drops	Sunspire*
	Licorice, Rasp./Straw. Bars	Panda
	Peppermint	Edward & Sons*
	Carob Malt Balls	Simple Snacks
	Carob Peanut Clusters	Simple Snacks
	Peanut Butter Cups	**Newman's Own**
	Yogurt Malt Balls	Simple Snacks, Sunspire
	Yogurt Raisins	Sunspire, Woodstock Farms
	Chocolate Peanuts	Planet Harmony, **Woodstock Farms**
	Milk Chocolate /Peanut Butter	**Endangered Species**
	Milk Chocolate Rice Crisps	**Endangered Species**

CEREAL

Description	Product	Brand Name
COLD	Banana-Os	**Erewhon***
	Orangutan-Os	**EnvrioKidz***
	Purely Os	**Cascadian Farms**
	Apple Struddle	**Erewhon***
	Corn Flakes	**Arrowhead Mills*, Erewhon, Nature's Path**

Description	Product	Brand Name
	Cocomotion	U.S. Mills*
	Cornfetti	U.S. Mills*
	Amazon Frosted Flakes	**EnviroKidz***
	Gorilla Munch	**EnvrioKidz***
	Koala Crisps	**EnvrioKidz***
	Cheetah Chomps	**EnviroKidz**
	Honey, Puffed	Kashi
	Wild Puffs, lightly sweetened	Barbara's Bakery
	Peanut Butter Panda Puffs	**EnvrioKidz**
	Peanut Butter Bumpers	Mother's
	Groovy Grahams	Mother's
	Raisin Bran	**Cascadian Farms, Erewhon, Nature's Path**
	Cocoa Bumpers	Mother's
	Cocoa Crispy Rice	U.S. Mills*
	Crispy Brown Rice	**Erewhon**
	Blueberries & Cream	Breadshop Granola
	Strawberries & Cream	Breadshop Granola
	Cinnamon Oat Crunch	Mother's
	Honey Nut'Os	**Cascadian Farms**
	Honey Round-Ups	Mother's
HOT	Instant Oatmeal	**Arrowhead Mills, Erewhon,** Mother's, Nature's Path
	Quick/Minute Oatmeal	Quaker Oats
	Rolled Oats, no additives	**Arrowhead Mills,** Quaker Oats, **Lundberg**
	Rice and Shine	**Arrowhead Mills**
	Cream of Rice	**Erewhon, Lundberg**

CHEESE (additive-free!)

WHITE (only)

Description	Product	Brand Name
	Cream Cheese, low-fat	Alta Dena, **Horizon*, Organic Valley***
	Cheddar, mild, reduced fat	Alta Dena, Cabot*, **Organic Valley Tree of Life**
	Cheddar, shredded	Cabot, **Horizon*, Organic Valley***
	Cheddar, sliced	Applegate Farms*, Cabot, **Organic Valley***
	Cheddar, sharp	Alta Dena, Cabot, **Organic Valley, Organic Creamery, Tree of Life**
	Cottage Cheese, low-fat	Cabot, Friendship (low fat only), **Horizon, Organic Valley**
	Goat Cheese, plain	Alta Dena, Chavrie, Ile de France, Montchevre
	Muenster, slices	Applegate Farms*, Cabot
	Monterey Jack	Alta Dena, Cabot, **Horizon*, Tree of Life***
	Monterey Jack, shredded	Cabot, Horizon*, **Organic Valley***
	Mozzarella	Cabot, Horizon*, Il Villaggio, Land O'Lakes, **Organic Valley,** Polly-O, Sorrento, **Tree of Life***
	Mozzarella, shredded	Cabot, **Horizon*,Organic Valley***
	Mozzarella, string/sticks	**Horizon*, Organic Valley*, Polly-O, Sorrento**

Description	Product	Brand Name
	Parmesan, grated	**Horizon**, Locatelli, **Organic Valley,** Tree of Life
	Parmesan, wedge	Assiago, Bel Gioioso, Grand Padano Regianno
	Provolone, slices/block	Applegate Farms*, **Organic Valley**
	Ricotta	Bel Gioioso, Sorrento
	Romano, grated	100% Imported, DiGiorno, Locatelli, **Organic Valley,** Tree of Life
	Romano, block	Di Giorno, Locatelli, Pecorino
	Swiss, slices/block	Applegate Farms*, Cabot, Land O'Lakes, **Organic Valley**
JAR	Nacho Cheese, mild	Enrico's
FROZEN PREPARED	Cheese Appetizers	Fillo Factory
	Mozzarella Sticks	Health is Wealth
CHICKEN (additive-free!)		
FRESH	All Cuts	Bell & Evans, **Organic Valley,** Rocky, **Rosie**
FROZEN	Bologna	Bell & Evans
	Buffalo Wings*	Health is Wealth
	Franks (hot dogs), uncured	Applegate Farm*, Bell & Evans, **Organic Valley,** Shelton's
	Legs, Kosher	Empire
	Nuggets	Applegate Farms, Bell and Evans* Health is Wealth
	Burgers	Bell & Evans
	Patties	Health is Wealth,* Harmony Farms
	Tenders (breast)	Bell & Evans
	Sausages (apple/maple)	Bell & Evans
	Chicken Sandwich Steaks	Bell & Evans
	Chicken Pot Pie	**Amy's, Shelton's**
CHIPS/STICKS		
CHIPS (baked)	Potato, 40% reduced fat	Cape Cod
	Golden Russet	Cape Cod
	Kettle-Cooked	Cape Cod, Kettle*, Michael's Seasons*
	Original	**Garden of Eatin',** Kettle*, Lay's Natural (sea salted)
	Sour Cream Potato Chips	Good Health Snacks*
	Baked Potato Chips	Kettle*
	Classic Potato Chips	Lay's Natural
	Ruffles, reduced fat	Lay's Natural
	Mesquite BBQ	Michael Season's*
	Potato Flyers	Robert's American Gourmet
	Potato Poppers	Simple Snacks
	Potato, all natural	Barbara's Bakery, Wise
	Original Corn	Fritos, **Garden of Eatin', Little Bear, Skinny Corn Chips, Tostito**
	Blue Corn	**Garden of Eatin',** Kettle, Little Bear, **R. W. Garcia, Tostito**

Description	Product	Brand Name
	Tortilla Chips	Little Bear, Kettle, Michael Seasons, Newman's Own, R.W. Garcia,
	Mini Rounds	**Garden of Eatin'**
	Frito Scoops	Fritos
	The Dud Chips (Corn Chips)	Robert's American Gourmet*
	Black Bean	**Garden of Eatin', Kettle, Simple Snacks**
	Red Chips	**Garden of Eatin'**
	Sesame Chips	**Garden of Eatin'**, Michael Season's*
	Tamari Chips	**Garden of Eatin'**
	Corn Chips, all kinds	Skinny Corn Chips*
	Cheese Puffs	Barbara's Bakery, **Little Bear, Michael Season's***
	Eat Smart Cheddars	Synder's of Hanvoer
	Cheddar Guppies	Good Health Snacks*
	Cheese Curls	**Michael Season's***
	Nacho Chips	**Little Bear, Newman's Own, Simple Snacks***, Skinny Sticks*
	Cinnamon Twists	**Sweet Organics***
	Personality Puffs	Robert's American Gourmet*
	Pirate's Booty	Robert's American Gourmet
	Veggie Booty	Robert's American Gourmet
	Garden Veggie	Skinny Sticks *
	Maui Wowie	Skinny Sticks*
	Onion	Skinny Sticks*
	Original Spud Snacks	Skinny Sticks*
	Broccoli, Carrot, Potato, Spinach, Tomato, or Veggies Stix, 3 0% less fat	Good Health Snacks*
	Soya, all flavors	Soya King*
	Plantain	Iselita's, Mariquitas

CHOCOLATE CHIPS (Please see BAKING INGREDIENTS)

CONDIMENTS

Description	Product	Brand Name
HOT SAUCE	Hot Sauce, mild	**Cholula**, Crystal's, Frank's, Louisiana, Sontava
MAYONNAISE	Canola Mayonnaise	Spectrum*
	Grape Seed Oil Mayonnaise	Vegenaise
	Mayonnaise	Duke's, Vegenaise
KETCHUP	Tomato	**Heinz**, Enrico, **Muir Glen,** Robbie's, **Tree of Life,** Westbrae
MUSTARD	Classic Yellow	**Eden's,** French's, **Tree of Life,** Westbrae
	Mustard, Dijon	Grey Poupon, **Tree of Life, Westbrae**

COOKIES

Description	Product	Brand Name
	Animal Cookies, van./choc.	**Country Choice***
	Brown Bear, vanilla/chocolate	Our Family Farm
	Wild Animal, vanilla	Our Family Farm
	Artic Bear Iced Lemon	Our Family Farm

Description	Product	Brand Name
	Snackimals, chocolate chip	Barbara's Bakery
	Arrowroot, vanilla	Healthy Time, Mi-Del, Newman's Own
	Chocolate Chip	Mi-Del Cookie Lovers, **Joseph's Sugar Free***, Newman Os, Tofutti, Westbrae
	Chocolate Chip, champion chip	**Newman's Own***
	Oatmeal Chocolate Chip	**Country Choice**
	Pecan Chocolate Chip	**Joseph's Sugar Free***
	Double Fudge Brownie	**Country Choice***
	Crème Supreme	Mi-Del Cookie Lovers*
	Crème Supreme, Chocolate	Mi-Del Cookie Lovers*
	Newman's Os, original	**Newman Os***
	Tops & Bottoms	**Newman Os**
	Cinnamon Grahams, alphabet	**Newman's Own**
	Cinnamon Honey Grahams	Mi-Del Cookie Lovers
	Oatmeal, wheat-free	Barbara's Bakery
	Peanut Butter	Mi-Del Cookie Lovers*
	Crispy Rice Bar	**EnviroKidz**
	Shortbread	Mi-Del Cookie Lovers*
	Chocolate Snaps	Mi-Del
	Ginger Snaps	Mi-Del
	Vanilla Snaps	Mi-Del
	Vanilla Wafers	**Country Choice**
	Monster Peanut Butter	**Tree of Life**
CRACKERS		
	Nut Thins, all flavors	Blue Diamond*
	Original Cheese Bites	**Barbara's Bakery**
	Cheddar Bunnies	**Annie's**
	Cheese Crackers	**Late July**
	Captain's Catch Baked Cheese	**Our Family Farm**
	Field Friends Baked Wheat	**Our Family Farm**
	Rite Light Rounds	**Barbara's Bakery**
	Classic Goldens, low-fat	**Tree of Life**
	Rice Crackers, plain	**Cedar's, Lundberg**
	Rice Cakes, apple/cinnamon	**Lundberg***
	Rice Cakes, butter caramel	**Lundberg***
	Rice Cakes, sesame tamari	**Lundberg**
	Rice Cakes, toasted sesame	**Lundberg**
	Oyster Crackers	Hain
DIPS		
SALSA	Salsa, mild	Desert Pepper, Enrico's, Jardine's, **Muir Glen,** Rio de Oro, Santa Barbara, Shot Gun Willies, **Walnut Acres**, Zapata
OTHER DIPS	Mild Nacho Cheese*	Enrico's
	Black Bean	**Bearitos** (fat-free), Desert Pepper, Enrico's
	Pinto Bean	Bearitos
	Onion Mix	Fantastic Foods*
	Veggie Bean, fat free	**Bearitos**

Description	Product	Brand Name

DRESSINGS, salad (Please see SAUCES / DRESSINGS / MARINADES)

DRINKS (please see WATER and SPRITZERS/SPORTS DRINKS)

EGGS

Description	Product	Brand Name
	Cage-free, DHA Omega-3	Gold Circle Farms, **Organic Valley**
	Cage-free, large	Eggland, Gold Circle Farms, Regional Brands , Tree of Life
	Grade A, large	Farmer's Pride, **Horizon*, Organic Valley,** The Happy Hen,
FROZEN PREPARED	Breakfast Munchies /cheese	Health is Wealth

FISH

Description	Product	Brand Name
FRESH!	Cod	Local Fish Store
	Haddock	Local Fish Store
	Halibut	Local Fish Store
	Salmon	Local Fish Store
	Sole	Local Fish Store
	Tuna	Local Fish Store
CANNED (Dolphin Safe!) Packed in water.	Tuna	Bumble Bee, Chicken of the Sea, Starkist
	Tongol Tuna, no salt	Tree of Life*, Miramonte
	Salmon	Bumble Bee, Chicken of the Sea, Miramonte, Natural Sea
FROZEN	Fish Sticks	Ian's Fish Sticks, Natural Sea
	Fish Fillets	Natural Sea
	Halibut	Ecco-Fish
	Mahi Mahi	Ecco-Fish, Omega Foods
	Salmon Burgers	Aquacuisine*, Ecco-Fish, Omega Foods
	Tuna Burgers	Aquacuisine*, Omega Foods

FRUIT

Description	Product	Brand Name
BARS	All Fruit Cobbler Flavors	Health Valley*
CANNED/JARS	Applesauce	Earth's Best, **Eden**, Motts (natural), **Santa Cruz**
	Apple Butter	**Eden**
	Mandarin Oranges	Dole, Geisha
	Pumpkin 100%	Libbys, Walnut Acres
DRIED	Banana Chips	Planet Harmony, Tree of Life
	Dried Cranberries	Ocean Spray (Craisins), Sun Sweet
	Raisins	**Pavich**, **Tree of Life**
FRESH FROZEN	Blueberries	Big Valley, **Cascadian Farms***, Dole, **Tree of Life***

Description	Product	Brand Name
	Dark Sweet Cherries	**Cascadian Farms, Tree of Life**
	Mixed Berries	**Cascadian Farms, Tree of Life**
	Mixed Fruit	**Tree of Life***
	Peaches	**Cascadian Farms***
	Strawberries	**Cascadian Farms**, Dole, **Tree of Life***
	All Store Name Brands, NO additives!	
JELS	All flavors	**Horizon**
JUICE (PURE) CONCENTRATES	Black Cherry	Knudsen, Tree of Life
	Grape	Knudsen, Tree of Life
	Wild Blueberry	Tree of Life
JUICE, 100% FROZEN	Apple	**Cascadian Farms**, Seneca
	Cranberry	**Cascadian Farms**
	Grape	**Cascadian Farms**
	Lemonade	**Cascadian Farms**
	Orange	**Cascadian Farms**, Minute Maid, Tropicana
	All Store Brand Names, NO additives!	
JUICE, 100% BOTTLED Best: not from concentrate	Apple Juice	After the Fall, Apple & Eve, **Knudsen**, Martinelli's, Tree of Life, Walnut Acres
	Oregon Berry	After the Fall
	Cranberry	Apple & Eve, After the Fall, Knudsen
	Grape Juice	Knudsen, Welch's
	Lemonade	After the Fall, Knudsen
	All Store Name Brands, NO additives, especially sugar!	
JUICE, 100% Refrigerated	Lemonade	Fresh Samantha*, Knudsen, Newman's Own Fresh
	Orange (calcium enriched!)	Dole, Florida Natural, **Horizon,** Indian River, Odwella*, **Organic Valley,** Tropicana
	Pineapple	Dole
	Tropical Fruit	Dole
	Desperately Seeking Susan	Fresh Samantha*
	Raspberry Juice	Fresh Samantha*
	Super Juice	Fresh Samantha*
	All Store Name Brands, NO additives, especially sugar!	
POUCHES/BOXES 100% juice	Koala Punch	After the Fall
	Oregon Berry	After the Fall
	Big Bird Apple Juice	Apple & Eve
	Bert & Ernie's Berry Juice	Apple & Eve
	Elmo's Punch	Apple & Eve
	Cranberry	Apple & Eve
	Very Berry	Apple & Eve
	Cranberry Grape	Apple & Eve
	Power Pouch	Apple & Eve
	Fruit Punch	Apple & Eve
	Juice Slam, all flavors	Hansen's (enriched)

Description	Product	Brand Name
FRUIT LEATHER	Great Grape	Stretch Island
	Chunky Cherry	Stretch Island
	Rare Raspberry	Stretch Island
	Sweet Strawberry	Stretch Island
PASTRIES Frozen	Apple Pie	**Amy's***, **Wholly Healthy Pies**
	Apple Turnover	The Fillo Factory*
	Blueberry, Cherry, Pumpkin	**Wholly Healthy Pies**
SPREADS/JAMS (no additives, no added sugar)	Blueberry	**Tree of Life,** Polaner, Sorrel Ridge, St. Dalfour
	Cherry	**Tree of Life**
	Grape	Polaner, Sorrel, Ridge, **Tree of Life**
	Raspberry, seedless	Polaner, Sorrel Ridge, **Tree of Life,**
	Strawberry	Polaner, Sorrel Ridge, St. Dalfour, **Tree of Life**
JELS	Juicy, All Fruit Flavors	**Horizon**

GRAVY MIXES (Please see SAUCES/DRESSINGS)

ICE CREAM, FROZEN YOGURT, FROZEN DESSERTS

Description	Product	Brand Name
	Chocolate Covered Bananas	Fruit Stix*
	100% Fruit Bars	Dole, **Natural Choices**, Welch's
	Lemon Popsicles	Cold Fusion*
	Pineapple Popsicles	Fruit Stix*
	Ice Cream, 100% reall	Ben and Jerry's, Breyer's, Haagen Daz, Julie's, **Stonyfield***
	Ice Cream Sandwiches	Tofu Cuties*
	Sorbet (no dyes)	Ben & Jerry's, Haagen Daz
	Yogurt, most are okay	Ben & Jerry's
	Waffle Cones	**Let's Do Organic!**

JAMS (Please see FRUIT, SPREADS/JAMS)

JUICE (Please see FRUIT/ BOTTLED, BOXED, FROZEN)

LUNCH BOXES

Description	Product	Brand Name
(Refrigerate)	Turkey Bologna	Applegate Farms
	Turkey Breast	Applegate Farms
	Pepperoni Pizza	Applegate Farms

MACARONI/PASTA and CHEESE

Description	Product	Brand Name
CANNED	All Stars	**Annie's***
	Bernio's	**Annie's***
	Cheesy Ravioli	**Annie's***
	Psghetti Loops	**Annie's***
	Arthur Loops	**Annie's***
BOXED	Shells & Wisconsin Cheese	**Annie's***
	Arthur's Mac and Cheese	**Annie's**

Description	Product	Brand Name
	Bunny Shaped Pasta/Cheese	**Annie's**
	Homestyle Macaroni & Cheese	**DeBoles**
	Mac & Cheese Meals (microwave)	**Annie's (single serving)**
FROZEN	Lasagna	**Annie's***
	Macaroni and Cheese	**Annie's***, **Cascadian Farms**
	Enchiladas, cheese	**Annie's***
	Lasagna, cheese	**Annie's***
	Lasagna, veggie	**Amy's**
	Ravioli, cheese	**Annie's***
	Toaster Pops, cheese	**Annie's***
	Spinach Cheese Appetizers	Fillo Factory*

MEAT (Please See BEEF, CHICKEN, OR TURKEY)

MILK

Description	Product	Brand Name
	Almond	Blue Diamond, Pacific
	Chocolate	**Horizon, Organic Valley**
	Coconut, lite	Native Forest, Thai Kitchen
	Cow's, 2% (reduced fat)	**Horizon, Organic Valley**
	Goat, chocolate	Oak Knoll Dairy*
	Rice, plain enriched	Harmony Farms, Rice Dream
	Rice, vanilla enriched	Harmony Farms, Rice Dream
	Rice & Soy	**Eden**
	Soy, plain enriched	**Eden**, Harmony Farms, **Pacific,** Soy Dream, Vita Soy
	Soy, vanilla enriched	**Eden**, Harmony Farms, **Pacific**, Silk
	Soy, chocolate	**Eden,** Vita Soy

NUTS/SEEDS (including NUT BUTTER)

Description	Product	Brand Name
BUTTER	Peanut Butter, creamy/crunchy	**Arrowhead Mills, Maranatha,** Smucker's (natural only), Spanky's, **Tree of Life***
	Almond Butter, creamy/crunchy	Kettle, **Maranatha**, **Tree of Life**
NUTS	Almonds, raw (chopped, ground, sliced, slivered, whole)	Blue Diamond*, Sunkist Nuts About Florida, **Woodstock Farms**
	Honey Roasted Almonds	Blue Diamond
	Almonds, tamari	**Tree of Life**, **Woodstock Farms**
	Peanuts in the Shell	Planters, Jumbo Jumbo
	Pecans, unsalted (chopped, shelled)	Blue Diamond, Nuts About Florida, Tree of Life, **Woodstock Farms**
	Pecans, ground	So. Georgia Pecan Company
	Walnuts, unsalted (chopped, ground, shelled)	Fisher's Chef, Nuts About Florida, Planter's, **Tree of Life, Woodstock Farms**
SEEDS Packaged	Pumpkin, raw	Nuts About Florida, **Tree of Life, Woodstock Farms**
	Sesame, raw	Arrowhead Mills, Bob's Red Mill, McCormick's, Tree of Life, **Woodstock Farms**
	Sunflower, raw	Nuts About Florida, **Woodstock Farms**

Raw nuts/seeds are found in bulk bins in many stores. Check ingredients!

Description	Product	Brand Name
OILS & VINEGARS		
OIL 100% Pure	Canola Oil	**Arrowhead Mills**, Hain, **Spectrum*, Tree of Life**
	Coconut Oil	Garden of Life**, Spectrum, Tree of Life**
	Flaxseed Oil	**Arrowhead Mills, Spectrum, Tree of Life**
	Olive Oil, extra virgin	Colavita, Da Vinci, Filippo Berio, **Gia Russa, Hain**, Pompeian, **Spectrum*, Tree of Life**
	Sesame Oil	Hain, Loriva, Spectrum*, Tree of Life
	Sesame Oil, toasted	**Eden**, Loriva, Spectrum*
NON-STICK SPRAYS (one second!)	Canola Spray	PAM, **Spectrum***
	Olive Oil Spray	PAM, **Spectrum***
VINEGAR (raw, unfiltered)	Apple Cider	Bragg, Hain, **Spectrum, Tree of Life,**
	Balsamic	Regina, **Spectrum***
PASTA (Please see MACARONI/PASTA AND CHEESE)		
BOXED	Angel Hair	**DeBoles, Venecia**
	Alphabet (vegetable)	**Eden**
	Bowtie	**DeBoles**, Hodgson Mills, **Venecia**
	Couscous, parmesan	Near East
	Elbows	**Bionature (gluten-free), DeBoles, Venecia**
	Fettucini	**DeBoles, Venecia**
	Lasagna	**DeBoles*, Venecia**
	Linguini	**Bionature (gluten-free), DeBoles, Venecia**
	Penne	**Annie's, Bionature (gluten-free), DeBoles*, Venecia**
	Ribbon	**De Boles**
	Rotini	**Annie's, DeBoles, Venecia**
	Shells	**DeBoles**, Hodgson Mills, **Venecia**
	Spaghetti	**Annie's, Bionature (gluten-free), De Boles**, Hodgson Mills, **Venecia**
	Ziti	**DeBoles, Venecia**
	Rice Pasta, wheat-free	**DeBoles**, Pasteriso, **Pinkyada**
	Spelt Pasta	Purity Foods, Vita Spelt*
	Whole Wheat	**Annie's, DeBoles, Hodgson Mills**
PASTA/PIZZA SAUCE (For canned tomato products, please see Tomatoes.)		
	Marinara	**Amy's**, Enrico's, **MOM's, Muir Glen, Walnut Acres**
	Tomato Basil	**Amy's**, Classico, Colavita, Enrico's, Garden Valley*, Gia Russa, **Muir Glen, Walnut Acres**
	Vegetables	Garden Valley
	Spaghetti	**Eden**, MOM's
	Roasted Garlic	**Enrico's**, Garden Valley*, **Muir Glen**
	Pizza Sauce	**Eden**, Enrico's**, MOM's, Muir Glen**

Description	Product	Brand Name
PIZZA		
FROZEN	Pepperoni Pizza	**Bravissimo**
	Pizza, cheese	**Amy's***
	Pocket Cheese Pizza	**Amy's***
	Spinach Cheese Pizza	**Amy's***
	Spinach Feta Pizza	**Amy's***
	Soy Cheese Pizza	**Bravissimo***
	4 Cheese Pizza	**Bravissimo**
	5 Cheese and Tomato	California Pizza Kitchen
	Tofu Pizza Munchies	Health is Wealth*
	Cheese Pizza Munchies	Health is Wealth
	Pizza Bagels	Health is Wealth
POPCORN		
POPPING	Original Popcorn, microwave	**Simple Snacks**
BAGGED	Buttery Popcorn	**Bearitos**
	White Cheddar	**Bearitos**
	Butter Popcorn Rice Cakes	Hain
	Plain Popcorn Rice Cakes	Hain
POULTRY (Please see CHICKEN or TURKEY)		
POWER SHAKE POWDERS		
PROTEIN	Strawberry	Atkins
	Vanilla	Atkins, ZONE
	Chocolate	ZONE
	Simply Natural (Spiruteen)	Nature's Plus
	Plain	ZONE
	Soy Essence (Fermented)	Jarrow Formula's
SUPER GREENS	Original	Greens+
PRETZELS		
	Alpha Pretzels	Good Health Snacks*
	Peanut Butter Pretzels	Good Health Snacks*
	Waffle Pretzels*	Good Health Snacks*
	Honey Pretzels	Henry's
	Sourdough Pretzels	Henry's
	Pretzels, all kinds	**Newman's Own**
	Classic Mini	**Synder of Hanover**
	Honey Wheat	**Synder of Hanover**
	Spelt Pretzels	Good Health Snacks*
FROZEN	Soft Pretzels	SuperPretzel
PRODUCE (for FROZEN please FRUIT or VEGETABLES)		
FRUIT	FRESH, All Kinds!	Organic, Local Farmers, Grocery Store, Regional/Local Brands, Dole

Description	Product	Brand Name
VEGETABLE	FRESH, All Kinds!	**Organic,** Local Farmers, Grocery Store, Regional/Local Brands, **Bunny Love**, Dole, **Earthbound Farms**, Fresh Express, New Star

PUDDING

Description	Product	Brand Name
	Rice	Kozy Shack, **Natural By Nature**
	Chocolate	**Horizon, Natural By Nature**
	Vanilla	**Horizon, Natural By Nature**

RICE (For Rice Cakes, please see CRACKERS)

Description	Product	Brand Name
BOXED	Rice Pilaf	Near East
BAGGED	Spanish Rice Pilaf	Near East
	Basmati Brown Rice	Cache River, Fantastic Foods, **Lundberg**
	Basmati White Rice	Cache River, Fantastic Foods, **Lundberg***
	Brown, short	**Arrowhead Mills**, **Lundberg,** Mahatma
	Quick Cooking, brown	**Arrowhead Mills**, Carolina's, Konrico, Uncle Ben's
	Risotto	Rice Select, **Lundberg***
	Risotto, tomato basil	Spice Hunter, **Lundberg***
	Risotto, creamy parmesan	Spice Hunter, **Lundberg***
	Kasmati	Rice Select
	Texmati, brown	Rice Select
	Texmati, white	Rice Select
	Sushi, white	**Lundberg**
	Sushi	Rice Select
	Rice may be found in bulk bins in many stores. Check ingredients!	

SALAD DRESSINGS (Pleases see SAUCES/DRESSINGS)

SALSA (Please see DIPS)

SAUCES/DRESSINGS (Please see PASTA/PIZZA SAUCE for SPAGHETTI SAUCE)

HOT SAUCE (Please see CONIDMENTS)

Description	Product	Brand Name
SALAD DRESSINGS/MARINADES		
	Balsamic	Annie's, Blanchards, Newman's Own, **Spectrum***
	BBQ	Bone Suckin'Sauce, Bubba's, Enrico's, **Muir Glen**, Robbie's, Shot Gun Willie's, Stubb's
	Bragg Liquid Aminos	Bragg
	Caesar	Cardini, Newman's Own, **Spectrum***
	Garlic Sesame	Premier Japan
	Creamy Garlic	**Spectrum***
	Ginger	**Eden,** Miko Sauces

Description	Product	Brand Name
	Ginger Garlic Vinagrette	**Spectrum***
	Pad Thai	Thai Kitchen
	Roasted Garlic Peanut	Miko Sauces
	Peanut Sauce, original recipe	San-J, Satay, Thai Kitchen
	Sloppy Joe	**Bearitos, Simply Organic**
	Ranch	Newman's Own
	Sweet & Sour	Robbie's
	Taco Seasoning Mix	**Bearitos**, Casa Fiesta
	Tamari	San-J
	Teriyaki	San-J
	Three Cheese & Italian Spices	Stone Oven
	Toasted Sesame	Miko Sauces, **Spectrum***
	Worcestershire	Robbie's
GRAVY MIXES	Brown	Hain, Natural Touch, **Simply Organic**
	Chicken	Hain, Lysander's, Natural Touch, **Simply Organic**
DESSERT	Chocolate Sauce	Ah!Laska*, Wax Orchards
SEASONINGS		
SALT	Sea Salt	Alessi, Baleine, Celtic, Eden, Fresh Atlantic, Hain,
	Salt, kosher	David's Kosher
	Seasoning Salt	Café Sole, Gomasio, Herbamare, Jane's, Crazy Mixed Up Seasonings, Mrs. Dash, Old Bay, Spice Garden Spike
HERBS/SPICES (Non-irradiated, only!)	BBQ	Stubb's Spice Rub
	Blackened Redfish Magic	Chef Paul Prudhomme's
	Blackened Steak Magic	Chef Paul Prudhomme's
	Cayenne	Frontier, Spice Garden, **Simply Organic, Spice Hunter**
	Cinnamon, ground	Frontier, Spice Garden, **Simply Organic, Spice Hunter**
	Garlic, dehydrated	Spice World
	Italian Seasoning	Spice Garden
	Meat Magic	Chef Paul Prudhomme's
	Mexican Seasoning	Frontier, Spice Garden
	Nutmeg, ground	Frontier, Spice Garden, **Simply Organic, Spice Hunter**
	Oregano	Frontier, Spice Garden, **Simply Organic, Spice Hunter**
	Paprika	Frontier, Spice Garden, **Simply Organic, Spice Hunter**
	Parsley	Frontier, **Simply Organic, Spice Hunter**
	Pizza/Pasta Magic	Chef Paul Prudhomme's
	Poultry Magic	Chef Paul Prudhomme's
	Poultry Seasoning	Café Sole, Frontier, Spice Garden
	Rosemary	Frontier, Spice Garden, **Simply Organic, Spice Hunter**

Description	Product	Brand Name
	Salad Herbs	Spice Garden
	Seafood Grill	Café Sole
	Tarragon	Frontier, Spice Garden, **Simply Organic, Spice Hunter**
	Veggie Magic	Chef Paul Prudhomme's
SOUPS		
BROTH		
	Beef , boxed	Kitchen Basics
	Beef Flavored, canned	Health Valley
	Chicken, canned	Health Valley, Shelton's, Walnut Acres
	Chicken, boxed	Imagine, Kitchen Basics, Pacific
	Vegetable, cubes	Morga, Vegex
	Vegetable, canned	**Amy's**, Health Valley, **Walnut Acres**
	Vegetable, boxed	**Imagine**, Kitchen Basics, Pacific
PREPARED CANNED	Chicken Noodle	Hain, Health Valley, Shelton's, **Walnut Acres**
	Chicken Rice	**Walnut Acres**
	Chicken Tortilla	**Shelton's**
	Minestrone	**Health Valley, Walnut Acres** Westbrae
	Split Pea	Hain, Westbrae
	Tomato Vegetable	**Health Valley**
	Cream of Tomato	**Walnut Acres**
	Tomato Tuscany	Westbrae
SOUR CREAM		
	Sour Cream	Alta Dena, Axelrod, Cabot, Daisy, **Horizon***, **Organic Valley***
SPRITZERS/SPORT DRINKS		
SPRITZERS	Cherry Cola	**Blue Sky,** Knudsen, Reed's
	China Cola	Reed's
	Cola	**Blue Sky**
	Lemon Lime	**Blue Sky**, Knudsen
	Ginger Ale	**Blue Sky,** Knudsen
	Apricot/Peach	Wild Fruitz*
	Orange Huckleberry/Blueberry	Wild Fruitz*
	Raspberry	**Blue Sky**, Wild Fruitz*
	Root Beer	**Blue Sky**, Hansen's, Reed's
	Sparkling Apple	Knudsen
	Sparkling Cranberry	Knudsen
	Sparkling Cider	After the Fall, Martinelli
	Sparkling Concord Grape	After the Fall
	Vanilla Cream	**Blue Sky**, Hansen's
SPORT DRINKS	Lemon	Recharge*
	Orange	Recharge*
	Tropical	Recharge*

Description	Product	Brand Name
SUGAR		
DRY	Brown Sugar	**Hain**
	Pure Cane Sugar, white, brown	Dixie Crystals, **Hain**
	Dehydrated Sugar	Esculent
	Date Sugar	Tree of Life
	Natural Sugar	Florida Crystals
	Fructose	Esculent
	Powdered Sugar (confectioner's)	Dixie Crystals, **Hain**
	Sucanat	Wholesome
	Turbinado, raw	Balance, Esculent, Hain, Sugar in the Raw
	Golden Natural Turbinado	Dixie Crystals
SYRUP	Honey,	Bee Natural, Joe's, Local Brands
	Honey, raw clover	Tree of Life
	Honey, raw orange	Tree of Life
	Honey, wild flower, unfiltered	Bee Natural
	Molasses, blackstrap	Plantation, Slow As, Tree of Life, Wholesome
	Barley Malt	**Eden**
	Brown Rice	**Lundberg**
	Maple, 100% pure	**Great Northern**, Maple Grove Farm of Vermont, **Shady Maple Farms**, **Spring Tree**, Tree of Life, **Upcountry**
SUPPLEMENTS		
	Vitamin C, Chewable	Natrol, N.F. Factors
	Yummi Bear , full line	Hero Nutritional Products *
	Yummi Bear Child Bright, am/pm	Hero Nutritional Products
	Rhino Vits	Nutrition Now*
	Essential Fatty Acids (EFAs)	Health From the Sun, Nordic Naturals, Spectrum, Tree of Life
	Flaxseed Oil, liquid	**Spectrum, Tree of Life**
	Grape Seed Extract	Orange Peel Enterprises
	Sea Buddies Multi Vitamins	Enzymatic Therapy
	Veggie Multi-Vitamin	Kid Bear*
	Kids Chewable Vitamins	Natrol
	Animal Friends, chewable	Twin Lab
	Baby Bear Vitamins with Bears	Yummy Bears*
	Vitamins and Minerals	Yummy Bears*
	Enzymes	Blue Bonnet, Rainbow Light
	Probiotic Cultures	BioK+, Kyolic, Natren, Nature's Way
	Dr. Vanessa's Formula	Dr. Vanessa's Formulas
	Zand's Supplements for Children	Zand Herbal Formulas
POWDERED (multi-vitamins)	Vitamin C (Super Orange Tangerine, Tropical)	Emergen C

PROTEIN SHAKES (Please see POWER SHAKE POWDERS)

Description	Product	Brand Name
READY TO DRINK	Vanilla.	Balance*, Imagine*, Zone
	Chocolate	Balance*, Imagine*, Zone
TACO SHELLS		
	Shells, corn	**Bearitos,** Casa Fiesta
TEA		
	Green Tea	Bigelow, Celestial Seasonings,
	Lemon Zinger	Bigelow, Celestial Seasonings,
	Peppermint	Bigelow, Celestial Seasonings
TOASTER POPS		
	All Fruit Flavors	**Amy's***
	Cheese	**Amy's***
TOMATOES (For spaghetti sauces, please see Pasta/Pizza Sauces)		
CANNED	Crushed	**Eden**
	Diced	**Eden**, Hunts, **Muir Glen**, **Walnut Acres**
	Paste	Contadina, Goya, **Muir Glen**
	Peeled, tomato/basll	Progresso
	Peeled, whole	Cento, **Delallo, Muir Glen, Walnut Acres**
	Puree	Contindina, **Muir Glen**, Progresso, **Walnut Acres**
	Sauce	Hunt's, **Muir Glen, Walnut Acre**
TURKEY (free-range!)		
DELI	Bologna	Applegate Farms*
	Franks (dogs)	Applegate Farms*
	Salami	Applegate Farms*
	Slices, roasted (pkg.)	Applegate Farms*
	Slices, roasted	Boar's Head (Golden Roasted ONLY), Dietz and Watson
FRESH CUTS	Ground	Bell & Evans, Shady Brooks Farms
	Tenderloin	Bell & Evans
FROZEN/ REFRIGERATED	Bacon	Applegate Farms*
	Breasts, boneless	**Organic Valley**, Shelton's*
	Bolonga	Shelton's*
	Burgers	Shelton's*
	Franks	Applegate Farms, Shelton's*
	Meatballs	Shelton's*
	Pot Pie	Shelton's*
	Sausage Links	Applegate Farms, Shelton's*
	Sausage Patties	Shelton's*
	Strips	Shelton's*
	Tenders	Bell & Evans*
	Turkey, whole	Bell & Evans, Diestel, Mary's, **Organic Valley, Shelton's***

Description	Product	Brand Name
VEGETABLES (For FRESH, please see PRODUCE)		
CANNED/JARS	Artichoke Hearts	Fanci Foods, Progresso, Reese, Vigro
	Bamboo Shoots	La Choy, Hoken
	Olives	Goya, Lindsay, Santa Barbara
	Water Chestnuts	La Choy, Hoken
FROZEN	Artichoke Hearts Broccoli Florets, Carrots Corn, Green Beans Mixed Vegetables, Peas String Beans, Spinach	Bird's Eye, **Cascadian Farms**, Green Giant, **Tree of Life**
	Potatoes (French Fries, Hash Browns, Oven Fries, Shoe String, Spud Puppies) ss	**Cascadian Farms, Tree of Life**
	ALL Store Name Brand Vegetables, No additives	
VEGGIE BURGERS/NUGGETS		
FROZEN	All American Burgers	**Amy's**
	Original Burgers	**Gardenburgers**
	Chicken Burgers	Health is Wealth*,
	Chicken Free Nuggets	Health is Wealth*, Lightlife
	Chicken Free Patties	Health is Wealth*
	Corn Dogs	Shelton's
	Fakin' Bacon, Smokey	Lightlife
	Smart Bacon	Lightlife
	Gimme Lean Sausages	Lightlife
	Pepperoni	El Burrito, Vegi-Deli*
VITAMINS/MINERALS (Please see SUPPLEMENTS)		
WAFFLES		
FROZEN	Gorilla Banana Waffles	**EnviroKidz**
	Mini Homestyle Waffles, original	**Van's***
	Mini Homestyle Waffles, chocolate	**Van's**
	Wheat-Free Waffles, apple	**Van's**
	Wheat-Free Waffles, blueberry	**Van's***
	Wheat-Free Waffles, cinnamon	**Van's**
	Chocolate Chip Mini Waffles	**Van's***
	Koala Chocolate	**EnviroKidz**
WATER!		
BOTTLED	Artesian Spring	Eden, Figi
	Genuine Spring Water	Crystal Springs, Eldorado Natural Springs
	Pure Spring	Deer Park
	Natural Spring	Crystal Geyser, Evian
	Spring	Aberfoyle Springs, Dannon Springs, Iceland Spring, Poland Springs, Volvic, Zehpyrhills

Description	Product	Brand Name
WATER!		
BOTTLED	Purified	Aquafina, Dasani
	All Vitamin/Sports Waters	Glaceau*
	All Smart Waters	Glaceau*
WHIPPED CREAM		
	Whipped Cream	Natural By Natural
	Sun Soy Whipped Cream	White Wave
YOGURTS		
(with live cultures)	Banilla	**Stonyfield***
	Banilla Blast	**Stonyfield**
	Blueberry, low-fat	Cascadian Fresh, **Horizon**, **Stonyfield**
	Lemon, low-fat	**Stonyfield**
	Maple, low-fat	**Stonyfield**
	Plain, low-fat	Axelrod, **Brown Cow**, Dannon, **Horizon, Stonyfield**
	Raspberry, low-fat	**Horizon, Stonyfield**
	Strawberry, low-fat	Cascadian Fresh, **Horizon**, **Stonyfield**
	Strawberries & Bananas, low-fat	**Horizon, Stonyfield**
	Strawberry Vanilla	**Stonyfield***
	Vanilla, low-fat	**Horizon, Stonyfield**
	Yo-Self, all flavors	**Stonyfield**
	Yo-Squeeze (peach, raspberry, strawberry)	**Stonyfield***
	Yo-Yos. low-fat, all flavors	**Horizon**
	Tubes, low-fat, all flavors	**Horizon**
	Tubes, low-fat, all flavors	**Horizon**
	ALL Store Name Brands, NO additives, especially sugar.	

NOTES:

The organic symbol (bold letters) means the product is 100% organic or partially organic. They have had to meet one of the four organic categories identified by the FDA.

Look for store brand name products that contain ingredients with no additives. Please read the labels.

Just because one product from a brand name collection is recommended, does not mean we recommend the rest of the line.

If your local supermarket does not stock any foods or drinks listed, ask them to do so. Most are available to them through their distributors. Use this Better Choices Grocery List for easy to prepare foods and drinks for your family.

It is your safety net. Your kids will like a lot of the foods from the above grocery list. These foods better meet the fueling requirements of growing children. Use this list and your kids won't be running on empty, anymore!

Grocery Update

Since the writing of this book, food manufacturers have begun to respond to the concern of increasing obesity and diabetes among children. As a result, some Better Food Choices are showing up on the grocery shelves. Please refer to the Web site, www.betterfoodchoices.com for updates.

14

Supplements: Vitamins and Minerals Kids Need Them

Chapter Quick Facts

- One in six children are seriously deficient in calcium. Thirty-three percent are deficient in iron. About 50 percent are deficient in zinc. Over 80 percent are deficient in magnesium. One in six lack vitamin A. Nearly 50 percent are seriously deficient in vitamin C. Nearly 33 percent are deficient in vitamin B^6. One in 7 are deficient in vitamin B^{12}.[168]
- Nutrients deficiency in kids may lead to illnesses such as autoimmune diseases, ADD, earaches, depression, and obesity.
- There are two kinds of vitamins: fat-soluble (A, D, E, K) and water-soluble (B, C, and more). All are important for a growing mind and body. So are EFAs.
- Minerals are both organic and inorganic compounds that support hard tissues (bone, teeth), and soft tissues (muscles, nerves) plus bodily fluids (blood).
- Not all supplements are equal. Reasons: lower-grade source, artificial ingredients, added fillers, added artificial sweeteners, packaging, shipping, and storage reduce potency.
- Good supplements are not a waste of money. They serve as health insurance.
- Bare minimum supplement recommendations for healthy kids: Multivitamin and mineral, EFAs (500 milligrams), and vitamin C (500 milligrams)

Supplements: Vitamins and Minerals Kids Need Them

When you look at the facts, it is clear that kids do need supplements. If you already accept this truth, then simply jump to the last page for recommended brand names of supplements for your kids. If you need convincing, read on!

Simply put, when kids are not supplying their bones, tissue, and organs with the vitamins they need, they become a target for vitamin-deficient illnesses. When kids are not supplying their tissue and organs with the amount of minerals they need, they are vulnerable to mineral deficient illnesses. The incidences of autoimmune diseases, diabetes, ADD, ADHD, asthma, ear infections, colds and flu, depression, and obesity are way up. Many other reported illnesses among children are on the rise. These days, kids are not eating the foods that supply them essential bio-available (easily digested) nutrients. Most of the foods eaten by the junk food generation contain few to none. Kathi Kemper, M.D., director of the Center at Children's Hospital in Boston said, "... studies show that kids don't eat healthy diets. Fewer than 1 percent meet their RDA (recommended daily allowance) for vitamins through diet." If kids would eat according to the traditional dietary guidelines, they would provide themselves with many needed nutrients. Three problems are a reality.

- Most kids do not eat according to any guidelines.
- The guidelines, themselves, are insufficient.
- Most were written for an average adult's needs, not a growing child's.

You know that your kids are not eating the number of servings suggested by the USDA Food Pyramid. Just know that you are not alone. We would bet that most kids are not aligned with our Food Circles™ recommendations either. (Please refer to Chapter One.) This is why your kids probably need supplements. Consulting a licensed health professional is advisable.

Kids Use Up A Lot of Vitamins and Minerals

All day, your son and daughter's body are gobbling up, using, and dispersing any nutrients they are eating, just to support their daily demands. Those involved in sports and the performing arts are particularly in need of a supporting pool of nutrients. When not enough vitamins or minerals are consumed to meet your kids' needs, their bodies turns to readily available fat, bones, and other tissues in order to keep their command centers humming, machines purring, and hearts ticking. A good example of the body supplying nutrients from its own resource shows up in a calcium deficiency condition. Your son or daughter's bones will actually sacrifice their contents in order to supply the calcium needed for the normal function of the muscles, including the heart. Yes, it will eat itself, taking what it needs for survival from wherever it can be supplied. And there is a second priority, ample nutrient availability needed to support healthy growth. If metabolized nutrients are not provided by the foods they are eating, they must be supplemented. If not, the growth of healthy bones, organs, and tissue will be sacrificed as time passes. Vitamin and mineral deficiencies can affect the growth of the body, negatively. Unhealthy organs create unhealthy kids. Sometime this shows up when they are children. Sometimes the collective damage does not show up until later in life, during adulthood.

Nutrient-Deficient Kids Suffer

The message, feed kids nutrient-filled fruits, vegetables, grains, fish, poultry, beef, and some good fats, is falling on deaf ears. The following facts are frightening:

Common Deficiencies in Children[1]

- One in six are seriously deficient in calcium.
- 33 percent of children are deficient in iron.
- About 50 percent lack sufficient zinc.
- Over 80 percent are deficient in magnesium.
- One in six lack vitamin A.
- Nearly 50 percent are seriously deficient in vitamin C.
- Nearly 33 percent are deficient in vitamin B^6.
- One in seven are deficient in vitamin B^{12}.
- One in five are deficient in folate (folic acid).
- Nearly 3 million, between six and seventeen years, suffer high blood pressure.

Please note that these facts were published in 1992. Eleven years later, the quality of food supply has continued to diminish so it is reasonable to assume that the number of kids suffering from nutrient deficiencies is higher. Isn't this hard to believe? Believe it.

It is staggering to note that almost all kids are deficient of magnesium. Magnesium builds bones, metabolizes blood sugar, monitors blood pressure, metabolizes vitamin C, calcium, protein, phosphorous, vitamin Bs and enzymes, strengthens the heart, protects arteries, nourishes and calms nerves, relaxes muscles, supports the immune system, makes DNA and RNA and regulates the body's temperature. Your kids' lives depend on this multitasked workhorse. Yet, over 80 percent of children are deficient in magnesium. Can you imagine the consequences? Magnesium is just one of the ten deficiencies listed. We, as a society, have a potential monstrous mental and physical health crisis in process. The shortage of nutrient consumption has been and will continue to take a toll on the health of kids organs and bodily systems. "Every study reveals deficiencies or sub-optimal intakes of many micronutrients. This is a large part of the reason why we have so much heart disease, cancer, osteoporosis and other life-shortening degenerative diseases. Diet and nutrient-deficiency related degenerative diseases kill more Americans than anything else."[2] Most diseases begin with poor eating habits during childhood. It is time to supplement.

What Are Supplements?

Our reliable wordsmith, Daniel Webster, defines supplements as "that with which anything is made full or whole; a filling up. Something added, especially to make up for a lack or deficiency."[3] In dietary supplements, that something added should be a nutrient that is well absorbed and utilized in the human body. Vitamins, minerals and other food factor supplements provide nutritional support for good health. They are available in tablet, capsule, powder, and liquid forms. Nutritional supplements for kids are designed to keep them from running on empty. They are meant to be helpful in filling them up! Plus, they are to assist in the prevention of every day viral illnesses (colds, flu), challenging bacterial infections (strep throat), and serious diseases such as cancer.

KIDS NEED SUPPLEMENTS. GOOD SUPPLEMENTS

When your son and daughter is not consuming enough nutrient-filled foods, careful use of supplementation, under the guidance of a licensed health professional, is advised.

Vitamins are Vital

Vitamins are organic compounds that your son or daughter needs for growth, maintenance, and repair. They are essential to the metabolism of all living organisms. Research to date, has identified up to seventeen vitamins. When they are not supplied through foods, supplements can save the day!

Below is a vitamin chart that includes some of their functions and sources. Please note that there are two groups of vitamins, fat- and water-soluble.

Fat-Soluble Vitamins are made biologically available for absorption in the body only when there is fat present upon digestion. They need to be consumed with meals.

Fat-Soluble Vitamins	Makes, Maintains, Strengthens
Vitamin A	Blood, bones, digestive tract, eyes, hair, immune system, lungs, hair, mucous membranes, skin, teeth. FOODS: Fish (cod, halibut, salmon, tuna), beef, yellow fruits and vegetables, white cheese, egg yolks, Vitamin-A fortified milk, dark-green leafy veggies (spinach), broccoli, carrots, yams, blueberries.
Vitamin D	Bones, immune system, muscles, teeth, thyroid, FOODS: Sunshine! Tuna, salmon, sea bass, swordfish, butter, fortified milk, egg yolks.
Vitamin E	Blood, cells, enzymes, heart, muscles, nerves, skin, tissues FOODS: Green leafy veggies, legumes (beans), whole wheat flour, nuts, wheat germ, vegetable oils (most), egg yolks, butter, seeds, spinach, yams.
Vitamin K	Blood, bones, gallbladder, liver FOODS: Dark-green leafy veggies (spinach), broccoli, cabbage, cauliflower, peas, potatoes, vegetable oils, most fruits.

Water-Soluble Vitamins are biologically available for absorption in the body in water. They should be taken when there is food present in the stomach to avoid indigestion.

Water-Soluble Vitamins	Makes, Maintains, Strengthens
Vitamin B[1] (Thiamine)	Digestive tract, heart, intestines, muscles, nerves, stomach FOODS: Blueberries, peas, nuts, rice, soybeans, lima beans, peanuts, oatmeal, whole grains, poultry, fish.
Vitamin B[2] (Riboflavin)	Adrenal glands, cells, digestive tract, eyes, hair, nails, skin FOODS: Blueberries, green leafy veggies (spinach!), asparagus, avocados, broccoli, brussels sprouts, whole grains, tuna, salmon, almonds, egg yolks, yogurt, cheese, milk, legumes (beans),mushrooms.
Vitamin B[3] (Niacin)	Blood, cells, hormones, nerves, skin, tongue FOODS: Poultry, fish (tuna, cod, halibut, salmon), beef, egg yolks, nuts, whole grains, peas, green beans, sunflower seeds, avocados, broccoli, carrots, dates.

Water-Soluble Vitamins	Makes, Maintains, Strengthens
Vitamin B^{6} (Pyridoxine)	Blood, digestive tract, immune system, nerves, skin FOODS: Avocados, spinach, green leafy veggies, broccoli, green beans, legumes (beans), nuts, potatoes, eggs, fish (tuna, halibut, salmon), oatmeal, sunflower seeds, walnuts, whole grains, bananas, soybeans, poultry.
Vitamin B^{12} (Cobalamin)	Blood, digestive tract, nerves, whole body FOODS: Poultry, fish (haddock, tuna), beef, lamb, egg yolks, milk, yogurt, cheese, sea veggies (mostly found in animal foods).
Biotin	Bones, digestive tract, hair, nerves, skin, sweat glands FOODS: Fish (haddock, halibut, tuna), chicken, lamb, eggs, dark-green leafy veggies, green beans, nuts, cauliflower, raspberries, oranges, grapefruit, legumes (beans), whole grains.
Folic Acid (Folate)	Cells, blood, genes, hair, liver, nerves, skin, whole body FOODS: Green leafy veggies (kale, spinach, beet greens), broccoli, brussels sprouts, sweet potatoes, asparagus, legumes (beans, especially black-eyed peas), salmon, egg yolks, oranges, bananas.
Vitamin B^{5} (Pantothenic Acid)	Digestive tract, hormones, sinuses, whole body FOODS: Fresh vegetables, fish (especially salt-water varieties), eggs, mushrooms, sweet potatoes, corn, soybeans, beans, nuts.
Vitamin C	Adrenal glands, blood vessels, bones, connective tissue, digestive tract, enzymes, gums, immune system, ligaments, nerves, skin, teeth, tissue FOODS: Citrus fruits, tomatoes, strawberries, blueberries, blackberries, cherries, guava, melon, dark-green leafy veggies (beet greens, collards, kale, turnip greens, spinach), green and red bell peppers, yellow potatoes, broccoli, parsley, watercress, cabbage, papaya, kiwi, asparagus, cantaloupe.

Minerals Are Essential

Minerals are both organic and inorganic compounds that are essential for hard tissues (bone, teeth), and soft tissue (muscles, nerves) plus bodily fluids (blood and tissue). Of the multitude of minerals existing, seventeen have been found to be necessary for optimal body functions. Minerals are difficult for the body to absorb, so it is best to take them with meals. Magnesium is the exception. We advise it to be taken with calcium before bedtime to help with relaxation, anxiety release, nervous disorders, and stress.

Minerals and Trace Minerals

Minerals	**Makes, Maintains, Supports**
Calcium	Blood, bones, cell membranes, enzymes, heart, immune system, muscles, nerves, teeth FOODS: Citrus fruits, dark-green leafy veggies (collards, kale, mustard, spinach, turnip greens), broccoli, legumes (soybeans), peas, salmon, nuts, broccoli, cabbage, sea veggies, dairy products.
Iron	Blood, cells, immune system, whole body FOODS: Egg yolks, green leafy veggies (spinach), peas, fish, potatoes, whole grains, poultry, red meat, legumes (beans, tofu).
Magnesium	Arteries, blood, bones, digestive tract, genes, heart, immune system, nerves, body temperature FOODS: Fresh green vegetables dairy products, most meats and seafood (salmon), nuts (almonds) soybeans, seeds, whole grains, potatoes, bananas, apples, milk.
Phosphorous	Bone, cells, digestive tract, genes, heart, kidneys, muscles, nerves, teeth. FOODS: Fish, poultry, meat, egg yolks, legumes (beans), peas, whole grains, dairy products (yogurt).
Potassium	Blood, cells, digestive tract, heart, muscles, nerves, kidney FOODS: Blueberries, citrus fruits, bananas, cantaloupe, avocados, broccoli, lima beans, meats, poultry, fish, nuts, seeds, milk, yogurt.
Zinc	Digestive tract eyes, hair, immune system, nails, nerves, reproductive system, skin, whole body FOODS: Seafood, poultry (dark meat), beef, egg yolks, whole grains (wheat bran, oatmeal), nuts, peas, carrots, spinach, sunflower seeds.

Trace Minerals	**Makes, Maintains, Supports**
Boron	Brain, bone, hormones FOODS: Spinach, fruits, veggies, salmon (canned)
Chromium	Blood, brain FOODS: Fresh fruits and veggies, legumes (beans), peas, whole grains, dairy products.
Copper	Blood, bone, cells, genes, hair, muscles, nerves, skin, tissue FOODS: Cherries, raisins, poultry, shellfish, nuts, whole grains, egg yolks, legumes (beans), peas, avocados.

Trace Minerals	**Makes, Maintains, Supports**
Iodine	Digestive tract, hair, nails, skin, teeth, thyroid FOODS: Seafood, iodized sea salt, Celtic salt, sea veggies.
Manganese	Blood sugar, bone, nerves, tissue FOODS: Spinach, egg yolks, avocados, blueberries, nuts (pecans, hazelnuts), seeds, sea veggies, whole grains.
Molybdenum	Cells, immune system, kidneys, liver FOODS: Dark-green leafy veggies, beans, legumes, peas, whole grains.
Selenium	Cells, immune system, skin, thyroid, whole body FOODS: Soybeans, nuts (Brazils!), pineapples, seafood, chicken, garlic, whole grains.
Silica (silicon)	Arteries, bone, hair, nails, skin, tissue FOODS: Beets, dark-green leafy veggies, brown rice, bell peppers, soybeans, beef, eggs.
Sodium	Blood, muscles, nerves FOODS: All foods.
Sulfur	Immune system, liver, skin FOODS: Eggs, seafood, cabbage, brussel sprouts, kale, garlic, soybeans, turnips.

This simple chart is designed so you may quickly and easily identify the body parts and the related general functions of the vitamins and minerals. More in-depth explanations of the functions are found in many books and on several Websites. Some books include: *Prescription of Natural Healing, The Nutrition Almanac, Nutrition Made Simple, The Real Vitamin & Mineral Book, Vitamin Bible, and Smart Medicine for a Healthier Child.*

EFAs (Essential Fatty Acids) Are Left Out

A category of food that is not mandated for identification by the FDA (Food and Drug Administration) is essential fatty acids. EFAs are necessary for proper cellular communication in the brain. They work to keep the neurons and cells healthy. Research has revealed that EFAs can actually increase the number of sending and receiving sites in the brain. This means that the capacity to send and receive information in the brain can increase. Great news for us parents, as well as for our kids who are striving students, artists, and athletes. Current research shows that EFA rich diets contribute to a healthy immune system. Some children who suffer from symptoms of ADD and ADHD are experiencing benefits from EFA rich foods and supplementation. EFAs encourage healthy levels of glucose in the blood and decrease insulin resistance. This is great news for kids who crave sweets, and for those who have diabetes. Since EFAs also help reduce inflammation and fatigue, they may be beneficial for your athletic or performing artist son or daughter.

Essential fatty acids are now available in supplement form. Usually they are found in liquid and soft gel capsule forms. Soft gel capsules are much easier for kids to swallow than most tablets. Since these supplements are healthy fats, they need to be consumed with meals for optimal absorption by the body. Most kids need anywhere from 300 milligrams to 500 milligrams per day. Kids can either start to eat more fish like cod, salmon, and tuna, use flaxseed oil on their food, or take EFA supplements. By the way, there are small amounts of EFAs in pumpkin seeds, walnuts, sesame seeds, and eggs! Regular grocery store eggs contain only 35 milligrams per egg. Some brands sell eggs rich in DHA, as much as 175 milligrams of pure DHA per egg! Ask your supermarket manager to carry them.

The five sources of good EFA supplements are Evening Primrose Oil (omega-6), Borage Oil (omega), DHA Fish Oils (omega-3), Flaxseed Oil (omega 3,6,9). Try to balance the intake of omega-3 oils with omega-6. Flaxseed oil is an all in one solution. The milder tasting flaxseed oil may be added to protein shakes, smoothies and/or used in salads. A few drops will power up the drinks. How many healthy fats a day do your kids eat? If the answer is little to none, supplement!

ENZYMES, Living Enzymes!

Living enzymes, found in raw foods, are necessary for digestion. So much of the food kids are eating today are void of enzymes. That is because so many of today's food products are subjected to heat exceeding 118 degrees, a process that kills living enzymes. A good full spectrum vegetable-based digestive enzyme is recommended for kids with a diet primarily filled with processed foods. They contain a wider range of digestive nutrients than animal-based enzymes. Also, these enzymes are gentler on the digestive systems of kids. Living enzymes, your invaluable digestive asset, insure the transfer of ingested nutrients throughout your kid's body!

Green Foods Are Life Savers!

Green foods are the easiest way to fuel your kids! Our favorite is Greens+. One tablespoon of these complete synergistic blends of living foods will fill your kids with about five (!) salad bowls of about 18 colors of vegetables and fruits, most of which they would not normally eat if their life depended on it! This magic food solution blends smoothly in juice or in vanilla soy/rice/almond milks, leaving little to no aftertaste. Advanced Greens offers real lemon/lime and cinnamon/spice flavors! Pour your chosen mix into a plastic opaque shaker with hole in the top, seal it, shake it vigorously, and serve it with a straw. This strategy eliminates the turn-off reaction to green liquids. Camouflage these nutrient-packed green powders in protein shakes. Start with small amounts. Every little bit counts! It is a bountiful way to start your kid's day.

Some brands of green food drinks ingredients offer only a single food, such as barley. Many brands can leave a grassy taste that turn off kids. This is why Greens+ is recommended for them. The synergistically blended combinations found in a product brand such as Greens+ is an ideal option for fueling your kids with super foods. Read the ingredients lists! Introduce them to greens with less than a half-teaspoon. After a few days, add more. Repeat this over time until you are up to one tablespoon.

Our own kids and their friends provide living proof of the power of green drinks. The before and after stories are impressive. One young boy was a carbohydrate-addicted kid who had frequent emotional vocal outbursts. His energy reached peaks and then dove down into valleys. Headaches were so frequent that he downed a form of aspirin daily. Then, at the age of eight, he began drinking a Greens+ shake daily. Today, at seventeen, he will tell you that gradually his energy level stabilized, his headaches diminished in frequency, and his craving for sugars dissolved. In addition, he will also tell you that when he does skip taking Greens+, he notices the difference in energy and mental acuity immediately. So you see, green foods do make a significant positive difference. Experience has taught us that super food green drinks are the easy ticket to health. They are a great way to get about five servings of vegetables into your kids a day!

Fiber!

Fiber is essential to the digestive system. Without it, nutrients and waste do not move through the systems properly, causing uncomfortable short term and serious long-term illnesses. Today's young generation is mostly eating processed fiber-less foods. The best way to meet fiber needs is to eat fresh fruit, vegetables, and whole grains. Apples, oranges, berries, beans, oats, the list is long. These foods are very available in your local supermarket. If all else fails, there are chewable fiber tablets.

Probiotics

These can be your best friend! Acidophilus and lactobacillus, the friendly bacteria, are found in yogurt, the good member of the dairy family. If your kids are not eating enough, give them a teaspoon or two from the refrigerated strawberry flavored liquid source or resort to the capsule. A critical time to do this is when you sense that your son or daughter is fighting a bug. Give them a spoonful of these good guys to get rid of the bad guys. Really, kids should be eating yogurt a few times a week to maintain a healthy digestive tract. Try to stay away from the heavily sweetened brands.

Not All Supplements Are Created Equal

Always consider the source. A common complaint is that you do not get your monies worth. This is often true. Some vitamins and minerals are prepared from natural plant food sources and excipients. Some natural plant food sources can be replicated in a lab and work well with your body's chemistry. These vitamins would include the B-complex family and ascorbic acid (vitamin C). Supplements like vitamin E should always be in a natural form. Look for D-Alpha tocopherols or Mixed tocopherols when purchasing vitamin E supplements. A "DL" prefix usually signifies a synthetically derived petroleum or turpentine source that has a lower biological activity rate in the body. A sure giveaway is the price. Natural vitamin E products always cost more than synthetic ones. They are worth it!

Unbeknownst to you, some ingredients used for vitamins and minerals stem from lower grade qualities than others. This means that they may be less potent. As in the manufacturing of foods, there are ways synthetic filler ingredients are camouflaged. The result is a vitamin or mineral whose ingredients may be an adulterated version of the real thing, providing little to no nutrient supplementation. Your money is then wasted. Research the brand that you are purchasing. Also look for standards of quality on the labels themselves such as USP (United States Pharmacopeia) or GMP (Good Manufacturing Practices). You may also contact the manufacturer directly and ask for assays and certification materials.

Some of the fillers used by manufacturers are aspartame (NutraSweet), polyethyleneglycol, coal tar, talc, also known as silicon dioxide, modified food starch, sodium, FDC and/or artificial colors (i.e. red #40, yellow #6), and flavors of any kind that are hidden in the phrase listed as "other ingredients" on the back of labels. These ingredients, especially the colors, can trigger a variety of allergies in some kids and are suspected of contributing to other health problems. Aluminum is still used in some supplements. Do not feed these to your kids. Aluminum is a toxic metal that can have many negative side effects. You see, some supplements fall into the same suspect category as some processed foods. Please read the ingredient lists.

Not all manufactured vitamins and minerals are bioavailable, meaning, not all can be absorbed during the digestive process. That's because digestive juices cannot break them down. The result is that the residues of some supplements go right through the body, ending up in the toilet bowl. No doubt you have heard the comments about expensive urine. In order to insure the consumer that their supplements are digestible, some brands list the disintegration time right on the label. This is your clue that the tablets or capsules in the body will most likely be absorbed and put to work in your kid's body.

Shipping and storage conditions affect the potency of vitamins and minerals. Heat can kill nutrients. Light can deplete nutrients of properties. Vitamins and minerals have a shelf life, just as living foods do (check expiration dates.). Supplements you buy are best bottled in containers that do not allow light inside. A good example of this is flaxseed oil. The best brands offer flax in a black plastic container for optimum protection. Pass by those vitamins and minerals displayed in or near the store windows! Be sure to keep your supplements at home in a dark cool cabinet. Refrigerate soft gels, green foods, colostrums, acidophilus, and oil products.

Enough is Enough

The other times vitamins and minerals end up in the toilet is when someone takes more than his or her body needs. Balance applies here as well. Enthusiasm for the benefits of iron as a blood builder should not persuade you to give more iron than is recommended to your kids. "When treating your child with nutritional supplements, you should be aware that if a formula appears to be helping support your body, it does not follow that 'more is not better.' Toxic overdoses of vitamins and minerals are rare, but they can occur, especially with products containing iron."[4] Please honor the biochemists' work and follow the recommended amounts for a healthy kid. Again, any questions should be referred to licensed health professionals.

The benefit of water-soluble vitamins is that when someone has taken more than they need, the excess is excreted through the urine. Bodies have their own check and balance system. This is a good thing. Those who are taking many more supplements than needed should adjust their intake per a health professional's advice.

Interpreting Supplement Labels

On food labels, the percentage of Recommended Daily Values (RDVs) of nutrients found in the product ingredients are identified. You ask, "What are RDVs?" The Food and Nutrition Board of the National Research Council from the National Academy of Science ... phew, initially established the Recommended Daily Allowances of nutrients back in 1941. The original purpose was especially important then. Nutrient levels were designed to reduce and prevent severe nutrient-deficient diseases that were more common at that time. Examples are scurvy which is brought on by the absence of vitamin C, Berberi, by the absence of vitamin B, and pellagra by the absence of vitamin B^3 (niacin). The government wanted to establish the minimum amount needed on a daily basis to prevent such illnesses.

Today, RDAs are now identified as Recommended Daily Values or RDVs. The vitamin and mineral recommended daily values, currently found on labels, are amounts that were updated in 1968 and 1989. Since then, as more research has identified more nutrients, addendums have been made. Again, it is believed that these amounts fall short of healthy requirements. Actually RDVs have only been created to provide the minimal amount of nutrients needed to prevent disease. The currently used Recommended Daily Value is based on the model of a person eating enough nutrient-filled food to provide fuel needed to burn 2000 calories a day to support optimal bodily functions. The results can invite improved energy levels, mental acuity, circulatory efficiency, and physical and mental overall performance. Not every body requires the same amount of fuel. Some bodies are bigger, some smaller, some older, some younger, some are more active, some are less active, and some have faster metabolisms. In addition, each child has his or her own specific body anatomical profile and growing needs. A six year old girl who likes to spend the afternoon playing with Barbie dolls has different caloric requirements than an eleven year old boy and girl who play soccer a few days a week. The kinds of nutrient sources of calories needed by each child may be different. Another challenge attached to the RDVs is the fact that they were established for groups of people (populations) not individuals, and certainly not for children. Thus, the amounts of nutrients recommended then and now are often inadequate for your kids. A consensus is that they do not provide kids with the daily needed nutritional supplementation.

"A tremendous amount of scientific research indicates that the 'optimal' level for many nutrients, especially the so-called antioxidant nutrients like Vitamin C and E, beta-carotene, and selenium, may be much higher than the current RDAs."[5] An example is that "the amount of vitamin C that prevents scurvy is 10 milligrams a day. The amount that helps prevent heart disease is at least 30 times that."[6] or 300 milligrams. The current RDV is 60 milligrams, too low for the average kid.

Research scientists and biochemists have been working on establishing vitamin and mineral recommendations more suited to today's nutritional demands, specifying amounts of adult, male and female, and for children, by ages. Many doctors, dietitians and nutritionists support this work. Below are our general recommendation:

- 1 Multivitamin and mineral formulated for kids
- Vitamin C, 500 milligrams
- EFA, 500 milligrams (minimum)

Add these when possible:

- Green Powder in a drink, one teaspoon (minimum)
- Probiotic cultures such as acidophilus or Bifidus
- Calcium/magnesium, chewable
- Digestive enzymes, add these when fresh foods are not being eaten.

A good children's multivitamin covers most of their supplemental needs. For those of you who want to more specifically address the needs of your student, artist, and/or athlete, please see a nutritionist, dietitian, doctor of naturopathy, or, pediatrician.

Doubting Doctors

For those health professionals who have told you that supplements are not safe, take a look at these facts. "According to the National Center for Health Statistics, 125,000 people died in 1992 as a direct result of drugs prescribed by doctors, while 9,000 people died in 1992 as a result of food poisoning. No one died that year due to the use of vitamin or mineral supplements."[7] For those health professionals who have told you that supplements are a waste of money, take a look at these facts. "Dietitians, the largest group of nutritionists in America, say that we don't need to supplement, yet a recent survey showed two-thirds of all dietitians take supplements. Cardiologists do not recommend supplements to their patients, yet two-thirds of them take antioxidants to protect their own hearts and arteries."[8] Doctors are beginning to notice the value of nutrition and supplementation.

Choose Wisely

Natural whole foods are the preferred way to nourish the body. Supplements are just something added to make up for a deficiency, a junk food deficiency. For kids who are not eating enough servings of whole foods, supplements help fill their nutrient drained bodies with a back-up, high-octane fuel.

Better Choices

- Multi Vitamins:
  - Blue Bonnet
  - Dr. Vanesa's Formulas
  - Emergen C (Alacer)
  - Enzymatic Therapy
  - Hero Nutrition Products
  - Natrol (chewables)
  - N. F. Factors
  - Nutrition Now
  - Twin Lab
  - Zand's Supplements for Children
- Protein Shakes:
  - Soy Essence (Fermented), Jarrow Formulas
  - Dr. Atkins (vanilla)
  - Nature's Plus: Spiruteen, Simply Natural
  - ZONE Perfect Protein Powder (plain, vanilla)
- EFAs Brands: (soft gels)
  - Health from the Sun
  - Nordic Naturals, DHA capsules
  - Spectrum Naturals
  - Tree of Life
- Enzymes:
  - Blue Bonnet
  - Rainbow Light
- Green Drinks:
  - Greens+

Probiotics:
- BioK+
- Kyodophilus
- Natren
- Nature's Way, Primadophilus Junior

Supplements serve as insurance for your kids' better health!

15

Quick and Easy Recipes Taste-Tested by the Kids

Chapter Quick Facts

- Each recipe had to meet the following requirements:
  - Take no longer than 15 to 20 minutes to prepare. Cooking may take longer.
  - Could be prepared in advance, refrigerated overnight, or frozen for future meals.
  - No more than 10 ingredients, preferably less.
  - Minimum of two different God-made colors.
  - Easy to read, simple directions.
  - Ingredients available at local stores.
  - Whole fresh foods used.
  - Clean ingredients, no additives or preservatives.
  - Few to no bad fats.
  - Reasonable amount of sodium and sugar.
  - No MSG or other lab-made sodium.
  - No fake sugar.
  - Kids have to like it!
- Recipes are organized by Breakfast, Lunch, Snack, and Dinner. In them, the Food Circles™ and God-made colors are counted. Also, find ingredients options, suggestions of what to serve with each recipe, and comments by kids and mothers. The layout of ingredients and accompanying directions is logical, making cooking easier for you. Look forward to many delicious meals that will fill up your kids!

QUICK AND EASY RECIPES TASTE-TESTED BY THE KIDS

Your copy of *Are Your Kids Running on Empty?™* includes a CD-ROM Cookbook with recipes tested and family approved. Homecooked meals are an important family tradition. Unfortunately the art of home-cooking has been lost to time restraints created by the crazy schedules governing so many families these days. Few of us have time to spend hours preparing meals, especially dinner. Yet, we know the value of preparing and serving well-balanced, well-sourced meals to our children. We have addressed this struggle by organizing kid-friendly recipes that will fit into the schedules of today's moms and dads.

For several Sundays and during some weekdays, spread out over many months, the Kid Kritics blind test tasted many recipes. Blind testing means the kids do not know what foods or drinks they are tasting. Regardless of whether they could identify the samples, their number one job was to decide if they liked the taste. There were no preconceived expectations, positive or negative. They were the masters of their own decisions. Numerous tested recipes were given thumbs down by the Kid Kritics. These have been tossed out! So have the ones that some kids liked and some did not. Usually the kids' votes were pretty united, for or against. The winning recipes have been given the Kid Kritics seal of approval, noted below by an asterisk.

The rest of the recipes found on the CD-ROM, *Mom, I'm Hungry, What's for Dinner?*, have been tested by kids but not under the formality of the Kid Kritics Taste Test. The difference is that mothers prepared them for their whole family to taste test. If kids did not like what was served, the recipe was tossed. Thus, you can be assured that most of the published recipes are liked by kids!

RECIPE REQUIREMENTS

We set recipe requirements with the whole family in mind. For emphasis they are listed again:

- Take no more that 15 to 20 minutes to prepare. Cooking time may take longer.
- Could be prepared in advance, kept overnight in the refrigerator, or, frozen for future meals.
- *No more than 10 ingredients, preferably less.*

- Minimum of two different God-made colors
- Easy to read, simple directions.
- Ingredients available at local stores.
- Whole fresh foods used.
- Clean ingredients, no additives or preservatives.
- Few to no bad fats.
- Reasonable amount of sodium and sugar.
- No MSG or other lab-made sodium.
- No fake sugar.
- Kids have to like it!

For you convenience, the recipes are organized so it is easy for you to find solutions for meal menus — Breakfast, Lunch, Snacks, or Dinner. In addition, at a quick glance you can see the number of different God-made colors and which Food Circles are found in each recipe. Instead of strictly adhering to the fact that counting colors refers to the phytonutrients found in fruits and vegetables, we have taken the liberty of counting every God-made color in all the foods, meat included. This may provide a greater incentive for your kids to eat from more food groups. The ingredients have been put in order of use along with the directions applying to them. How many times have you forgotten to include ingredients in recipes because your eyes missed one as they jumped up and down from ingredients to directions and back up to ingredients? OPTIONS are included for ingredient variations that may appeal to your kids. The number of servings is based on the formula that one serving is equivalent to a medium handful per person. Of course hand sizes vary so the estimates are not perfect. In order to help you with a menu, we added Serve With ideas. We also thought you would enjoy reading some comments made by kids and their moms who taste-tested these recipes. Along the side of each recipe you will find an ingredient grocery list. At a glance, you can see whether you have to run to the grocery store. Below, the Grocery List is a customized Food Circle highlighting the food groups found in the recipe.

For your convenience, we have put the *Mom, I'm Hungry, What's for Dinner?* cookbook on a CD-ROM, which is located in a sleeve in the back cover of this book. It is full of breakfast, lunch, snack, and dinner recipes. You can put this CD in your computer at work or at home and quickly find recipes that will work for your family. Print them out when needed. We have chosen a favorite recipe, the *Rius Breakfast Burrito,* to use as an example of what you will find on this CD-ROM. It is simple, meets nutritional needs, and tastes great!

RIUS BREAKFAST BURRITOS

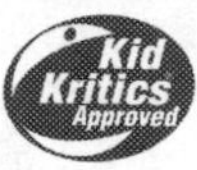

Preheat: burner, medium temperature
toaster oven, medium temperature
(or use microwave)
Pan: skillet, medium size

6 eggs, large
1/3 cup turkey bacon, crumbles or chopped
1 tablespoon green chilies, mild, finely chopped
Beat together in bowl. Pour into non-stick sprayed (1 second!) pan. Cook, stirring a few times, until eggs are firm.

¼ cup white cheddar cheese, low-fat, grated
3-4 tortillas, medium size
Place egg mixture over half of tortilla, sprinkle cheese on top. Roll up tortilla tightly, Place in toaster oven or microwave. Warm until cheese is melted. Serve.

Number of Servings: 3-4
Serve with: Bottled water, 100 percent fruit juice, or smoothie
Comments: Kids, *"This is really good!"*

Grocery List

✓ eggs
✓ turkey bacon
✓ green chilies
✓ white cheddar cheese
✓ tortillas

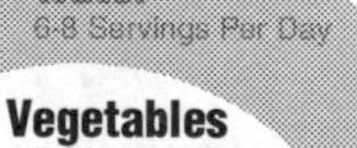

4 Colors: white, orange, brown, green

Food Circles: eggs, poultry, vegetables, dairy, grains

16

Fast Foods For Thought

Chapter Quick Facts

- About half of most people's hard-earned food money is spent at restaurants, mostly fast food restaurants.
- "Every month, about 90 percent of American children between the ages of three and nine visit McDonald's."[1]
- Fast food is everywhere: restaurants, service stations, malls, and even hospitals!
- To enhance their budgets, school administrators cut deals with fast food chain, soft drink, and junk snack food companies. Many deals fall into the six-figure category. In schools, young students, with developing taste and eating habits, are an ideal target market. This is a perfect environment for influencing short and long-term consumer loyalty.
- Fast food is high on anti-fuels. Sub sandwiches are one of the few fast foods which kids eat with veggies such as lettuce!
- When you have no options but to eat on the run, fuel up on the Better Choices.

Better Burger: Wendy's, plain
Better French fries: Wendy's, small
Better Pizza: Papa John's, cheese
Better Fast Food Restaurant: Subway
Better Chicken Nuggets: Wendy's
Better Sub: Subway, roast beef/Swiss cheese
Better Bagel: Bruegger's, sesame seed
Better Smoothie: Jamba Juice

FAST FOODS FOR THOUGHT

This last chapter was supposed to be short and succinct ... FAST! After learning that about half of the money a family spends on food today is spent at restaurants, mostly fast food restaurants, it became apparent that we needed to spend more time researching your options. Do you realize that about half of your hard earned food money is mostly spent on fast food fat, sugar, sodium, and man-made additives. Less is spent on food filled with the vitamins and minerals, needed by your children for their mental and physical development.

The fast food restaurant business has infiltrated the American culture, beginning with a focus on the kids. For emphasis, we are repeating this mind-boggling quote. "Every month, about 90 percent of American children between the ages of three and nine visit a McDonald's"[2] Odds are, your kids have been there at least once this month. If McDonald's reaches its goal of having every American within four minutes of one its restaurants, as was recently reported by the *New York Times*, you may be spending more time and money in a McDonald's than you are now. Already, this fast food giant is well on the way toward reaching this goal. According to Eric Schlosser, author of *Fast Food Nation*, they open almost two thousand a year. McDonald's is not the only game in town. How many times this month have your kids eaten at a Burger King, Wendy's, Chic-Fillet, Subway, Blimpee's, Pizza Hut, Checkers, Taco Bell or Arby's? How many times have you been to a "take-out" such as Dunkin Doughnuts, Domino's, or KFC (Kentucky Fried Chicken)? The number of fast food restaurant companies and locations is growing with the fast demands of today's working moms (about 66 percent of you, and this number is growing) who must cope with their kids' nearly impossible schedules.

SWIFT, SPEEDY, QUICK, RAPID, HASTY...FAST! NOW

How fast can we buy or cook it? How fast can your kids eat it? Your kids want their food to be served the minute they are hungry. They want it to take minutes to eat. Kids want to have finger food at their fingertips. They want their taste buds jumping with satisfaction immediately. Kids want one-minute meals that satisfy their desires instantly!

Instant gratification is the name of their social order. This attitude makes it difficult to be a mom. The need for instant solutions is even greater for working mothers. This is why about 50 percent of weekly meals are not prepared or eaten at home. This is why the fast food restaurants are billion dollar businesses. This is why prepared frozen and deli foods occupy such a large percentage of grocery stores square footage. Microwave ovens are the number one fast cooking appliance sold to consumers. Gas stations are no longer just gas stations. They are "service stations" with food courts. Car seats replace kitchen chairs as today's kids munch on wheels. Crunching, munching, and gulping snacks, breakfast, lunch, and dinner in cars is so common that some car manufacturers are entertaining the idea of putting mini iceboxes and microwave ovens in them!

Let's not kid ourselves; the fast food lifestyle is here to stay.

Fast Food Positives and Negatives

Positives

Convenience. They are everywhere, from airports to highways, from malls to a few miles from your home.

Price. For just a few dollars you can feed your kids burgers, fries, and a drink. No fuss, no muss. Such a deal!

Taste. The food additive industry is masterful at artificially recreating "flavors" in a laboratory for fast food restaurant foods and drinks. Flavors are invented to make your kids' mouths water.

Popular. Television, radio, and magazine marketing have made their fast food the food to eat and their restaurants the place for kids to be. The message: your kids gotta go there. So you better take them.

Instant gratification.

PARENTS:	KIDS:
No meal planning	Menu selection is kid driven
No grocery shopping	Packaging and environment are kid friendly
No cooking	Food tastes good
No dishes to wash	Eat what they want
Meet schedule crunches	Great toys
Low price fits the budget	Playgrounds, too!
Kids eat what they want	It's FUN!
Kids are HAPPY!	It's fast!

Negatives

Price. We all know you can't get something from nothing. Around 20 percent of the cost of a fast food item is the ingredients. Ask yourself, what quality of ground beef and hamburger bun could you buy for that price?

Nutrients. Not many. Sure, these meals fill tummies, but they do not meet daily vitamin and minerals quotas.

Artificial Ingredients. In order to entice kids to eat fast foods, and eat more of it, artificial ingredients are used to stimulate their taste buds, sense of smell, and visual appeal. The formula for drawing in repeat consumers is a well-researched science. The preservation formula is so perfect that bugs won't even eat this stuff!

Deep-Fried Foods. Fries, oh those French fries, the number one vegetable eaten by kids. They are usually drenched in oils that have been heated to hot temperatures, creating toxic trans fatty acids. This cooking formula spells trouble.

Absence of God-made foods. Naturally occurring foods are seldom seen in fast food restaurants. How often do you see fresh fruit such as apples at these restaurants? Where are the natural colors of nature? Where are the phytonutrients?

Advertising sends the message that low-nutrient "fake" junk foods are a BLAST to eat, again, and again, and again! However, being ill with diabetes, heart disease, cancer, or depression is hardly a blast to experience. It may take twenty years, it may take less. At some point, your kid's body will become compromised by a fast food, junk, diet. Why go there?

Let's Get To The Fast Facts

As reported by the *Washington Post* newspaper, Eric Schlosser author of *Fast Food Nation* noted that, in the year 2000, Americans spent $110 billion on fast food. That adds up to a $104 billion dollar increase over these past thirty years. "Americans now spend more money on fast food than on higher education, personal computers, computer software, or new cars. They spend more on fast food than on movies, books, magazines, newspapers, videos, and recorded music—combined."[3] When combining the fact that French fries are the number one vegetable eaten by kids, and 90 percent of kids aged three to nine eat at McDonalds monthly, it is fair to say that kids are eating many pounds of fast food fries a year. Even at fast food prices, the amount of money spent on low cost, nutrient-void, additive-filled fries is mind-boggling.

When not spending money at fast food restaurants, prepared foods are filling freezers and cupboards. "About ninety percent of the money that Americans spend on (grocery) food is used to buy processed food."[4] Does this mean that Americans are only spending ten percent of their food budget on fresh, God-made food?

Fast Food Is Everywhere

Fast food restaurants used to be stand-alone buildings, only. Now they are located in other buildings, too. You can find them in service stations, malls, discount stores, office buildings, airports, train stations, bus terminals, theme parks, sports stadiums, movie theatres, entertainment centers, cruise ships, colleges, universities, high, middle, and lower schools, and even hospitals. In most every city, town, and village of America, a fast food chain restaurant is situated along at least one street. Suburbia is cluttered with fast food restaurants. These recognizable structures and signs have cluttered the landscape of America.

Two categories of locations should raise your ire: hospitals and public schools. As we have alerted you, ingredients found in some fast foods are known to cause serious illnesses. What in the world are hospital administrators thinking when they put fast foods into hospitals, even if it is just the cafeteria? (We all know that patients are often brought cafeteria food up to their rooms.) Why in the world are public schools putting fast food restaurant foods into their cafeteria? The answer is simple, MONEY, and plenty of it.

Schools Are Paid Big Bucks

School administrators, on local and regional levels, cut deals with fast food chain companies. Schools receive income for advertising space on school facilities such as sports venues. Even your kids' teaching materials may be marketed to schools by the fast food chains. Franchise arrangements are made so kids can buy chicken McNuggets or other fast foods for lunch. McDonald's, Pizza Hut, Taco Bell, Subway, Domino's and others are infiltrating the public schools. Channel One, a closed-circuit school television channel airs fast food chain commercials in the classrooms where there are monitors. This medium reaches millions of middle and high school students daily. Wow, that's better coverage than MTV.

Soda companies use the school marketing opportunities the same way as fast food companies. For distribution, they position vending machines around the campus of most every public school. Over $750 million annually is spent on vending machine sales, alone, bringing huge dollars into the school coffers ... Top sellers are soft drinks, coffee, juice and pseudo-juice drinks, candy, chips, pretzels, cookies, and even French fries.[5] Deals are negotiated on a per bottle sale, based on quotas met. It pays for schools to encourage kids to drink liquid candy, sodas, during the school day, morning and afternoon. No wonder kids can't focus and be productive in their classes.

Fast junk food marketing in schools is a high-stakes game. "'Influencing elementary school students is very important to soft drink marketers," an article in the January 1999 issue of *Beverage Industry* explained, "because children are still establishing their tastes and habits.' Eight-year-olds are considered ideal customers; they have about sixty-five years of purchasing in front of them."[6] Schools have the young bodies on campus and in their buildings five days a week. Soda companies have the drinks. The school sells your kids as captured consumers to the soda companies and other vendors for the money. This is an outrage. Remember, a continual diet of soda leads to diabetes, obesity, high blood pressure, heart problems, autoimmune deficiency diseases and numerous other mental and physical illnesses. Are you are mad, now? You should be. Ask your neighboring school about the contracts they may have with fast food and soda companies. They may respond by saying they need the money to buy educational materials for your kids. Fine. Tell them to make deals with manufacturers of Better Choices Grocery List™ foods and drinks. Can the sodas and fake junk fast food. Your children are invaluable.

Size, Another Fast Food Phenomenom

We have the fast food industry to thank for impregnating kids with the perception that bigger is better. Super Size, Super, Whopper, Double, Triple, Big, Bid Xtra, and King are the big buzzwords for, you deserve big! Billions of advertising dollars are spent to send this message. Serving sizes are larger than they used to be. Today's small size is as big as the former medium size, the medium size is as big as the former large sizes and what is labeled as large size did not exist a few years ago. In the 1980s, McDonald's large French fries had about one third the calories as today's super size. Today, some "small" sodas contain 22 ounces of "liquid candy". That equals almost three cups of the artificially colored sugar water. A large soda can contain 44 ounces or about five and a half cups of liquid sugar, dyes, and bubbled gas. Collectively, that is enough sugar to invite insulin shock within hours. No wonder "Adult-onset" diabetes among children is on a dramatic rise.

"Children eat more if they are served more," says Brian Wansink, director of the Food and Brand Research Laboratory, University of Illinois. He goes on to say the "People can often eat about fifty percent more of hedonistic foods like candy, chips, and popcorn when they come in bigger packages. With other foods, the increase is usually about twenty-five percent."[7] The movie theatres sure capitalize on these facts. The sizes of candy bars, soda servings, and popcorn buckets are enormous. So are the sizes of the refreshment stands, theatres, and even the seats. That's because kids and adults are bigger, too. Remember, in a former chapter, you learned that today's classroom desks and chairs are bigger because kids could no longer fit into the chairs used by kids of the same age not too long ago? True fact.

Bigger almost always means more fat, more sodium, more sugar, and more unused caloric energy for our couch and computer potatoes. Take a look.

Burger King:

Cheeseburger (5oz.)	380 cal.	19 gr. fat	770 mg sodium
Double Cheeseburger (7.5oz.)	600 cal.	36 gr. fat	1060 mg. sodium
Double Whopper with Cheese (13.2oz.)	960 cal.	63 gr. fat	1420 mg. sodium

Notice, the sodium count is extremely high, ranging from about 800 milligrams to 1400 milligrams. Your kids need sodium, but only about 500 milligrams a day. Imagine what the extra 200 to 900 milligrams of sodium in one meal are doing to the blood vessels of you son or daughter? On average kids should consume about 20 grams of good fats a day, depending on their age, height, and activity. One Double Whopper with Cheese significantly exceeds the desired amount of fat for you son or daughter. Think of how many more fat grams are consumed when adding their breakfast, snack, lunch, or dinner trip to Burger King? Bigger is not better.

Coca Cola:

12 ounces has about 9 teaspoons of sugar
32 ounces has around 25 teaspoons of sugar

That is a heap of sugar in one sitting. Two teaspoons is enough on one day. Now do you wonder why kids have a hard time focusing and sitting still? It has been reported that a startlingly large number of two-year olds are drinking sodas. If you look around in a fast food restaurant, this will not surprise you. You know that fast food restaurants are not imposing a drinking age for cokes or any other sodas. Yet, it is known that excessive sugar can promote addictive behavior. By the way, diet soda is worse since it has substituted sugar with lab-made additives. Water, juice or milk is what our kids should be drinking at fast food restaurants. Notice, none are offered in supersizes. Water should be.

Media, Big Money

Fast food chains and junk food manufacturers bet megabucks on the fact that your kids will eat a lot of their food and drink products. Big thinking applies here as well. Kelly Brownell, professor of psychology, epidemiology, and public health at Yale University, is quoted as saying, "The food industry spends billions of dollars each year on advertising and promotion to create an environment that constantly pressures us to eat."[8] The key phrase here is "create an environment that constantly pressures us to eat." It is reported that kids watch five, seven or more hours of television a day. How many times do you think your kids have seen a McDonald's ad for happy meals with happy toys for the happy family? How many pizza ads tell the story of fun friends having fun fooling around while feasting on pizza dripping with cheese? It's pizza party time, all the time! Britney Spears, and other idolized stars before her have clearly convinced kids that drinking Pepsi gives you the moves; its cool! Friends and fun go with Coke. It goes on and on and on. These ads are also on the radio airwaves, in pages and pages of kid magazines, and in the schools. Kids want to experience all the social benefits implied by these ads, constantly. They are impressionable, and they fall for it, big time.

Make This Cultural Phenomenom Work For You

Advertising only works when the consumer buys into it. The way to vote NO is to not buy the products advertised. The way to move kids to vote NO is to tell them the truth about the ingredients in the foods. The many kids we have talked to verified that when told the facts kids will make better choices. Educate yourself and your kids. Start with knowing what to look for in the fast food industry.

Food Source Can Be a Problem

Sickening Stories. The factual stories of deaths and impairments caused by the presence of *E. coli* 0157:H7 and salmonella in fast foods, particularly in ground meat and chicken, are heartbreaking.

> About five percent of children who develop HUS (hemolytic uremic syndrome) caused by *E. coli,* are killed by it. Those who survive are often left with permanent disabilities, such as blindness or brain damage ... *E. coli* 0157:H7 is now the leading cause of kidney failure among children in the United States.... Every year in the United States, food tainted with salmonella causes about 1.4 million illnesses and five hundred deaths The CDC (Center for Disease Control) now estimates that roughly 37,000 Americans suffer food poisoning each year from non-0157 strains of *E. coli,* about 1,000 people are hospitalized, and about twenty-five die".[9] Young bodies are particularly vulnerable.

E. coli is more commonly found in beef. However, there is a greater chance of exposure to the *E.coli* or another bacteria, giardia, be it from beef or poultry, when it has been ground. Some meatpacking and distribution companies follow good safety measures. Some do not. In short, the sanitary conditions of feedlots, alone, often invite the contamination of bacteria. So do many processing facilities and sloppy procedures. When one infected animal leaks into the processing system, it can potentially contaminate thousands of pounds of ground meat. One fast food burger can be comprised of many different animals and may be open to contamination. This system sets up unsettling odds. It only takes one.

Employees Do Make a Clean Difference. Low-paid employees usually are the connection between you and the food your kids are eating. Unfortunately, some are not inclined or motivated to maintain a clean facility or practice sanitary procedures when preparing and serving your kids food. Food dropped on the floor may be circulated back into servings. Hands, a major transportation network for viruses and bacteria, are not always washed properly. There have been incidences of insect infestation. This is reality in today's society. Depressed? Disappointed? Turned Off? All of the above? You aren't alone. So what do you do? When you walk into a restaurant, scan the part of the kitchen and serving area you can see. Check out the bathrooms. If either are dirty, so may be your food. Clearly, if there is evidence of little pride and interest in sanitary conditions, you do not want your kids eating the food served there.

Well-cooked meat, please. In all clean restaurants, make sure all the meat is cooked thoroughly, well done. This greatly reduces the odds of your kids ingesting active *E. coli* or salmonella bacteria. In fact, it is always advisable to serve well-cooked meat. This is a health insurance policy in our imperfect world. Rare and raw meat, poultry, and fish open the door to bacteria.

Look for the Anti-Fuels: fat, sodium, and sugar. Ask for the Nutrition Facts on menus and review the amounts of fat, sodium and carbohydrates (sugar) in the foods that your kids like to eat. If these facts are not available in the restaurant, they are posted on most fast food restaurant chain Websites (Example: SEARCH, Jack in the Box restaurants.)

FAT. Fat is a staple of fast food. It is a cheap ingredient that gives food that smooth "mouth-feel" and the stomach a full feeling. Traditional fast food is filled with it, covered with it, and often cooked in it. Sometimes the fat is from animals; the storage tissue for toxins, and some is from corn, safflower, cottonseed or soybean oils. Sometimes they are mixed. Trans fatty acids created while deep-frying fats are sometimes reused. If kids are eating more than twenty grams of fast food fat in one meal or snack, it is very likely that they will overdose on fat that day. Unfortunately, it is easy to overdose.

McDonald's	Big Mac: 31 grams of fat Large fries: 22 grams of fat Total fat: 53 grams
Wendy's Jr.	Cheeseburger: 13 grams of fat (bigger ones: more!) Biggie (French fries): 23 grams of fat. Total fat: 36 grams
Taco Bell	Beef Burrito Supreme: 23 grams of fat Nachos, alone: 18 grams of fat.
Subway	6" Hot Meatball Sub: 16 grams of fat 6" Hot Subway Melt: 12 grams of fat

You can see that when ordering a meal at most any fast food restaurant, it does not take long for your kids to exceed their recommended daily intake of fat. Most kids are not active enough to burn up this amount of fat so it collects in their bodies where it is stored in all the wrong places.

SODIUM. Sodium is an ingredient that is disguised under many names and is used excessively by food manufacturers. Sodium takes care of taste appeal and encourages repeat sales, that very day! Something about sodium makes you want more. It makes your kids feel thirsty. So, they reach for soda that also makes them feel thirsty. Then they eat more fries that add to the need to quench their thirst. Yes, your kids are caught up in the vicious cycle of sodium thirst addiction.

Kids need just about 500 milligrams of sodium in one day. Somebody forgot to share this health fact with the fast food companies.

Wendy's	Jr. Bacon Cheeseburger: 830 milligrams of sodium
Taco Bell	Bean Burrito: 1100 milligrams of sodium
Subway	6" Subway Melt: 1746 milligrams of sodium
McDonald's	McNuggets, 6 pieces: 510 milligrams of sodium Super fries: 390 milligrams of sodium
Pizza Hut	One slice of stuffed crust pepperoni pizza: 1120 milligrams of sodium

Not only do these sodium numbers add up quickly, their source is cause for concern. Most include varieties of monosodium glutamate (MSG). As you recall, MSG is an excitotoxin of the brain cells and can cause nervous disorders. At fast food restaurants, kids usually eat more than double the amount needed in one day. When anyone ingests up to 18 grams (1800 milligrams) of sodium, danger lurks. Two slices of Pizza Hut cheese pizza are filled with around 2200 milligrams of sodium or 22 grams, sending your kid's body beyond the danger zone and into the red alert.

SUGAR. Your number one source of sugar at fast food restaurants is soda. At around seven teaspoons of sugar per eight ounces of soda, it adds up quickly. You may be surprised to learn how many carbohydrates (All sugars are carbohydrates, some simple, some complex.) are found in hamburgers and fries. McDonald's medium French fries, at around 57 grams (over 14 teaspoons) of carbohydrates, have more than a cheeseburger, which has about 35 grams (almost nine teaspoons). Potatoes are filled with starchy carbohydrates. One slice of cheese pizza may have between 21 and 71 grams of carbohydrates. Flour products, including bread and buns have a significant amount of carbohydrates in them. Few if any are complex carbohydrates. Again, it is the collective amount from a meal of fast foods that adds up to excess, especially when you add desserts and breakfast foods to the mix. fast food manufacturers liberally use sugar to insure their foods will be well liked by kids. The naturally occurring complex carbohydrates found in God-made foods, especially vegetables and fruit provide all the sugar kids need. Trouble is, kids are not eating these foods. They are gorging on refined and fake sugar. Now you see why adult-onset diabetes among children is rising at a disturbingly rapid rate. Let's not forget that unused sugar is stored as fat, a fact that significantly contributes to the current epidemic of obesity. These stirring facts have been repeated throughout this book for emphasis.

Look For Better Choices

Better is not best but it really beats the bad choices. Some in the fast food industry are beginning to show some interest in including better foods. A couple of restaurant chains are beginning to offer alternatives to the traditionally high fat, sodium, and sugar foods.

Nutrition Facts and Ingredients

Nutrition Facts are helpful facts listing the quantities of nutrients found in foods. Some fast food companies make these available at their restaurants or on their Websites. Look for them. Ingredient lists are harder to come by. Some fast food chains, such as Subway, offer this helpful information at the restaurants. Some lists of ingredients can be found on Websites. Some may be requested from a company by calling its customer service number. Some companies will not reveal their ingredients to you, no matter how many times and ways you ask for them. This is a particularly interesting notion since some of their competition shares all.

Though Nutrition Facts may give you pertinent information about the food you are eating, until you know the source, you cannot be sure of the food value. It pays to know the ingredients of the foods you kids are eating.

FAST FOOD INGREDIENT WISH LIST

- **Food without additives, fresh food!**
- Baked French fries
- 100% beef hamburgers, grilled or broiled
- 100% chicken, grilled or broiled
- 100% albacore or tongol tuna
- Less sodium
- No MSG additives
- White real cheese
- White cheese sauces with real cheese and not additives
- Baked potatoes with real butter or canola spread
- Sweet potatoes with real butter or canola spread
- Salad dressings made of clean ingredients ... no artificial flavors or additives
- Fresh cold cut veggies with clean tasty dips (mild salsa)
- Fresh breads, bagels and dough without preservatives
- Whole grain breads, pita, bagels or crackers

- No sodas
- Large glasses or bottles of water
- Low-fat milk, additive free
- 100 percent fruit juices
- Shakes made with real fruit and milk
- Good, low sugar smoothies made with real fruit
- Lower fat mayonnaise without additives
- Ketchup with little sugar
- Pickles without additives, such as dyes
- Fresh fruit, whole and cut up as fruit cup served in its own juice
- Lower fat, lower sodium bean tacos and burritos, made without additives
- Lower fat and lower sodium chili made with beans, turkey and sauces without additives
- Spaghetti with clean tomato sauce made with vegetables
- Soups! Cleanly made soups: chicken noodle, tomato, carrot, sweet potato, pureed vegetable
- All sandwiches include lettuce and other choices of veggies such as diced celery and tomatoes
- Desserts made with real ingredients, not lab-made, flavored, and colored ingredients

Be an advocate for your kids. Tell a company your wish list. Send it to them via an email or call customer service. Company contact numbers are easy to access by typing in the name of the company into the Search box on your internet home page. Since few people do this, your email will be noticed. Of course, the more they hear from their consumers, the better.

The Kid's Menu

The Dataessential Research, Inc. "studied kids menu items (out of over 37,000 total menu items) offered at the nation's top 500 chain restaurants (full service and quick service) and found that French fries are the most frequently listed food, with 710 mentions.... Salads top the veggie category, appearing a paltry eleven times among 1,937 menu items."[10] This is the list of what foods are most to the least available for kids as listed on Kids' Menus.

Item	Percentage
French fries	37
Chicken	19
Ice cream	13
Burgers	12
Pasta	10
Grilled cheese	7
Hot dogs	7
Pizza	6
Fish	3
Cookies	3
Shrimp	2
Pancakes	2
Shakes	1

Kids usually choose from their narrowed suggested menu options ... the power of suggestion. As you can see, salads did not even show up on this survey as the incidence of finding them on a menu is about less than one percent. It is important to note that this survey reflects "Kid Menus" only. When eating at a regular restaurant, extend your son and daughter's choices by also reading from the adult menu. Unfortunately, the above food list reflects the trend of most favorite foods ordered by kids at restaurants. Because fast food limited choices are a reality, an option available to us as parents is to patronize the fast food restaurants which serve the "cleanest" version of these food categories. There is a trend toward offering better foods. This is encouraging.

Better Choices

We have made a list of better fast food restaurants choices for several food categories. The purpose of this list is to guide you to the safer version of hamburgers, sub sandwiches, pizza, bagels, and other fast foods available.

The Kids Kritics were asked which were their favorite fast food restaurants, plus which foods they liked to order. By the way, the Kid Kritics revealed a very interesting fact. The only fast food restaurant where kids consistently eat vegetables is a sub sandwich restaurant. Almost all of the kids put at least lettuce in their sub. Many add tomatoes. A couple kids had eaten the McShake salad and only one mentioned eating a Wendy's salad from the salad bar. So, right off the bat, it appears to be best to take your kids to a sub sandwich shop for protein, vegetables, and grains. TIP: Some wheat bread is simply white bread with added coloring such as caramel coloring. In this case, it is better to eat plain white bread if your kids won't eat the multi-grained offered in a few restaurants.

Our BETTER list of popular fast food categories are as follows:

BETTER Burger: Wendy's, better with little to no white cheese
BETTER Chicken nuggets: Wendy's (or none)
BETTER French fries: none
BETTER Chicken Sandwich: Wendy's, grilled, OR, Subway's, roasted chicken breast
BETTER Turkey and Cheese Sandwich: Subway's (better without the cheese)
BETTER Tuna Sandwich: Subway's on whole grain
BETTER Sub: Subway's Roast Beef with Swiss cheese, and chopped veggies
BETTER Pizza: Papa John's, Cheese with Thin Crust (better to ask for half the cheese)
BETTER Baked Potato: Wendy's, with or without Sour Cream and Chives

BETTER Salad: McDonald's Salad Shaker, Grilled Chicken, Newman's fat-free Vinaigrette dressing
BETTER Taco: Taco, Soft, Grilled Chicken or Steak (no ground beef). Easy on the cheese (ask for white) and sauce. Add some chopped veggies.
BETTER Burrito: Taco's Bean Burrito Supreme (once in awhile)
BETTER Bagel: Bruegger's, Sesame Seed or Everything. (Go light on the cream cheese).
BETTER Breakfast: Einstein Bros. Bagels, eggs and bagel (turkey sausage!)
BETTER Smoothie: Jamba Juice
BETTER Drink: Bottled or Filtered WATER!
BETTER All Around fast food Restaurant: Subway, read the ingredients!

Not only does Subway do a good job in their food selection and preparation, they are also willing to reveal all the ingredients to every interested consumer. You may read them yourself on their Web site, www.subway.com. Not all of their menu items are Better Choices. Some are too loaded with sodium, fat, or additives. Read the food facts before ordering. Subway is chosen above Wendy's because kids put chopped veggies in the food they order! Blimpee's actually is a close second. They have several subs that closely compare to Subway's in quality. Again, we favor the sub sandwich restaurants, as that is where kids do add some chopped fresh veggies to their meal.

There are many very welcomed new fast fresh-food restaurant chains surfacing. Some that are more regional may be more national when you read this. Each one deserves your patronage as they offer an elevated selection of quality foods, usually better than those offered by the larger chains. Also, some of the larger chains are responding to the consumer trend of demanding better quality food choices. McDonalds recently announced that they have made a deal to use Newman's salad dressings, offering a significant improvement over their versions. Keep a discerning eye out for "new and improved" versions of meat and chicken dishes, and, salads.

When it is time to eat on the run, fuel up on Better Choices!

Glycemic Index Guide

The Glycemic Index identifies carbohydrates according to their rate of absorption into the body. The lower the index, the longer it takes for sugar to enter the bloodstream after the food is eaten. This is good. The result is balanced productive energy that lasts longer.

We have abbreviated this index to include only the low to moderate foods that are the Better Food Choices™. We encourage you to use it to monitor the amount of sugar your kids are eating.

LOW

Bread
None

Cereals
None

Bakery products
None

Grains
None

Crackers
None

Dairy
Whole milk
2% milk
Low fat milk
Skim milk
Yogurt, plain low-fat
Cheese
Cottage cheese
Sour cream
Cream
Butter

Fresh fruit
Cranberries (no sugar added)
Blackberries
Blueberries
Raspberries
Strawberries
All other berries
Cherries
Grapefruit

MODERATE

Bread
Pita
Pumpernickel
Rye
Sourdough
Stone-ground whole wheat
Whole grain
Whole wheat

Cereals
Granola, some
Grape nuts
Life
Muesli, some
Oatmeal, rolled oats

Grains
Barley
Brown rice
Bulgur
Couscous
Rolled oats
Rye
Whole wheat

Crackers
Stoned wheat thins

Dairy
Ice cream, low-fat

Fruit, fresh
Apple
Apricot
Cantaloupe
Grapes

LOW

Fresh fruit
Plum
Tomato

Vegetables
Asparagus
Artichokes
Broccoli
Brussels sprouts
Celery
Cucumber
Eggplant
Garlic
Green beans
Kale
Lettuce, all kinds
Mushrooms, all kinds,
Onions, all kinds
Peppers, all kinds
Radishes
Spinach
Zucchini

Legumes (beans)
Soy beans
Butter beans
Lentils

Animal protein
Beef
Fish
Poultry
Eggs

Fats
Olive oil
Canola oil
Sesame Oil

Sweetener
Stevia

Herbs and Spices
Almost all

MODERATE

Fruit, fresh
Kiwi
Mango
Orange
Papaya
Peach
Pineapple
Watermelon

Vegetables
Peas
Sweet potatoes
Yams

Nuts
Almost all

Legumes
Adzuki beans
Baked beans
Black beans
Black-eyed peas
Chickpeas (garbanzo)
Kidney beans
Lima beans
Navy beans
Pinto beans
White (Haricot)

Other
Pasta, all kinds
Pizza
Popcorn
Potato chips
100% pure jams

Web Sites We Recommend

We have sorted out some credible and informative Web sites for you that relate to the subject of this book. Most grocery stores and food/drink manufacturers have a Web site. Simply type their names in the Search window or try typing www. the name, and then .com. Knowledge is a powerful tool. Enjoy learning and keeping up to date with these sites.

www.altmedicine.com (Alternative Medicine News Online)
www.ama-assn.org (American Medical Association)
www.ams.usda.gov/nop/ (National Organic Program, USDA)
www.askdrsears.com (Dr. Sears, pediatrician)
www.aspartametruth.com (aspartame link)
www.blonz.com (Ed Blonz, Ph.D., M.S., F.A.C.N.)
www.centerforfoodsafety.org (Center For Food Safety)
www.cetos.org (Center for Ethics and Toxics)
www.cfsan.fda.gov (Department of Health and Human Services)
www.checnet.org (Children's Health Environmental Coalition)
www.citizens.org (Citizens for Health)
www.cspinet.org (Center for Science in the Public Interest)
www.dadamo.com (Dr. D'Adamo, Blood Type Diet)
www.drwhitaker.com (Dr. Julian Whitaker)
www.earthsave.org (EarthSave)
www.eatright.org (American Dietetic Association)
www.ewg.org (Environmental Working Group)
www.fatsforhealth.com. (Karlene Kerst, B.Sc, R.D.)
www.fatsthatheal.com (Udo Erasmus, Ph.D.)
www.fda.gov (Food and Drug Administration)
www.feingold.org. (Feingold Association – families and physicians)
www.foodallergy.org (Food Allergy and Anaphylaxis Network)
www.geaction.org (Genetic Engineering Action Network)
www.global-reality.com (Campaign for Food Safety)
www.gefoodalert.org (Genetic Engineering Food Alert)
www.healthyeating.net (Nancy Frawley)
www.healthyfood.org (American Frozen Food Institute)
www.healthlettertufts.edu (Tufts University)
www.healthwell.com (New Hope Natural Media)
www.kidseatgreat.com (Christine Wood, M.D., C.L.E.)
www.mercola.com (Joseph Mercola, M.D.)

www.nancymarkle.com (aspartame and Monsanto)
www.navigator.tufts.edu (Tufts University-nutrition)
www.nih.gov (National Institute of Health)
www.nutritionaction.org (Center for Science in the Public Interest)
www.olen.com/food (Food Finder-Olen Publishing)
www.organicconsumers.org (Organic Consumer Association)
www.ota.com (Organic Trade Association)
www.pcrm.org (Physicians Committee for Responsible Medicine)
www.pric-pottenger.org (Price-Pottenger Nutrition Foundation
www.rodale.com (Rodale Publisher)
www.supplementinfo.org (Dietary Education Alliance – all age groups)
www.tinytummies.com (Sanna Jame Delmonic, M.S., R.D.)
www.truefoodnow.org (GMO and non-GMO food list – Greenpeace)
www.ucsusa.org (Union of Concerned Scientists)
www.usda.gov (United States Department of Agriculture)
www.valupage.com (Catalina Marketing Corp.)
www.vm.cfsan.fda.gov (Center for Food Safety and Applied Science)
www.vrg.org (Vegetarian Resource Group)
www.5aday.com (Better Health Foundation)

References

Chapter One

1. *Webster's New World Dictionary of the American Language, College Edition*, New York: The World Publishing Company, 1959, p. 562.
2. Eric Schlosser, *Fast Food Nation,* New York: Houghton Mifflin Company, 2000, p. 121.
3. Paul A. Stitt, *Beating the Food Giants,* Manitiwoc, Wisconsin: The Natural Press, 1993, pp. 126, 127.
4. Fred Pescatore, M.D., *Feed Your Kids Well*, New York: John Wiley & Sons, 1998, p. 15.
5. Paul A. Stitt, *Beating the Food Giants,* Manitiwoc, Wisconsin: The Natural Press, 1993, pp. 127, 128.
6. Carol Simontacchi, *The Crazy Makers,* New York: Tarcher/Putnam, 2000, p. 2.
7. *Consumer Reports,* Des Moines, Iowa, December 1997, p. 13.
8. *Newsweek*, New York July 3, 2000, p. 43.
9. Joseph C. Piscatella, *Fat Proof Your Child*, New York: Workman Publishing, 1997, p.121.
10. *Nutrition Action Newsletter*, Center of Science for the Public Interest, Volume 28/1,Jan,/Feb. 2001, p. 3.
11. Judy Mazel and John E Monaco, M.D., *Slim & Fit Kids:* Deerfield Beach, Florida: Health Communications, Inc., 1999, p.13.
12. www.5aday.com/html/research/consumptionsstats.php, p. 4 of 4.

Chapter Two

1. "Nutrition Labeling - Applicable Foods", The Food Label, www.cfsan.fda.gov/label.html, May 1999, p 2. www.cfsan.fda.gov/label.html
2. Ibid.
3. Russell L. Blaylock, M.D., *EXCITOTOXINS, The Taste That Kills*, Santa Fe, New Mexico: Health Press, 1997, pp. xx, Introduction.
4. Judy Mazel, John E, Monaco, M.D., *Slim & Fit Kids*, Deerfield Beach, Florida: Health Communications, Inc., 1999, p. 34.
5. Fred Pescatore, M.D., *Feed Your Kids Well*, New York: John Wiley & Son, Inc., 1998, p. 5.
6. Sam Graci, *The Power of Superfoods,* Ontario, Canada: Prentice Hall, 1999, p. 126.
7. Fred Pescatore, M.D., *Feed Your Kids Well*, New York: John Wiley & Sons, 1997, p. 67.
8. Mitch Lipka, "Fibbing on Food Labels, an easy crime," Sun Sentinel, Vol.42, #137, September 9, 2001, p. 1A.
9. *USA Today*, "A Better Life: Study finds peanut allergens go unlisted", April 5, 2001, 10D.
10. Mitch Lipka, "Labeling: Many Nutritious Labels Erroneous," Sun Sentinel, September 2, 2001, p. 22A.
11. Bonnie Liebman, "Ingredient Secrets", Nutrition Action Newsletter, July/August 2001, pp. 8,9.
12. "The Most and Least Trusted Industries", *USA Today,* Money Section (B), July 2, 2001, p. 1B.

Chapter Three

1. *The Human Body and How it Works*, New York: Exeter Books, 1979, p. 293.
2. Susan T. Borra, R.D., President of the American Dietetic Association, Speech to the New Jersey School Nurses-D.C. Day, Washington, D.D., Thursday, June 14, 2001, www.eatright.org/Public/GovernmentAffairs/98_childhoodobesity.cfm
3. Susan Kalish, *Your Child's Fitness, Practical Advise for Parents*, Champaign, Illinois: Human Kinetics, 1958, p.63.
4. Albert C. Goldberg, M.D., *Feed Your Child Right*, New York: M. Evan and Company, New York, 2000, pp. 44, 45.

Chapter Four

1. Carol Simontacchi, *The Crazy Makers*, New York: Tarcher/Putnam, 2000, p. 116.
2. Brandon Loomis, "Kraft pledges to fight obesity with healthier recipes", Fort Lauderdale, Florida: Sun Sentinel, July 2, 2003,p.3A.
3. Paul Pitchford, *Healing With Whole Foods*, Berkeley, California: North Atlantic Books, 1993, pp. 149, 150.
4. Carolyn Dean, M.D., N.D., *Sweet Conspiracy*, Natural Health, Salt Lake City, Utah: Weider Publications, January/February 2001, p.125.
5. "Diabetes in Children and Adolescents", Bethesda, Maryland: National Institutes of Health, National Diabetes Education Program, www.ndep.nih.gov, Februrary 202, p.1.
6. Robert Hass, *Eat To Win For Permanent Fat Loss*, New York: Harmony Books, 2000,p. 75.
7. "Type II Diabetes – Kids' Epidemic", Andhra Pradesh, India: Centrex Technologies, Ltd. (Internet Portal on Diabetes), www.diabetovalens.com, May 6, 2003, p.1.
8. Keith Mulvihill, "CDC makes dire diabetes prediction for US children", New York, New York: Reuter's Health, www.reutershealth.com, p.1.
9. Anita Manning, "Kid obesity tips scales toward diabetes epidemic" *USA Today,* McLean, VA. Gannon Co. June 13, 2000, p. 8D.
10. Barbara Reed, Ph.D, *Food, Teens & Behavior*, Manitowoc, Wisconsin: Natural Press, 1983, p. 55.
11. *Prevention Magazine*, September, 2000, p. 82.
12. Phyllis A. Balch, C.N.C. & James F. Balch, M.D., *RX Prescription for Cooking and Dietary Wellness*, Greenfield, Indiana: P.A.B. Publishing, Inc., 1993, p. 177.
13. *Food Resource*, Oregon State University, Corvallis, OR., July, 2001. http://food.orst.edu/.
14. Dr. Michael Gazsi, N.D., Alternative and Complimentary Medicine, www.webman.att.net, July 2001.
15. Paul;A. Stitt, *Beat the Foods Giants*, Manitowoc,Wisconsin: The Natural Press, 1993, p. 132.
16. Joseph C. Piscatella, *Fat-Proof Your Child*, New York: Workmans Publishing, 1997, p. 121.
17. Gayla J. Kirschmann, John D. lirschmann, "Weights and Measurements", Nutrition Almanac, New York: McGraw-Hill, 1996, p. 391.
18. Carol Simontacchi, *The Crazy Makers,* New York: Tarcher/Putnam, 2000, p. 21.
19. Doris Sarjeant, Karen Evans, *Hard to Swallow*, BC Canada: Alive Books, 1999, p. 8.
20. Harvey and Marilyn Diamond, *Fit for Life,* New York: Warner Books, 1985, pp 125, 126.
21. Robert Hass, *Eat To Win for Permanent Fat Loss*, New York: Harmony Books, 2000, p. 74.
22. Eric Schlosser, *Fast Food Nation*, Boston: Haughton, Mifflin Company, 2001, p. 54.
23. Bonnie Liebman, Jayne Hurly, "The Juice Jungle," *Nutrition Action Newsletter,* Washington, D.C.: Center for Science in the Public Interest: June, 1999, pp. 14, 15.
24. Fred Pescatore, M.D. *Feed Your Kids Well*, New York: John Wiley & Sons, 1997, p. 48.
25. Dr. Marshall Gilula, Norm Shealy, M.D., Ph.D. "*Aspartame Health Warning! 'Nutra Sweet', 'Equal', & Spoonful"*,World Envrionmental Conference and the Multiple Sclerosis Foundation Conference speech,,Internet Communations, January 20, 1999, pp. 4, 5.
26. `H. Leighton Steward, M.D., Morrison C, Bethea, M.D., San S. Andrews, M.D., Luis A. Balart, M.D., *Sugar Busters*, New York: Ballentine Books, 1995, p. 59.

27. Joseph C. Piscatella, *Fat-Proof Your Child*, New York: Workman Publishing, 1997, p. 115.
28. Joseph C. Piscatella, *Fat-Proof Your Child*, New York: Workman Publishing, 1997, p. 115.
29. Joseph C. Piscatella, *Fat-Proof Your Child*, New York: Workman Publishing, 1997, p. 118.
30. Joseph C. Piscatella, *Fat-Proof Your Child*, New York: Workman Publishing, 1997, p. 118.
31. Paul A. Stitt, *Beat the Food Giants,* Manitowoc, Wisconsin: The Natural Press, 1993, p. 135.
32. "Is There Salt In Your Pepper?", Boston: Tuft's University Health and Nutrition Letter, June 2001, p. 3.
33. Carol Simontacchi, *The Crazy Makers,* New York: Tarcher/Putnam, 2000, p. 96.
34. Russell L. Blaylock, M.D., EXCITOTOXINS, Sante Fe, New Mexico: Health Press, 1997, pp. 255, 256.
35. Fred Pescatore, M.D., *Feed Your Kids Well*, New York: John Wiley & Sons, 1998, pp. 62, 63.
36. Sam Graci, The Power of Superfoods Canada: Prentice Hall, 1999, p. 128.
37. Udo Erasmus, *Fats and Oils*, BC Canada: Alive Books, 1986, pp. 84-89.
38. Joseph C. Piscatella, *Fat-Proof Your Child.*, New York: Workman Publishing, 1997, pp. 105.
39. National Center for Health Statistics, http://www.cdc.gov/nchs/fastats/overwt.htm., p. 1.
40. Joseph C. Piscatella, *Fat-Proof Your Child*, New York: Workman Publishing, 1997, p. 161.
41. Stephanie Beling, M.D., "*Olestra, oh, no!*, Your Health, October 1998, p. 13.
42. "Milk: No Longer Recommended or Required", Washington, D.C.: Physicians Committee for Responsible Medicine, www.pcrm.org., November 16, 1998, pp.1-3.
43. Julian Whitaker, M.D., "Milk is 'Udder' Nonsense", Heal & Healing, Potomac, Maryland: www.drwhitaker.com., October 1998, pp.2-3.
44. Fred Pescatore, M.D., *Feed Your Kids Well*, New York: John Wiley & Sons, 1998, p. 102.
45. Margo Whooten, "Don't Say Cheese", www.cspinet.org/new/cheese.html, February 6, 2001, p.1.
46. "Don't Say Cheese", Nutrition Action Newsletter, Washington, D.C., CSPI Press Release, February 6, 2001, p.15.
47. Ruth Winter, M.S., A Consumer's Dictionary of Food Additives, New York: Crown Trade Paperbacks, 1994, p. 96.
48. Fred Pescatore, M.D., *Feed Your Kids Well*, New York: John Wiley & Sons, 1998, pp. 39, 101.
49. Harvey and Marilyn Diamond, *Fit For Life,* New York: A Time Warner Company, 1985, p. 122.
50. Catherine Monahan, "Nix Your Fix," www.healthwell.com/delicious, November 4, 2003, pp. 5,6.
51. Robert Haas, M.S., Eat to Win For Permanent Fat Loss, New York: Three Rivers Press, 2000, p. 85.
52. "Caffeine, The Inside Scoop", Nutrition Action Newsletter, www.cspinet.org., November 21, 2001, pp. 1, 2.
53. The Organic Report, News & Trends, March 2001, p. 6.
54. Michael Pollen, "Discover How Your Beef is Really Raised", Schaumberg, Illinois: www.mercola.com, April 24, 2002,p.2.
55. Ronnie Cummins, Ben Lilliston, "Beef Hormones, Irradiation, & Mad Deer: America's Food Safety Crisis Continues", Food Safety News # 19, www.global-reality.com, June 4, 1999, p.
56. Ruth Winter, M.S., *A Consumer's Dictionary of Food Additives*, New York: Crown Trade Paperbacks, 1994, p. 183.
57. "Adverse Effects of Inactive Ingredients", Riverhead, New York: www.feingold.org, Feingold Association, pp.1-2.
58. Dr. Titus Venesa,Ph.D., Sc.D., research scientist, Orlando, Florida: Forever Young Natural Products, October 2002.
59. Eric Schlosser, *Fast Food Nation*, New York: Houghton Mifflin Company, 2001, p. 126.
60. Eric Schlosser, *Fast Food Nation*, New York: Houghton Mifflin Company, 2001, p. 122.
61. Eric Schlosser, *Fast Food Nation*, New York: Houghton Mifflin Company, 2001, p. 126.

62. Eric Schlosser, *Fast Food Nation*, New York: Houghton Mifflin Company, 2001, pp. 125, 126.
63. Eric Schlosser, *Fast Food Nation*, New York: Houghton Mifflin Company, 2001, pp. 126, 127.
64. Ruth Winter, M.S., *A Consumer's Dictionary of Food Additives*, New York: Crown Trade Paperbacks, 1994, p. 7.
65. Janet Zand, O.M.D., Rachel Walton, R.N., Bob Roundtree, M.D., *Smart Medicine for a Healthier Child,* Garden City, New York: Avery Publishing Group, 1994, pp. 42, 43.

Chapter Five

1. "Why Water", www.aquaid.co.uk/lb/htm
2. Dr. Michael Colgan, *Optimum Sports Nutrition,* New York: Advances Research Press, 1993, p. 19.
3. Jack L. Groppel, Ph.D., Les Knight, Ph.D. and The Florida Hospital Sports Nutrition Team, *The Winning Edge of Sports Nutrition*, Orlando, Florida: Florida Hospital Nutritional Services, p. 1.
4. "Why Water". www.aquiad.co.uk/lb/htm
5. Sam Graci, *The Power of Superfoods*, Ontario, Canada: Prentice Hall, 1999, p. 76.
6. Janet Zand, LaC,OMD, Rachel Walton, RN, Bob Roundtree, MD, *Smart Medicine for a Healthier Child,* Garden City, New York: Avery Publishing Group, Garden City Park, New York, 1994, p. 48.
7. Dr. Michael Colgan, *Optimum Sports Nutrition*: New York: Advance Research Press, New York, 1993, pp. 21, 22.
8. Phyllis A. Balch, C.N.C., James F. Balch, M.D., *Rx Prescription for Cooking & Dietary Wellness,* Greenfield, IN., P.A.B. Publishing, Inc., 1992, p. 184.
9. Han, Kugeler, Ph.D., "More Than 50 Toxins That Accelerate Aging," Journal of Longevity, Vol # 6, No.7, p. 25.
10. "On Whether Drinking 8 Glasses of Water a Day is Really Necessary," Boston: The Tufts University Health and Nutrition Newsletter, January 2001, p. .
11. Sam Graci, *The Power of Superfoods*, Ontario, Canada: Prentice Hall, 1999, p. 17.

Chapter Six

1. James A. Joseph, Ph.D., Daniel A. Nadeau, M.D., Anne Underwood, *Color Code,* New York: Hyperion, 2002, p. 8.
2. Stephanie Beling, M.D., *Power Foods*, New York: Harper Perennial, 1997, p. 45.
3. James A. Joseph, Ph.D., Daniel A. Nadeau, M.D., Anne Underwood, *Color Code*, New York: Hyperion, 2002, p. 15.
4. Doris Sarjeant, Karen Evans, *Hard To Swallow,* BC, Canada: Alive Books, 1999, p. 9.
5. Paul A. Stitt, Beating the Food Giants, Manitowoc, WI: Natural Press, 1993, p. 117.
6. "FDA Urged to Improve Labeling of or Ban Carmine Food Coloring", Center for Science in the Public Interest New Release, Washington, D.C. www.cspi.org/new/carmine, August, 1998, p.1.
7. Carol Simontacchi, *The Crazy Makers,* New York: Putnam Publishers, 2000, p. 119.

Chapter Seven

1. Alexander Schauss, Arnold Meyer, and Barbara Friedlander, *Eating for A's*, New York: Simon and Schuster, 1991, p. 18.
2. Jean Carper, *Your Miracle Brain*, New York: Harper Collins, 2000, pp. 48, 49.
3. Jean Carper, Boost Your Brain, Washington D.C.: USA Weekend, March 3-5, 2000, p. 7.
4. Jean Carper, *Your Miracle Brain*, New York: Harper Collin Publishers, 2000, p.68.
5. Jean Carper, *Your Miracle Brain*, New York: HarperCollins, 2000, pp. 162.
6. Jean Carper, *Your Miracle Brain*, New York: HarperCollins, 2000, pp. 113,114.

7. Robert Haas, *Eat To Win For Permanent Weight Loss,* Carson, California: Harmony Books, 2000, p. 134.
8. Jean Carper, *Your Miracle Brain*, New York: Harper Collins, 2000, p.245.

Chapter Eight

1. Dr. Michael Colgan, *Optimum Sports Nutrition*, New York: Advance Research Press, 1993, p. 284.
2. Daniel Gastelu, Dr. Fred Hatfield, *Dynamic Nutrition for Maximum Performance,* Garden City Park: Avery Publishing Group, 1997, p. 63.
3. Dr. Micheal Colgan, *Optimum Sports Nutrition*, New York: Advanced Research Press, 1993, p. 19
4. Jack L. Groppel, Ph.D., Les Knight, Ph.D. and The Florida Hospital Sports Nutrition Team, The Winning Edge of Sports Nutrition, Orlando, Florida: Florida Hospital Nutritional Services, p. 1.
5. Nancy Clark, M.S., R.D., Ready Set Grow, www.oxygen.com, p.2.
6. Gayla J. Kirschmann, John D. Kirschmann, *Nutrition Almanac,* New York: McGraw-Hill, 1996, p. 142.
7. Dr. Michael Colgan, *Optimal Sports Nutrition,* New York: Advanced Research Press, 1993, pp. 27, 28.
8. Alexander Schauss, Barbara Friedlander Meyer, Arnold Meyer, *Eating for A's,* New York: Simon and Schuster, 1991, pp. 229, 230.
9. Daniel Gasteau, Dr. Fred Hatfield, *Dynamic Nutrition for Maximum Performance*, Garden City, New York: Avery Publishing Group, 1997, pp. 98, 99.
10. Nancy Clark, MS, RD, Sports Nutrition Guidebook, Champaign, Illinois: Human Kinetics, 1997, p. 262.
11. Dr. Michael Colgan, *Optimum Sports Nutrition*, New York: Advanced Research Press, 1993, p. 74.

Chapter Nine

1. *Webster's New World Dictionary of the American Language*, New York: The World Publishing Company, 1959, p. 83.
2. *Webster's New World Dictionary of the American Language,* New York: The World Publishing Company, 1959, p. 1326.
3. David S. Sobel, M.D., Robert Ornstein, Ph.D., *The Healthy Mind Healthy Body Handbook,* New York: Patient Education Media, Inc., 1996, P. 70.
4. David S. Sobel, MD, Robert Ornstein, Ph.D., *The Healthy Mind Healthy Body Handbook,* New York: Patient Education Media, Inc., 1996, p. 69.

Chapter Ten

1. Nanci Hellmich, "Many Kids Are Eating (too much) in Front of TV", *USA Today,* February 14, 2001, p. 9D.
2. Shirley Dobson, *Focus on the Family*, "Coming Home," November 2000, p. 6.
3. Nancy Hellmich, "Many Kids Are Eating (too much) in Front of TV," *USA Today,* February 14, 2001, p. 9D.
4. Copyright 1997 CSPI. Reprinted/Adapted from Nutrition Action Healthletter.

Chapter Eleven

1. Michael Pollan, "Naturally", *New York Times Magazine*, New York: New York Times Company, May 13, 2001, p. 36.
2. *Organic Food is More Nutritious, The Journal of Alternative and Complementary Medicine*, Larchmont, New York, Mary Ann Liebert, Inc., 2001; 7 (2): 161.

3. "USDA and Biotechnology", Washington, D.C., United States Department of Agriculture,www.usda.gov/agencies/biotech/gaq.html,p. 5.
4. "Genetically Engineered Crops", *Mothers for Natural Law,* Fairfield, Iowa: www.safe-food.org, 2000, p.1.
5. Jeff. M. Smith, *Seeds of Deception*, Fairfield, Iowa: Yes! Books, 2003, p. 245.
6. Martha Herbert, M.D., "Genetically Altered Foods: We are Being Exposed to One of The Largest Uncontrolled Experiments in History", *Chicago Tribune*, September 3, 2000, p. 1.
7. Jeffrey M. Smith, *Seeds of Deception*, Fairfield, Iowa, Yes! Books, 2003, p. 69.
8. Jeffrey M. Smith, *Seeds of Deception*, Fairfield, Iowa, Yes! Books, 2003, pp. 83, 84.
9. Doris Sargeant, Karen Evans, *Hard To Swallow*, Burnaby, BC, Canada: Alive Books, 1999, pp. 111, 112.
10. Philip J. Regal, Ph.D., "Declaration of Philip. J. Regal. PhD", United States District Court for the District of Columbia, Civil Action No.98-1300 (CKK), p. 1.
11. Steven M. Druker, Legal & Scientific Critique of FDA's "No Labeling, No Safety Testing" Policy on GE Foods, public comment letter, May 2, 2001, p.3.
12. Doris Sargeant, Karen Evans, *Hard To Swallow*, Barnaby, BC, Canada: Alive Books, 1999, p.115.
13. Martin Teitel, Ph.D., Kimberly A. Wilson, *Genetically Engineered Food: Changing the Nature of Nature*, Rochester, Vermont: Park Street Press, 1999, p.39.
14. William W. Crist, "Waiter, there's a flounder in my fruit.", Vegetarian Times, Glen Allen, VA, November 1996, p. 22
15. ABC News Poll on GE Foods, "93 Percent want Labeling!", www.thecampaign.org, June 22, 2001, p. 14.
16. "Genetically Modified Crops and Food: Worldwide Regulation, Prohibition, and Production." www.centerfor foodsafety.org., October 7, 2003.
17. Doris Sargeant, Karen Evans, *Hard To Swallow*, *The Truth About Food Additives,* Burnaby, BC, Canada: Alive Books, 1999, pp. 130, 131.
18. Doris Sargeant, Karen Evans, *Hard To Swallow*, T*he Truth About Food Additives,* Burnaby, BC, Canada: Alive Books, 1999, p. 130.
19. Doris Sargeant, Karen Evans, *Hard To Swallow*, *The Truth About Food Additives,* Burnaby, BC, Cananda: Alive Books, 1999, pp. 128, 129.
20. Michelle Marcotte, *Labeling Regulations for Irradiated Foods,* www.food-irradiation.com/labeling, p. 2.
21. Dr. Joseph Moorman (Chaplin) *Safe Food News,* Fairfield, Iowa, Mothers for Natural Law of the Natural Law Party, 2000, p. 30.

Chapter Twelve

1. Stu Mittlemean, Katherine Callan, *SLOW BURN*, Harper Resource, New York, New York, 2000, p. 243. (Reference to beer, wine, coffee and tea were not included due to the inappropriateness for kids. Some herbal teas would be the exception.)

Chapter Fourteen

1. Phyllis A. Balch, C.N.C., James F. Balch, M.D., *RX Prescription for Cooking & Dietary Wellness,* Greenfield, Indiana: PAB Books Publishing Co., 1992, p. 45.
2. Robert Crayhon, M.S., *Nutrition Made Simple,* New York: M. Evans Company, Inc., 1994, p. 79.
3. *Webster's New Universal Unabridged Dictionary*, The World Publishing Company, New York, 1979, p. 1465.
4. Janet Zand, LAc, OMD, Allen N. Spreen, MD, CNC, James B LaValle, RPh, *ND Smart Medicine for a Healthier Child*, Garden City Park, New York: Avery Publishing Group, 1999, pp., 48,49.

5. Michael T. Murray, N.D., *Encyclopedia of Nutritional Supplements*, Rocklin. CA.: Prima Publishing, 1996, p. 9.
6. Robert Crayhon, M.S., *Nutrition Made Simple,* New York: M. Evans and Company, Inc., 1994, p. 83.
7. Robert Crayhon, M.S., *Nutrition Made Simple,* New York: M. Evans and Co., New York, 1994, p. 80.
8. Robert Crayhon, *Nutrition Made Simple,* New York: M. Evans and Company, Inc., 1994, p. 80.

Chapter Sixteen

1. Eric Schlosser, *Fast Food Nation*, New York: Houghton Mifflin Company, 2001, p. 47.
2. Ibid.
3. www.washingtonpost.com/wp-srv/style/longterm/books/chap1/fastfoodnation.htm, p. 2 of 9.
4. Eric Schlosser, *Fast Food Nation*, New York: Houghton Mifflin, 2000, p. 121.
5. Carol Simontacchi, *The Crazy Makers*, New York: Penguin Putnam, Inc., 2000, p. 147.
6. Eric Schlosser, *Fast Food Nation*, New York: Houghton Mifflin, 2000, pp. 53, 54.
7. Bonnie Liebman, *The Pressure to Eat*, www.cspinet.orsg/nah/7_98eat.htm, p. 5 of 6.
8. Bonnie Liebman, *The Pressure to Eat*, www.cspinet.org/nah/7_98eat.htm, p.1
9. Eric Schlosser, *Fast Food Nation*, New York: Houghton Mifflin, 2000, pp. 199, 200, 222.
10. Kids' meals full of fries, lacking vegetables, *USA Today*, A Better Life, Health, Education & Science, March 14, 2001, p. 5

INDEX

B

D

E

F

M

N

O

P

T

U

V

W